Postmodernity and the Fragmentation of Welfare

360 Cf

CORNWALL COLLEGE
LEARNING CENTRE

Postmodern ideas have been vastly influential in the social sciences and beyond. However, their impact on the study of social policy has been minimal. *Postmodernity and the Fragmentation of Welfare* analyses the potential for a postmodern or cultural turn in welfare as it treats postmodernity as an evolving canon – from the seminal works of Baudrillard, Foucault and Lyotard, through to recent theories of the 'risk society'.

Already disorientated by globalisation, new technologies and the years of new right ascendancy, welfare faces a significant challenge in the postmodern. It suggests that, rather than universality and state provision, the new social policy will be consumerised and fragmented – a welfare state of ambivalence.

With contributions from authors coming from a variety of fields offering very different perspectives on postmodernity and welfare, *Postmodernity and the Fragmentation of Welfare* also keeps social policy's intellectual inheritance in view. By exploring ways in which theorisations of postmodernity might improve understanding of welfare issues in the 1990s and assessing the relevance of theories of diversity and difference to mainstream and critical policy traditions, this book will be an essential text for all students of social policy, social administration, social work and sociology.

John Carter is a Senior Lecturer in the School of Social Sciences, University of Teesside.

D0279450

Postmodernity and the Fragmentation of Welfare

Edited by John Carter

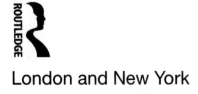

London and New York

First published 1998
by Routledge
11 New Fetter Lane, London EC4P 4EE

Simultaneously published in the USA and Canada
by Routledge
29 West 35th Street, New York, NY 10001

© 1998 John Carter, selection and editorial matter;
individual chapters, the contributors

Typeset in Times by M Rules, London

Printed and bound in Great Britain by
Creative Print and Design (Wales), Ebbw Vale

All rights reserved. No part of this book may be reprinted or
reproduced or utilized in any form or by any electronic,
mechanical, or other means, now known or hereafter
invented, including photocopying and recording, or in any
information storage or retrieval system, without permission in
writing from the publishers.

British Library Cataloguing in Publication Data
A catalogue record for this book is available from the British Library

Library of Congress Cataloging in Publication Data
Postmodernity and the fragmentation of welfare/edited by John Carter.
        p.   cm.
    Includes bibliographical references and index.
    1. Great Britain—Social policy—1979-.   2. Public welfare—
Great Britain.   3. Welfare state.   4. Postmodernism—Great Britain.
I. Carter, John, 1961–   .
HN390.P59 1998
361.6′1′0941--dc21   97–26563
                        CIP

ISBN 0-415-16391-9 (hbk)
ISBN 0-415-16392-7(pbk)

Contents

Contributors

Stephen J. Ball is Professor of Sociology at King's College London.

Peter Beresford works with the Open Services Project, is Reader in Social Policy at Brunel University College and is a member of Survivors Speak Out.

Robin Bunton is a Principal Lecturer in Social Policy at the University of Teesside.

Roger Burrows is Assistant Director of the Centre for Housing Policy at the University of York.

Jean Carabine is a Lecturer in Social Policy at Loughborough University.

John Carter works in the School of Social Sciences at the University of Teesside.

John Clarke is Senior Lecturer in Social Policy at the Open University.

Allan Cochrane is Dean of the Faculty of Social Sciences at the Open University.

Suzy Croft works with the Open Services Project and is a Social Worker with the St John's Hospice.

Barbara Fawcett is a Lecturer in Social Work at the University of Bradford.

Brid Featherstone is a Lecturer in Social Work at the University of Bradford.

John R. Gibbins is a Principal Lecturer in Social Policy at the University of Teesside.

Norman Ginsburg is Professor of Social Policy and Administration at the University of North London.

Paul Hoggett is Professor of Politics at the University of the West of England.

Brian D. Loader is a Co-Director of CIRA at the University of Teesside.

Kirk Mann works in the Department of Social Policy and Sociology at the University of Leeds.

Sarah Nettleton is a Lecturer in Social Policy and Social Work at the University of York.

Martin O'Brien is a Lecturer in Sociology at the University of Surrey.

Sue Penna is a Lecturer in Applied Social Studies at Lancaster University.

Chris Smaje is a Lecturer in Sociology at the University of Surrey.

Simon Thompson is a Senior Lecturer in Politics at the University of the West of England.

Acknowledgements

This collection's callow youth was as a conference, held at the University of Teesside in September 1996. Thanks therefore are particularly due to Jo Brudenell, Robin Haggart and Brian Loader at Teesside, who acted as fellow organisers. In addition, Sue Brown, Barbara Cox and Liz Simpson provided vital assistance at the event – as did other Teesside colleagues who chaired sessions and the like. The tolerance of Fiona Bailey and Heather Gibson at Routledge is also worthy of mention.

By their very nature conferences do not always hatch into good books. However, in this case, contributions by writers working at the top of their form have created what is hopefully an interesting treatment of postmodernity and welfare.

Chapter 1

Preludes, introductions and meanings

John Carter

INTRODUCTION

Postmodern ideas and attitudes have been rattling around the social sciences and humanities for a number of years now. Thus far, however, they have gained little purchase on the field of academic welfare, particularly in the United Kingdom. That domain has seemed at once both resistant and indifferent to what has elsewhere become intellectually established and influential. Not surprisingly this collection seeks to question that situation and argues that indifference is no longer an option. A non-engagement with significant ideas smacks of isolationism and limits the topics of conversation we can enter into with adjacent intellectual disciplines. Social policy then should at least explore the postmodern – but in doing so should subject it to a *critical* gaze. Recognising the need for a cultural turn in welfare does not imply that that literature be awarded the status of biblical text. Moreover, any sortie between social policy and the postmodern must keep the former in view as a developed intellectual field with its own concerns and constructs. Such a debate therefore needs to be conducted in both directions and may serve ultimately to enrich our conceptions of both welfare *and* postmodernism.

Throughout, the volume addresses the diverse and contested meanings of postmodernity and the postmodern. These include of course the contributions of Lyotard, Foucault, Derrida and others who, over the last thirty years, created what should properly be understood as a new perspective. Their value has been not only in the addition of specific new theoretical insights, but in critiquing and expanding the very notion of theorisation itself. Yet just as postmodernity did not begin with, say, Lyotard's *The Postmodern Condition* (1979), neither did it end there. Writers such as Giddens, Beck and Bauman continue to map our present condition and so feature heavily in this volume.

Mention of Beck and Giddens leads on to a parameters question. These writers would not necessarily regard themselves as postmodernists but might prefer to say that they are charting the later reaches of modernity. This sits happily and easily within the scope of the book which is really the wider 'epochal thing' rather than just the ideas of those authors who claim the title of 'postmodernist'. Indeed the often contradictory mix of the late and post-modern to be found in recent welfare reforms is a substantive theme of the volume.

Of course the book is also about social policy itself – how it theorises, how it understands a changing world and how it meets intellectual and political challenges. The issue of whether postmodernity and its associated concep-tions of power and identity can act as the midwife of a new, radical welfare politics is taken up by a number of contributors. In an age where real people are increasingly poor and exploited this is a far from abstract question.

Nevertheless, abstract and conceptual issues *are* posed for social policy by postmodernism. Even without ruling on the 'late' versus 'post'-modernism conundrum we should note that what we used to call the welfare state has passed through *something*. We are no longer living in the crisis years of the 1970s wherein welfare capitalism ground to a halt (more with a bang than with a whimper). Neither for that matter are we quite at the epicentre of Conservative and new right responses here and abroad – the 1980s – though of course the process of creative destruction still rumbles on. That which we also used to call reality has moved on as conservatives from Thatcher to Blair seek to translate globalising (and other) forces into a new welfare set-tlement. Despite any lingering emotional and indeed occupational attachment we might feel, that world has vanished up its own contradictions. It belonged to an earlier conjunction of political, economic and cultural forces. Anyway it has become commonplace to point out that the welfare of Beveridge and of our own social administration tradition was marbled through with its own conservative assumptions and hierarchical power rela-tions. We are of course reminded quite forcefully that this was no golden age by the postmodernists.

What then is the new world in social policy – a subject constructed and developed amid the apparent certainties of modernity and the twentieth cen-tury? To what extent should we assume that all bets are off and that a postmodern welfare template has been forged for the new age of anxiety? Not surprisingly the different authors included here offer different answers and vary in their interpretation of the new times. They also come at this from dif-ferent directions and from diverse disciplinary backgrounds. This issue of intellectual allegiance is itself significant. It may be that those outside of the social policy tradition feel able to apply postmodern ideas to that realm in a reasonably direct and clear way. For those writers working in welfare, the directional dynamic may be somewhat different. Their problem is one of matching postmodern predictions and propositions with an existing canon of welfare writings and a subject that has developed its own intellectual and political concerns over the years. There may therefore be a relationship between disciplinary background and conclusions drawn on 'postmodernity and welfare' (reflected in a creative tension which runs throughout this book).

STRUCTURE OF THE BOOK

Postmodern frameworks and social policy

We begin Part I with my chapter's view that the very notion of a postmodern social policy itself needs to be deconstructed, contextualised and understood as an interaction between established intellectual communities. Of these, social policy has rightly been criticised in the past for its narrow focus and theoretical calcification. Whilst this is less valid now, academic welfare has demonstrably failed to parley with the postmodern. This in turn reflects a shortcoming on the part of the postmodernists, in failing to consider *what social policy is* and the conceptual tools it has developed. Ironically, though, the very construction of welfare as a field of study may itself have erected barriers against the cultural realm and thus a postmodern turn.

A more wholehearted account of postmodernity's potential role in social policy is offered by John R. Gibbins. He particularly promotes the possibilities of a poststructural and deconstructionist variant for welfare – itself a creature of the Enlightenment. Against traditional notions of academic 'coherence' stand ambivalence, eclecticism and diversity – postmodernity's Holy Trinity. Taken together, these not only open up new theoretical possibilities but also hint at a new thought style for social policy.

Martin O'Brien and Sue Penna are similarly upbeat about the postmodern, which they display as a diverse field of meanings. Their chapter distinguishes between the different conceptual strands which make it a contested but dynamic intellectual endeavour. This perspective is deployed to critique the modernist assumptions that underpin 'anti-oppressive practice' in social work and training.

Finally in this part, Barbara Fawcett and Brid Featherstone focus on the postmodernism located within feminist analysis. However, notions of quality assurance and evaluation (as currently used in social work) actually form part of a modernist project applied in a postmodern era. In this, the large confidences of the past are supplanted by the 'small certainties' of modernism in an effort to try to retain fixed points of reference within the fluidity of the postmodern scene. This is illustrated through a case study of the supports provided for a disabled woman and her family.

Critical social policy and postmodernity

Kirk Mann turns the tables on the post- and late modernists, suggesting that they have things to learn from academic social policy. This can be seen in the works of Bauman and Giddens, which display an overly traditional and limited conception of welfare itself. Contrary to received wisdoms, the 'orthodox' welfare tradition has of late converged with its more radical cousin, critical social policy. Anyway, the latter has itself raised interesting questions about identity politics and the operation of power. This in turn challenges the presumed newness and uniqueness of the postmodern critique of welfare.

Ambiguity about the postmodern case also characterises the contribution of Suzy Croft and Peter Beresford. At first glance, by its very nature, a post-modernist position appears to offer opportunities for users' groups and other marginalised and previously unheard welfare voices. However, these same groups are interpreted rather than engaged with in postmodern discourses – a process of tokenisation. In this way, ironically, the postmodernists repeat one of the failings of 'orthodox' social policy.

Social divisions and social exclusion

By way of a contrast, Jean Carabine sees a more positive role for the post-modern in debates about social exclusion. She argues that sexuality should be used as a theoretical framework in social policy rather than simply as a bolted-on extra topic to study. In particular, Foucault's notions of normali-sation and regulation illuminate the inequalities and assumptions that have created a heterosexual welfare logic. This logic in turn interacts with and reinforces the other social divisions of gender, race, age and disability.

Chris Smaje notes that postmodern critiques undermine the normative universality of older philosophical traditions, but finds this problematic as a way of advancing debates about race and identity politics. Accordingly he is less keen to abandon all aspects of modernist thought and particularly revis-its Richard Titmuss's notion of the 'gift relationship'. This typifies an approach to be found in many of these contributions: responding to the cat-alyst of postmodern analysis, we need not abandon our intellectual past, but can instead reinterpret and retune it.

Drawing on the work of Beck and Giddens, Sarah Nettleton and Roger Burrows smuggle the concept of reflexive modernisation into social policy debates. In an era of economic insecurity, reflexive modernisation illuminates a society dominated by uncertainty and the search for 'ontological security'. Various policy instruments have served to privatise forms of risk and have emphasised the choices that individuals must make to secure their own well-being. This is particularly evident in the realms of housing and health.

Governance and new technologies of control in the new social policy

John Clarke develops the notion of *managerialism*, to be distinguished from the idea of management as a neutral 'skill' or tool. Managerialism acts to transform welfare structures, provision and relationships and thus to realise that which the various narratives of socio-economic change only sketch or imply. Indeed Clarke expresses concern that analytic frameworks such as Fordism/post-Fordism and now modernism/postmodernism are expressed as simple developmental binaries. Such a framing may serve to encourage 'post-modernism wars' in social policy in which contributors are forced into 'for' or 'against' positions.

Stephen J. Ball also reveals the unevenness of actual development. Recent educational changes in the UK have left the system perched between modernity and postmodernity, an uneasy mix of the old and the new. Ball uses Lyotard's notion of performativity to organise what would otherwise seem to be random trajectories in educational management – the disciplinary rise of the market, total quality management, inspection, forms of self-evaluation, etc. Collectively these are aspects of the shift from a welfare state to a competition state.

The theme of unevenness and epochal boundaries is developed in Robin Bunton's account of the changing management of drug use. In this, he charts a shift from the addiction model to more flexible forms of governance centred on the body and the regulation of habit. Drawing on Foucault he suggests that the pertinent transition here is not necessarily or directly from modernity to postmodernity. Instead, drugs policies and approaches indicate a move between different modernist disciplinary regimes.

Brian D. Loader considers the significance and impact of the explosion of new information and communication technologies. From their origin in the private sector they show signs of invading both the organisation and provision of welfare and of creating more 'self-serviced' forms. This adds to general individualising tendencies in social policy and to the fragmentation of public services. However, the progress of these new technologies is not yet determined and will be played out on the palette of welfare's social divisions.

Citizenship amid the fragmented nation state

Paul Hoggett and Simon Thompson seek to combine the universalism of old labour with the particularism of the new social movements. Drawing on Hirschman's distinction between exit and voice they assess the potential of the new 'associationist vision'. These new ways of coming together – at present putatively represented by the voluntary sector – may over time become the primary sources of welfare and social policy. Moreover, they contain more inclusive and participatory possibilities and could serve to reanimate welfare's pre-collectivist tradition.

Beginning with Marshall's seminal account of post-1945 social policy, Allan Cochrane goes on to consider the possibilities of a local welfare citizenship amid conditions of globalisation. In this context he also acknowledges that the new associationalism appears to have radical possibilities. However, these forms of 'intermediate government' are far removed from present conditions in which the apparatus of local democracy has been dismantled as opposed to reconstructed. How we can move from here to there is accordingly an awkward tactical and political question.

Norman Ginsburg concludes the volume at the supra-national level. Just as the domestic welfare state was an essentially modernist leviathan, so too was the original vision of a social Europe – a vision of social cohesion based upon class. Ginsburg detects the fading of this Delors dream and signs of a post-modern turn in recent European Union policy documents. This is particularly so in the recognition of non-traditional family structures, but can also be seen in the way that labour flexibility has been deployed of late. However, interpretative caution is still in order and it may be that this reflects no more than the reassertion of capital.

SOME DEFINITIONS

This section seeks to introduce the very notion of the postmodern and its attendant concepts – particularly to those for whom this is relatively new territory. Further explorations of this material can be found in John Gibbins's chapter and indeed in a number of texts which present and chart the postmodern. Of these, Bertens (1995) is particularly useful and readable.

As much as anything my purpose here is one of reassurance. Those new to these debates may feel they have failed to catch hold of a totalising definition of postmodernity or even some neat and comforting encapsulation. Yet this is the very nature of what has become an increasingly prominent but amorphous beast. Whilst it does contain specific and important ideas from seminal thinkers, postmodernity has transmuted as it has extended into more and more intellectual fields (and indeed into wider public parlance). It now stands as both a generalised motif *and* an incisive framework for academics. In these circumstances we will all have to learn to live with definitional ambiguities. We are therefore faced with the same problems as Uspensky's policeman: 'Quickly I seized the rascal by the collar! But what do I see? The confounded fellow has no collar!' (Luxemburg 1970: 78).

Of course this background does not make postmodernity definitionally untouchable. One point of entry is the way in which the term has been used as a form of periodisation or epochal shorthand. In this way writers in different fields have deployed modernity and postmodernity as somewhat reductionist organising concepts, to distinguish between historical eras and patterns. Of course these same authors see different dates and turning points and some prefer 'late-modern' to postmodern as a label for the present. Nevertheless treating postmodernity as an account of historical change allows access to many important issues produced under that wider canon. The following sketch is therefore an attempt to present the main aspects of that case and to set out the general postmodern position. It is presented without critique (for the moment) and may therefore cause opponents of the very idea to bristle. My own powder remains fairly dry, however, and I allow myself no more than the ghost of a cynical smile as I type:

Modernity was a child of the Enlightenment (Science 1, Superstition 0) which developed through the industrial revolution to reach its highpoint in the twentieth century. This 'victory' saw its predominance in the structures and thought systems of western societies and, at least from the perspective of Max Weber, was near universal. The story for non-western cultures is more complex – with regard to both modernity and postmodernity – but is not really the subject of this book (which might be sub-sub-titled 'our little corner of globalisation'). The essential characteristics of twentieth-century modernity begin with widespread industrial and economic development. These in turn have been supported by different types of planning regime or, to be more specific, the belief that things *can* be planned. Organisationally, this saw the predominance of the bureaucratic-hierarchical form and a belief in the rational ordering of human affairs. Society itself was separated along a number of fault lines (gender and class most notably), though these divisions were presumed to be objective and stable. The identities clustered around region, religion or even race were taken to be hangovers from the pre-industrial era that would fade under the march of progress. In Britain this produced a particular kind of class politics and saw labourism fill in for socialism. Socialism itself largely shook off its pre-industrial and Utopian origins and became an 'ism' of modernity in the twentieth century. Other ideologies too made their peace with the machine age, the secular and the scientific. This optimistic view of history was of course challenged by world war and the vileness of totalitarianism, but seemed still resilient into the second half of the century. Modernity believed the truth was out there, if only the scientist or philosopher could look in the right place and use the right tools.

How we got from all of this to the 1990s is of course a long story. From today's vantage point the premises of modernity appear naive and almost quaint, in ways that do not need to be elaborated here. Expectations have been dashed, particularly with regard to technology; problems remain unresolved and the only political 'ism' that thrives is nationalism. Similarly, modernity and all of its works have been challenged positively by feminism and the new social movements, by environmental critiques and by a range of intellectual positions.

But what *is* postmodernity? As Bertens (1995) shows, the term developed within various artistic and cultural debates in the 1950s. Since then it has spread virally to the humanities, social disciplines and beyond, making it more difficult to pull out core meanings and absolute definitions. However, we can identify strands, claims and tendencies – particularly the issues that most impinge on the social sciences.

A starting point is the view that the 'truth' has gone out of fashion. At its most fundamental, postmodernism asks questions about the way we see the world and denies that something called reality actually exists in a form that can be directly and simply observed. In Baudrillard's term, reality is a constructed simulation, a 'Disneyworld' representing the victory of the image.

Everywhere is irony – reality is done by mirrors – and truth is what you make it. Ideologies, philosophies and grand narratives that seek or are premised upon ultimate notions of truth or justice are not only flawed but dangerous – 'terroristic' even. There is no universal design and the watchmaker is dead. Nature itself may be less patterned than scientists from Newton onwards have assumed and the cosmos is chaotic.

This fraying of the old certainties is particularly evident in the decline of the nation state and in processes of economic globalisation. These in turn are both facilitated and promoted by the rise of new information and communication technologies beyond the control of any one government. The same technologies are implicated in the valorisation of 'flexibility' as the totem of the new order, particularly in the workplace. New production techniques and organisational styles – post-Fordism – serve to reject the rigidities and failures of bureaucracy. The customer is empowered and sovereign and comes in diverse packages unrecognised in the mass production era. The successful enterprise therefore is that which can respond quickly and imaginatively to this supposed new consumerism.

People themselves are also less predictable and are no longer tethered to permanent or absolute identities. The postmodern self is multifaceted and collaged from a person's multiple locations and attributes. Moreover, these identities are also subjective constructions – designer lifestyles – chosen by the wearer rather than imposed by the sociologist or policy planner. Our vision of 'society' is thus affected, if the term survives at all. Rather than an obvious entity composed of definite and established groups, it becomes a web of shifting communities, coalitions and individuals. Politics too is transformed and no longer plays out economistic battles over resources centred on the workplace.

Although set out without comment, this intentionally generalised presentation of postmodernity as a historical trajectory still needs to be slightly unpicked at this point. It was indeed valid to exhibit this as an emergent paradigm, one which has moved osmotically into the different branches of academia over the last thirty years. Indeed, it has now achieved the status of truism and is at least the starting point for many debates in the social sciences. Ironically, postmodernism has become something of a fixed point in the study of human affairs, just as it has become almost impossible to debate issues in entirely modernist terms (though perhaps social policy has thus far kicked its heels on the sidelines of all of this). However, it would be wrong to suggest that postmodernity was conjured out of nothing by a band who called themselves 'the postmodernists' to the exclusion of all other badges. In fact social scientific postmodernism owes much to the French poststructuralist influences of Foucault, Derrida, Baudrillard and others. Indeed, one reading would be that postmodernism is really poststructuralism with its name changed by deed poll (plus a liberal dose of feminism).

In a general introduction of this kind it would be unwise to get into arbitration questions as to what is and what is not postmodernism. However, its relationship to poststructuralism is a live issue. Hans Bertens (1995) is keen to separate the two traditions out, whilst the majority position in this volume is probably that poststructuralism should be regarded as a school or variant *within* postmodernism. This is certainly contestable and one could just as easily describe the relationship the other way round. That, however, can safely be left to those who delight in chicken-and-egg debates.

A more pertinent issue regards the definitional shape of this foreign body as it begins to enter social policy discourses. For some, postmodernity is composed of several highly specific and incisive arguments and critiques, some of which were sketched above. For others, though, it is primarily a state of mind – a sceptical approach to truth claims and to grand narratives. Yet others deploy the word to do little more than indicate the newness of 'new times' in Britain and beyond. In other words postmodernism is a composite term – a rolling stone that has gathered moss aplenty over the years. It comes down to us as both a reductionist appellation, a dense ball of complex meanings, and also an exploded term in which definitional clarity has been lost. Different levels of conceptual coherence are therefore compounded in a single word. At times it can feel like walking through a multihued fog in which you occasionally bump your shin on a sharply defined object. Some of these objects are depicted in the following extended glossary.

Poststructuralism

Poststructuralism's provenance is more easy to trace – the 1970s French theorisings of Foucault, Lyotard, Derrida, Barthes, etc. Unlike postmodernism it can be seen in rather specific terms; it developed as a response to what had been the orthodoxy of structuralism. The latter perspective had claimed that under the surface of everyday life lurked structures and realities which intellectuals could ultimately discover. Though often covert and concealed by ideology and other obfuscations, these frameworks determined life chances and social outcomes. A clear distinction could therefore be made between the notional human freedoms assumed in 'everyday life' and the ultimate constraints imposed by these fundamental structures.

Poststructuralists of course rejected the key assumptions of their structuralist predecessors. The search for these frameworks of power and social organisation just out of everyday sight was illusory. Indeed, the very notion that a single veil could be lifted or that existence could be dualised into 'surface' and 'reality' was rejected. Derrida preferred *meaning* to reality and argued that meanings and interpretations were themselves multifaceted, contingent and contested. Thus significant spadework was done for postmodernism.

Post-Fordism

The eponymous Ford Motor Company typified the mass production techniques that dominated much of the twentieth century. These were based upon
a high division of labour, hierarchical factory discipline and the existence of
mass markets. However as these methods reached their economic limits in the
1960s and 1970s new approaches were developed across the industrialised
world – post-Fordism. This established changed working practices, facilitated by the arrival of new technologies. Decentralised and less openly
hierarchical workplace structures were accompanied by more discrete mechanisms of control inherent in things like the 'quality' movement. Producers
were thus able to provide an increased range of goods for the new niche markets and to respond rapidly to changed circumstances and fluctuating
levels/types of demand. Post-Fordism, then, announced the arrival of a workplace and marketplace flexibility, but also that capitalism had sought to
reinvent itself after the economic and industrial shocks of the 1970s. Some
writers take this point further and see post-Fordism as a change in the state
itself, and as its new way of regulating the economy and labour process.

Postindustrialism

Postindustrialism is also a loose coalition of ideas and shares some of the
assumptions of the post-Fordist case (on the development and diversity of
postindustrial models see Kumar 1992). Its origins are in the 1960s and 1970s
contributions of writers like Daniel Bell and Alvin Toffler, who brought the
concept to a wider audience with works like *Future Shock* (1970) and *The
Third Wave* (1981). The key premise is again one of historical transformation – that we are seeing the decline/demise of the industrial society which
produced 'things' using physical resources.

   The emergent era is to be a postindustrial or information society. Its central
resources are data and knowledge, the new raw materials. Greater information flows are central to the operation of commerce and manufacturing and
enable rapid responses to customers and competition. This revolution needed
the development of the microprocessor to speed up the exchange of data but
does not end with it. Further momentum is provided by the Internet and
other globalising technologies, which add a belated reality to Marshall
McLuhan's notion of the 'global village'.

   The consequences of this shift are various. The rise of new sectors and
processes based on information technology heralds a changed industrial
structure. Firms and indeed whole industries unable to adapt face threats to
their very existence. Similarly, companies no longer need to be 'all in one
place' and can use the new technologies to achieve a greater degree of functional decentralisation or disaggregation. In practice this adds further to
globalising tendencies and the ability of firms to chase cheap labour costs.

People too are not immune and we are already seeing the emergence of the information rich and information poor. How this new social divide maps onto and interacts with existing societal divisions is a pressing question for policy makers.

Deconstruction

The notion of deconstruction is very much associated with Jacques Derrida. It relates to things as essential as writing, reading, communicating and the production of meaning. For deconstruction is about the process by which we use language and produce text. For Derrida these were not simple questions of authorial intent – what s/he 'intended to say'. Instead, to write is to deploy existing meanings developed by earlier authors in a constant process of accretion, to be subjectivised further by the interpretations the reader brings to the exercise. As a result of this 'intertextual weaving', the work is freed from the intentions of the writer whose name appears on the dust jacket – what Barthes called the 'death of the author'. Discourse therefore becomes a process of interaction and development, a collage of the different texts that have shaped the 'actual' text that confronts the reader. Moreover, the messages produced appear through an essentially unstable interaction of earlier works rather than some stately or formalised genetic inheritance.

If deconstruction itself has a message, it is one of sceptical readership, particularly when confronted by truth claims of a moral or political nature. Deconstruction is a process of laying bare and, in a very specific sense, a political act itself – perhaps the only meaningful postmodern political act.

This sceptical gaze connects with Michel Foucault's conception of power as a discursive strategy. The different ways that groups of people are represented serves to include or marginalise them. So just as conventional histories are said to be written by the victors, deconstructionist archaeologies can bring the excluded back into focus by revealing how they were initially peripheralised. Deconstruction therefore can have radical applications, whilst steadfastly rejecting the modernist categories with which the earlier left was constructed.

Normalisation

Foucault's concept of normalisation continues this same train of thought (for a fuller account see Jean Carabine's chapter in this volume). It relates to the process by which people come to be regarded as full members of society and argues that this process is not reducible to the concrete mechanisms of policy and legislation. Nations and communities use different techniques to differentiate between and designate behaviours/lifestyles as normal or abnormal. These discursive strategies create models through which certain attributes such as heterosexuality become normalised, whereas others achieve the status of deviant.

This elides with Foucault's arguments about power/knowledge – that the way academics and others organise knowledge about different groups is actually a form of power. Classification itself adds to normalisation and thus to the panoply of controls and exclusions that are deployed.

Performativity

At one level performativity merely relates to the word 'performance' and operates in a fairly direct way. However, it had a more specific use in systems theory and indicated that which was needed to orientate an organisation to its environment. This was therefore about matching inputs to outputs and creating functionally stable operations. It arrives with us via Lyotard, who used the idea in his analysis of the postmodern condition (and is debated here by Stephen Ball). His objective was to identify the control technologies, the forms of governance that were emerging in these new conditions. In postmodernity, these fly under the flag of the 'new managerialism', with total quality management, charters, mission statements and the like. This apparent shift to more decentralised ways of working actually represents a new locus of control built upon self-monitoring and attitudinal change.

BIBLIOGRAPHY

Bertens, H. (1995) *The Idea of the Postmodern: A History*, London: Routledge.
Kumar, K. (1992) 'New theories of industrial society', in P. Brown and H. Lauder (eds) *Education for Economic Survival: From Fordism to Post-Fordism?*, London: Routledge.
Luxemburg, R. (1970) *Rosa Luxemburg Speaks*, New York: Pathfinder Press.
Lyotard, J.-F. (1979) *The Postmodern Condition: A Report on Knowledge*, Manchester: Manchester University Press.
Toffler, A. (1970) *Future Shock*, New York: Random House.
Toffler, A. (1981) *The Third Wave*, New York: Bantam Books.

Part I

Postmodern frameworks and social policy

Chapter 2

Studying social policy after modernity

John Carter

INTRODUCTION

Writing in that most politically symbolic of years for the UK, 1979, John Baker sought to expose social policy's intellectual and moral soul, with a survey of its undergraduate reading lists. This was an ideal way of isolating the subject's essence – revealing its orientation and the way in which it was packaged for students. In this fashion he demonstrated the ongoing vitality (and indeed predominance) of what he called the 'social conscience thesis' (Baker 1979). With this the welfare community retained a longstanding, benevolent view of the state, which itself responded to an unproblematic flow of information about social need, inspired by a warm and comforting idealism. The welfare state itself was evolutionary and irreversible and moved in the direction of ever greater generosity. The reading lists studied also confirmed this world view by what they did and did not recommend. The only works to be found in more than half of these documents were, of course, Marshall's *Social Policy in the Twentieth Century* (1970), Titmuss's *Social Policy: An Introduction* (1974) and his *Essays on the Welfare State* (1958) (if anthropomorphised into a *Desert Island Discs* guest, social policy would choose the last of these as its lone book to spend eternity with).

Baker himself criticised this mind set, called for more critical and realistic research strategies and, in essence, painted the picture of a complacent academic subject. These, however, were the last days of Rome and complacency was not a viable option in the 1980s. Even those who had been blind to the gendered and racialised interests maintained and reinforced by the 'benevolent' state were to be shaken by the political, discursive and programmatic batterings of the Thatcher years.

Moving ten years on, Fiona Williams used an influential textbook to assess the state of academic social policy further. From this vantage point of late Thatcherism she too provided a retrospective critique of the older social administration tradition and found it to be empiricist, idealist, overly focused on the state and with too much faith placed in experts and professionals (Williams 1989: 8–9). Social administration in turn had been confronted by

the rise of feminism and a new political economy in the 1970s and subsequently by the emergent new right. However, the result of these challenges,
circa 1989, was a reformulation and updating of the older tradition, rather
than a truly new conceptual design. In particular it had failed to incorporate
the social divisions of gender and race into its core theoretical frameworks or
its thought collective.

This kind of critique was well made and has probably gained widespread
acceptance within the social policy community. It noted theoretical deficien-
cies and illustrated the social biases inherent in a major field of academic
endeavour. The present chapter moves on to the most recent charge made
against the social policy community – that it has failed to take account of that
which is, somewhat reductively, referred to as postmodernity. It argues that
the 'postmodernity and welfare' debate already shows signs of collapsing
into a for-or-against, accusatory discourse in which boundaries are reinforced
rather than permeated. Ostensibly, I appear to accept the substantive arguments of both sides: social policy *does* need to treat with both the substance
and the deconstructive, sceptical body language of postmodernity. However,
it also has to keep in view that which is distinctively its own and which distinguishes it from other academic fields. Up to this point the juxtaposition of
these two positions – the debate – has merely acted to disinter that old chest-
nut of a conundrum: what *does* happen when the seemingly irresistible force
of postmodernity meets the apparently immovable object of social policy?
Mired up to the axles in this paradox we therefore need to go beyond the
apparently simple and direct question, 'What can social policy learn from
postmodernity?', towards an analysis of the terms and conditions of such a
debate. All too often the much-vaunted interdisciplinarity of the social sciences begins to resemble truculent neighbours shouting at each other over the
garden fence. For this not to happen here, family traditions and perspectives
must be mutually respected and contributors adopt a self-reflective approach.
This point will be returned to in due course.

In similar vein, it would be unwise to leave our historical sketch of social
policy as pencilled above. Anyone already disposed to see the subject as
backward and ossified could take from this a picture of academic welfare still
living in the Pathe News reels, imbued with the spirit of Harry Enfield's
Messrs Grayson and Cholmondley-Warner. The range of papers presented
each year to the Social Policy Association conference, however, illustrates a
broadening of that which welfare academics study (also to be seen in the subject's literature – for example, Cahill 1994; Erskine 1996; Huby 1995). This
moving beyond the 'five main services', at least by implication, re-raises
some important questions about the nature and parameters of scholarly
social policy (issues raised yet more forcefully through the catalyst of postmodernity). Moreover, social divisions beyond class have been brought in
from the conceptual cold and are now objects of study and analytical frameworks in welfare research. Indeed, as Mann has argued (this volume), it is

now misleading to present the critical and 'orthodox' traditions as separate and distinct. The former has both influenced and enriched the latter.

This reinvigoration and updating of the subject was also noted by Wilding (1992), who showed how the 1980s undermined the comfortable, statist assumptions of the subject. In that same decade he detected a number of new trajectories, including:

1   a growing interest in state theory;
2   a developed and mature feminist analysis in and of welfare;
3   the shift from studying racial disadvantage per se towards the use of race and ethnicity as key analytic variables;
4   a nascent environmental critique of welfare, which questions the effects of economic growth and the central position it has been afforded within social policy accounts.

This historical detour is an unavoidable starting point from which to consider social policy's potential postmodern turn. It reminds us that previously the subject did have a rather narrow focus and bore a strong resemblance to its extended family of statism, familism, labourism and bureaucracy (Williams 1989). These intellectual and indeed ethical and political weaknesses have, however, been the subject of a vigorous internal critique from members of the social policy fellowship. Consequently, debates have moved on and new ideas developed, though this has not always been recognised by critics beyond the welfare fringe. Postmodernity is not the first challenge to welfare orthodoxy, and the way it responds will in part be shaped by previous encounters and skirmishes. That these exchanges are not just of *ideas* but are between self-interested intellectual *communities* should also not escape our attention.

SOCIAL POLICY AND POSTMODERNITY: THE STORY SO FAR

The other social sciences and humanities largely had their postmodern makeovers in the 1970s and 1980s. But have these tricky Gallic and American ideas reached the shores of 1990s social policy? One way to assess this would be through a laborious content analysis of journals and texts. Fortunately, an idler's methodology exists in the form of BIDS – the Bath Information and Data System. This electronic abstracting and indexing service allows us to chart the appearance of various concepts in the different journals. The approach I have taken is to do a simple electronic search for words and names that might indicate the social policy community is at least engaging with postmodern propositions. Specifically, I have scrutinised significant journal contributions – those pieces carrying a full abstract – and have scanned only *titles*, *abstracts* and author-provided *key words*. By way of justification I would suggest that for an idea or theme to be genuinely influential in an article it would feature in one of these locations. A search of the full text and references might throw up other mentions of the postmodern canon, but these are likely to be incidental or peripheral appearances (in fact very few extra references are thrown up by such a wider net-casting anyway). This is therefore a conscious attempt to avoid the 'monkeys-and-typewriters effect' and a way of only catching real and significant usages of postmodernity in welfare. So, in what is essentially a quantitative study, this might be seen as the quality threshold that words and phrases have to pass in order to qualify as a 'hit'. This is not then a study with any great methodological pretentions, but one which might still reveal the fossil evidence of social policy's post-modern dalliance.

The following figures cover the five full years 1992–6 and show sightings of postmodernity within the search criteria described above (they list the number of articles in which mentions were made rather than the total number of individual mentions). In the *Journal of Social Policy*, of the eighty-one articles covered only four made reference to postmodernity. Of these, three were, to a large extent, responses to an earlier piece on postmodernity. When the search was widened to include all of the 'post-literatures' (modernism, Fordism, structuralism and industrialism) the number of hits only rose to five. In the same period the *Journal of Social Policy* did not have a single reference to deconstruction. Similarly there was only a single appearance for Foucault, and none at all for Lyotard and Giddens (chosen not necessarily as paid-up postmodernists, but as indications that articles which cite them are drawing on that whole theoretical realm – litmus indicators are, I believe, neutral but display the colour of that in which they are dipped).

If this record indicates a certain indifference to the postmodern, it looks almost garrulous in comparison to *Social Policy and Administration*. That journal also had eighty-one abstracted pieces – but not a single reference to postmodernity. When the wider category of post-literatures was assessed this ballooned to two mentions (in both cases by writers from outside of the UK), though deconstruction was still off the menu. Foucault, Lyotard and Giddens were similarly absent.

By way of contrast, the *British Journal of Sociology of Education* was also scanned. Its 119 articles saw a relatively modest five outings for the post-modern, but thirteen usages of the full set of 'posts'. Deconstruction appeared in four pieces and there were also two references to Foucault and three to Giddens.

Some might object to this comparison by arguing that the last journal is, by definition, a more theoretical organ and that this accounts for the increased visibility of postmodern concepts and authors in its pages. That line, however, implies that it is permissible for the social policy lot to take a *less* theoretical line or that welfare need not elide its own concerns with recent strands of social theory. Acceptance of this argument would immediately restrict the subject's horizons and future development, and finds no sympathy here.

What this mini-survey does suggest is that postmodern ideas have been practically invisible in the pages of the central social policy journals – as research tools, theoretical frameworks or even the subject of negative critique. This position may be changing slowly (with, for example, the present volume), though here again the operative word is 'slowly'. Relatively speaking then, welfare's postmodern period – if it happens at all – is much later and less wholehearted than that seen elsewhere. This in turn betokens a certain isolationism from what has been one of the most significant intellectual movements of the last thirty years or so. I take it as self-evident that such a situation is not very healthy for welfare and that the subject should at least engage with and consider postmodern propositions and challenges. Regardless of conclusions drawn, it cannot be a very good idea simply to *ignore* a de facto intellectual revolution. Again, though, it is important to be clear about my charge. I am not making some sort of patronising claim that welfare writers just do not read the right stuff – they are as likely as anyone to have read Foucault, Derrida, Lyotard, Beck *et al*. However, we are still somewhat the prisoner of our history and of the political and academic foundations of our subject. This itself seems to have created intangible but definite barriers around a particular vision of welfare – encompassing what it is and is not, who provides it and in response to which kinds of force. In this way social policy can appear like a tightly walled city from which the inhabitants have found it hard to establish intellectual trade routes (or, for that matter, allow strangers into).

Carrying all of this baggage, we are inevitably left with a more complex question than simply whether social policy should go postmodern. It therefore demands a more considered and self-reflective approach to what is ultimately a question of interdisciplinarity: how *should* social policy respond to ideas developed almost entirely outside of its own borders?

PINNING DOWN THE POSTMODERN

This is not the place to debate the neatness of postmodernity's break with modernity or indeed whether we should be talking about late- as opposed to postmodernity. However, in a volume on postmodernity an iconoclastic starting point is probably in order. Whilst there has clearly been a discernible shift of direction and tempo in many fields, we are still unambiguously in the century of *modernity*. Artistically, Stravinsky, the Bauhaus, Picasso, Moore, Woolf, Lloyd Wright *et al*. have provided the essential components of our cultural vision. Even in the 1990s their influence remains immeasurably greater than the things Damien Hirst does to animals. Moreover, the appearance of postmodernity's supposedly ironic and self-referential art would have been impossible without the very modernist avant-gardes that they are supposed to critique and replace. It is therefore not always useful to draw up restrictive boundaries between cultural epochs, and often it is better to explore the actual lineage of ideas and influences. All too often the 'new' in fact takes the form of renovation, redecoration and extension rather than the building of entirely new structures. We therefore need to be cautious about those post-modernities premised on the death of the past. This is of course as true in the social sciences as it is in the arts and humanities.

A further entanglement regards the word 'postmodernity' itself, which, as Bertens (1995) shows, was adopted at quite different periods in the various artistic and academic fields. Its different usages in architecture, dance, literary criticism and so on tend to collide in important ways (most notably with regard to timescales and the question of just when the modern became post-modern). However, it is usual to note that postmodern is typified by an approach that rejects the supposed modernist emphasis on the purity and autonomy of art (Lynton 1989: 339).

In the social sciences too the term has become both contested and con-gested and now conflates a wide range of insights and arguments – something of a problem when trying to assess its utility and applicability for social policy. Consequently it is wise to begin with the *kinds* of guise in which post-modernism is at large in academia and beyond, rather than some absolutist and therefore exclusive definition. This is therefore not an attempt to con-struct a typology, more an almost random illustration of the levels of definitional coherence to be found.

The first of these is the well-established social scientific usage of 'post-modernism', which traces its lineage back to poststructuralism. This was founded on the deconstruction of Derrida (1967, 1970) and a rejection of the notion that language simply represents reality. It also encompasses Foucault's power/knowledge axis (1977, 1980) and his exposure of the oppressions wrapped in discourses. For good measure this package might also be said to contain the death of both the author (Barthes 1977) and the grand narrative (Lyotard 1979). Of course, those of a forensic nature might want to argue that this designation of a poststructuralist postmodernism actually conflates a number of quite discrete ideas and epistemologies. My point, however, is that this collection of insights has over time gathered itself into what has become a focus for postmodern debates.

The second level at which postmodernism has become a common currency is along the academic/political boundary. This has seen scholarly critiques of class and other supposedly modernist monoliths extended and utilised into the politics of identity and the 'new social movements'. In this approach – most notably in *Marxism Today* – the artistic, cultural and commercial realms are the terrain on which identities are expressed and reformulated (Hall and Jacques 1989). Postmodernism here is seen as a way of transcending the fix-ities and impositions of labourism, patriarchy and nationalism.

A third and more explicitly popular usage (if such a specification is now admissible) is the postmodernism of the Sunday supplements. This has seen the term used in every feature on subjects from chaos theory to cookery and from multimedia to Madonna. Journalists, advertisers and lifestyle gurus seem determined to convince us that human history thus far ended around 1979 and that we have since entered a brave new world – of choice. In turn, this is overlaid with the political victory of the right and the valorisation of the consumer. The yuppies may have been the vanguard of this particular postmodernist charge, but the new share- and home-owners were its unwitting quartermasters.

Do any of these general visions provide a new inspiration and impetus for the study of social policy? Not surprisingly I am keen to lose this third account (whilst recognising its political and symbolic significance), which seems to have merged so closely with the discourse of the new right that they now share a common DNA pattern. This is a celebrationist, Saatchi-style postmodernism, commodified to the gills – regardless of whether the shopping is done in the mall or cyberspace. It sidesteps disparities in wealth just as a group of advertising executives might circumnavigate a homeless beggar on their lunchtime return to the office. In this way it ignores the differential ability of groups to become active consumers and bestows full human status only on those able to choose. Its designation of gender and ethnicity and the like as merely lifestyle choices misses the point that these are also social divisions and still significant sites of inequality. This then is a complacent and selfish postmodernism which, with its hyper-commodification of the cultural realm, serves to exclude the poor just as efficiently as any caste system in history.

Even someone lacking my gut reaction to this 'Visa-Access' postmodernism might have some difficulty applying it in any direct way to welfare. It is really quite difficult to see the Child Support Agency as a 'playful artefact' or to present the Jobseekers Allowance as 'self-ironising'. Moreover, however traumatised social policy provision has been in the UK, it has emphatically *not* been transformed into a consumer-sovereign bazaar. In education, for example, the rhetoric has been of the parental choice and the market. The reality, though, has been government pressure to *close* schools and a steady rise in both overt and covert *selection* (Carter 1997).

The first and second postmodern sketches outlined above are, however, more promising. Potentially, they offer a radical critique of power and indeed of academic knowledge itself. This in turn might expunge the remaining bureaucratic, hierarchical and conservative social assumptions that lurk in social policy's unconscious. However, simple osmosis is not enough; welfare's potential cultural turn needs to be both constructed and constructive.

THE POSTMODERNISTS VERSUS THE WELFARE LOYALISTS: THE PROBLEMS OF CIRCLE SQUARING

We now need to explore the precise ambiguities and difficulties involved in creating a postmodernity/social policy dialogue. This requires a critical if often paradoxical interaction with what are effectively two opposed camps.

As a strategy this might appear like a cautious but painful bout of fence-sitting. However, the circumstances of the debate thus far require just such an elaboration of what have been little more than initial manifestos.

As noted earlier, there has been precious little that addresses postmodernity and social policy per se. The pages of the *Journal of Social Policy* have seen three contributions promoting the postmodern in welfare (Fitzpatrick 1996; Hillyard and Watson 1996; Penna and O'Brien 1996), which in turn were largely responses to an earlier contrary article by Taylor-Gooby (1994). Other occasional treatments of welfare themes can also be found in the wider and generic literature on postmodernity. These, however, are treated in Mann's contribution to this volume and so will not be covered here.

The postmodernists

An underlying theme in these pro-postmodernity contributions is, of course, new times – that global restructuring has undermined traditional beliefs in the state and its role in social amelioration. Fabian conceptions of governance are accordingly outdated and the state itself should be seen as 'disconnected and erratic' (Hillyard and Watson 1996: 338). In addition, an intellectual revolution has taken place beyond the shores of social policy – the different post-literatures – which offers an alternative interpretation not only of the world, but also of the very idea of academic knowledge. Furthermore, the works noted above go beyond the general orientations of postmodernity and dangle specific insights that are said to have implications for social policy.

Initially this argument begins with a call for conceptual widening and for the subject to move beyond merely political and economic accounts of change. As a result, it aspires to bring cultural and discursive practices to the centre stage of welfare study (Fitzpatrick 1996; Hillyard and Watson 1996; Penna and O'Brien 1996). This can be seen as the key postmodernist challenge to social policy, a challenge to use new tools and a fresh explanatory and conceptual syntax. From and by this, much of the remaining case either follows or is implied. Taken in outline, it is that welfare academics should move beyond the old fixities and embrace notions of fluidity and difference in their approaches to identity and social relations. They therefore need to escape from the central binary orderings (man/woman, gay/straight, etc.) that have existed as misleading and false dichotomies (Hillyard and Watson 1996: 333). Moreover, the very notion of universality, so central to both analytic and normative social policy analysis, becomes increasingly redundant in the new particularistic cosmos.

Looming over this call for a postmodern social policy is of course the figure of Michel Foucault. These writers remind us that power and knowledge imply each other (Penna and O'Brien 1996: 52–3) and that power should be seen as a strategy with disciplinary and biological variants (Hillyard and

Watson 1996: 326–9). For good measure, the Foucauldian notions of normalisation and surveillance are proposed as central constructs for the study of social policy. Again, the message is that welfare needs to utilise fundamentally different implements and reconceptualise its own field as a result. This is in essence a call for intellectual revolution rather than the sharpening of old tools or a reworking of moribund ideas.

It is difficult to disagree with much of this. These strands of postmodern thinking serve to challenge what remains of social policy's complacency in such areas as the state, stratification and identity. They also suggest an analytical attitude to power that is at once both more sceptical and richer than that found in traditional welfare fare. However, for these ideas to influence social policy they need to appear as *operational* and *utilisable* constructs for that subject. Interdisciplinary debate does not happen without constructive effort on both sides, and ideas need to be encouraged to cross the intellectual species barrier. Unfortunately the postmodern agenda for social policy has not yet been transmitted in a way that facilitates reception by its target audience. The following critique is of the wider literature that claims to have welfare implications, but will be illustrated here with reference to Hillyard and Watson.

The general approach of these works is to lay out large swathes of social and cultural theory, often quite well-known Foucauldian analysis. This is then followed by a rather casual sentence or two along the lines of 'this formulation might have relevance for social policy' (1996: 339). Alternatively, there may be some notion that the analysis is pertinent to the study of 'single parents' or 'community care', but no attempt to set out in any detail the legislation or policy developments that might now be better illuminated. Indeed, it is not always clear whether the argument is that postmodernity might add to the study of that which can be specifically understood as 'social policy' or to the wider category of 'public policy'. Alternatively, the very notion of 'policy' remains ill defined in these works and in fact the substantive interest appears to be 'the social' itself. All of these are of course proper objects of study, but the lack of specification does little to advance the notion that social policy per se should embrace the postmodern.

This charge can be expanded into a yet more problematic area – that postmodern accounts of social policy do not actually define what they *mean* by social policy. In other words, there is no recognition that this is inherently contestable and that different traditions (Fabian, Marxist, feminist, etc.) have operationalised quite diverse interpretations of welfare itself. The very act of defining maps out the institutions, processes and social divisions to be studied and thus frames the objects of analysis. This is as true now as it was in the era of the 'social conscience thesis'. Without paying attention to the different meanings and types of welfare one might reasonably assume that postmodernist writers, ironically, are operating with a highly traditionalist picture. If social policy needs no introduction it is presumably no more than state welfare – the 'welfare state'. This would not be the first time that an overly restrictive and reductive account of welfare had been provided by writers largely outside of the social policy tradition (on the post-Fordist welfare state thesis see Burrows and Loader 1994; Carter and Rayner 1996; Taylor-Gooby 1997).

This slightly casual approach to welfare in the postmodernity literature fails to address two particularly relevant concepts that have been developed in the social policy field:

1   The *mixed economy of welfare* notion reminds us that welfare is also provided outside of the traditionally understood public services, particularly the private and voluntary sectors. It also highlights the semi-submerged iceberg of familial welfare through which partners, parents and other relatives care and cope. Given the supposed proximity of postmodern analysis and feminism, one might have expected more attention to be paid to these different locations of welfare. Without these we can only guess whether postmodern themes and motifs are proceeding smoothly and equally in the various social policy arenas.

2   The older *social division of welfare* thesis is similarly absent from postmodern accounts. It also moves beyond the visible spectrum of the welfare state and notes other mechanisms through which the state distributes advantage, benefit and security. From Titmuss (1958) onwards, the social policy community has recognised that the *occupational* and *fiscal* systems not only contribute to personal and collective prosperity but also are types of welfare. Are recent changes in the tax structure or the increased availability of employment-based private health to be seen as postmodern? Possibly they are open to such an interpretation, though no attempt has yet been made to show how and indeed why this might be the case.

It is perhaps worth reiterating my argument here. I am not particularly concerned that those proposing a postmodern welfare have failed to take on board every nuance and detail of policy change from the last twenty years or so. This is still a small literature, composed as it is of general mentions in the canonical postmodernity writings and the more dedicated works noted above. Indeed, criticisms delivered in a 'you haven't looked at that' tone can sound negative and carping. Yet we do have a duty to point out a more general and important failing – an unwillingness to engage with the very essence of academic social policy. This can be summarised as a failure to discuss what social policy *is* and the fragmented locations in which it is *generated*. Without such a specification, ironically, the implication is that welfare is created in monolithic, homogeneous and even universalistic packages. Postmodernists, of course, *cannot* believe that to be so, as those very categories are oxymorons of postmodernity itself. However, the postmodernists' own welfare excursions fail to consider the diversity and fragmentation that have long been present in social policy as practised and studied.

A yet further barrier to a postmodernity – welfare rapprochement comes with the tendency of the former to be a bit rude about the latter. Hillyard and Watson (1996) dally in the insulter's foothills, painting a picture that may have been accurate once but is now something of an exaggeration. In this, social policy was 'founded on the idea of the expert ... based on linear notions of progress ... [which] in its universalism cannot take account of local and differentiated effects' (p. 324). Presumably they have not heard of critical social policy? They then pick up steam by noting the 'general reluctance of the social policy community to acquaint themselves with the tidal wave of postmodern thinking' (p. 321). In other words you just have not been reading the right things. Finally, 'fascinating' postmodern inspired work in the field of geography stands as a 'stark contrast to the social policy arena' (p. 334). Telling people they are a bit thick is not necessarily the best way to build intellectual bridges. Moreover, it reduces the likelihood that the genuinely important critique provided by the same authors will have an effect on the study of welfare.

The loyalists

In assessing the response of the social policy gang (which, if prodded with a stick, I would be forced to claim membership of), I am left with a similar mixture of sympathy and concern. These retorts come in two varieties – explicit and implicit.

There are in fact precious few direct treatments of postmodernity in works produced by scholars working unambiguously in the welfare milieu. Of these, Taylor-Gooby's (1994) article stands out. In this he suggests that the postmodern focus on diversity and differentiation ignores the universalising advance of market liberalism and commodification of the last twenty years. Postmodernism in welfare is an ideological smokescreen and (the subtitle of his piece) a 'great leap backwards'. There is of course a pertinent and timely warning here: a postmodern gaze can act to peripheralise the poor – an argument that elides with my earlier rejection of 'celebrationist' postmodernisms. It also reminds us that the right, in power domestically and beyond, have consciously sought to recreate inequality through choice and ersatz markets.

A problem, though, is that such a rejection of postmodernity in welfare acts as a conversation stopper. By implication if not design it can be taken as a generalised rejection – which walls off debates about difference and diversity from academic social policy. In highlighting the weaknesses of the postmodern case on welfare it implies that there cannot *be* a postmodern welfare – an 'end-of-story' stance. This might ultimately be a position like King Canute's, though, in danger of being ultimately overtaken by Hillyard and Watson's 'tidal wave'. Instead, a critical engagement with the postmodern position – which equally seeks to sustain the social policy agenda – might be more productive in the long run.

CORNWALL COLLEGE
LEARNING CENTRE

The second welfare reply to postmodernity, strangely enough, does not refer to postmodernity at all. For this is the actual construction and orientation of social policy as an academic subject – a far more significant barrier to a postmodern engagement than is represented by Taylor-Gooby's repudiation of particular arguments. This will be illustrated by way of two brief examples rather than a review of the whole field.

Glennerster wrote in 1988 regretting the reinvention of the Social Administration Association as the Social Policy Association. This, he suggested, was due to a collective lack of self-confidence and a desire to repackage the subject in such a way that new research funding and prestige could be found. Moreover, it abandoned any attempt to understand how local institutions and bureaucracies worked and, in turn, disengaged us from the realities of welfare as experienced and lived. Succinctly, Glennerster argued that 'if we had worried less about critical theory and more about clearing people's rubbish we would have served humanity better' (Glennerster 1988: 84).

Glennerster may or may not be right in the specifics of this, and Wilding's (1992) review of the 1980s in social policy actually noted an increased interest in organisational matters. But, as a call for a more socially and politically committed approach, Glennerster's case has much to commend it. One can forget how two decades of demoralisation have eroded the strong link between analysis and action that existed in the easily derided social administration era (though both the critical social policy tradition and the postmodernists would rightly raise the essentially paternalistic relationships this involvement was founded on). Glennerster's contribution does, however, raise issues of greater relevance to the arguments of this chapter. First and incidentally, he reminds us that social policy has indeed embraced developments in social and critical theory and in doing so shifted from its 'drains and sewers' heritage. Second, though, his desire to get back to refuse disposal hardly holds out a hand of friendship towards the postmodernists. Lyotard does not easily fit into a wheelie bin and the deconstructed refuse sack can leave one hell of a mess.

In similar vein, Spicker uses a recent textbook to mark out social policy's territory as a field of study. This too, at least by implication, erects defences against the postmodern intellectual 'other'. He begins by distinguishing social policies from their socio-economic backdrop, saying there are many contexts but that 'the study of the context is not social policy in itself ... social policy is not a subject which studies class, the family, race or gender in their own right' (Spicker 1995: 6). Social policy, then, studies welfare.

Many in social policy would just about hold with this – it marks out a distinctive set of concerns and points the way towards the designation of themes like poverty, altruism and stigma as 'belonging' to social policy (Spicker 1995: 8). Following on from the earlier analysis, we might also want the postmodernists to acquaint themselves with that which defines the field. However, the further distinctions Spicker draws have the effect of precluding the very notion of a postmodern social policy and are thus problematic. The first of these arises from his discussion of Cahill's (1994) text, *The New Social Policy*, which seeks to extend welfare analysis into areas such as communicating, shopping and viewing. Spicker agrees that these are components of well-*being* but argues that wel*fare* is more specific. The latter only relates 'to certain kinds of collective provision' and therefore Cahill is 'really interested in a different subject area' (Spicker 1995: 5). In effect this distinction – a listing of what can and what cannot stand under the social policy banner – nudges out the study of consumption practices (and thus a key component of postmodern analysis vanishes).

Second, Spicker considers social policy's relations with its near neighbours and thus how it is composed as a field of study. He lists the concerns that each adjacent discipline has in common with social policy and those which are distinctly their own. With regard to the study of *culture*, he classifies this as a sociology-only topic and not something that social policy has even a shared interest in. In these circumstances it is hard to envisage social policy making a 'cultural turn'. Consequently a further point of potential contact with the postmodernists is ruled out of court.

Again, contradictions are ever-present. Many of us welcome attempts to map out the territory of social policy and that which makes it more than the sum of its parts. However, that very act of specification can add to a mind set that locates postmodernity and all of its works beyond our borders. In extreme cases (not Spicker), this can sound like Eurosceptics banging on about sovereignty as an excuse for not wanting to talk to foreigners.

CONCLUSION: TALKING TO THE NEIGHBOURS AND USING MAPS

Thus far, then, the debate has been characterised by a rolling and cumulative ambiguity. We need postmodern accounts of social policy but should be worried at the rather nonchalant picture of welfare (as both studied and practised) painted in these works so far. Therefore, we have to maintain social policy as a discrete intellectual area, but should also be concerned that attempts to do precisely that can harden into a Maginot line against postmodernity. Any successful and convincing postmodern account of welfare is likely therefore to be found at the eye of these various storms.

Why then has the debate so far been, effectively, a non-debate? And why has such a gap emerged between social policy and sociology/cultural studies (the carrier disciplines of the postmodern position)? The answer to this is probably quite mundane and invokes the sociology of knowledge as much as it does the intellectual content of the debate itself.

John Baker was faced with a similar conundrum in 1979 when seeking to explain the continued dominance of the social conscience thesis. He emphasised the practical issues which had produced a particular bearing in the social policy community. Most notably, its social work links and practice orientation had conspired to create an overly positive view of the state and its role in welfare (Baker 1979: 190–7). Bringing this kind of analysis up to date, it does not at all follow that social policy's training connections should have narrowed the subject and made it resistant to the postmodern virus. However, in passing, we might note that other aspects of the organisation of welfare teaching might have created a certain image problem. In particular, social policy staff tend to find themselves teaching across a wide range of courses rather than on a dedicated single honours programme (see, for example, CNAA 1990). Linked to this tendency to service teaching is a diverse pattern of staff organisation. Some social policy specialists work in eponymously titled groups, though more often they find themselves as numerically junior partners in larger outfits. The usual linkages here are with social workers, sociologists and political scientists.

In such circumstances, then, social policy experts can find their own teaching is fragmented and shaped by the demands of outside professional bodies. Moreover, these same conditions may conceivably contribute to the apparently low regard in which social policy is held by some outside of the field. An (entirely false) perception may therefore be that a subject still tied to the training function and to something called the 'welfare state' can have no theory of its own. It consequently needs to receive conceptual Red Cross parcels from elsewhere, and the charitable donors need not worry too much about the specific dietary needs of the recipients. The political economy of academia may have produced rather specific terms of engagement between welfare and other disciplines.

There is of course a danger of exaggerating this point, and clearly many academics in the welfare field work both constructively and productively with sociologists and others. Interdisciplinary work in general can be rewarding, as it brings together ideas usually found in different contexts. This can have a catalytic effect and may serve to generate new ventures and revitalise old debates. However, interdisciplinary work can also be problematic. As Turner argues, *unreflective* interaction can 'produce a fragmentary pastiche of disciplines rather than intellectual integration' (Turner 1990: 1). Hence the very externality of the postmodern canon to the subject of social policy is a hurdle to be overcome. In similar vein Kemeny suggests that attempts to apply ideas to adjacent intellectual realms require a 'prior anchoring' in those disciplines (Kemeny 1992: 11). This might be understood as reaching a kind of anthropological understanding of other subjects, which in turn facilitates debate and intellectual trade. It may be, however, that the postmodernists have not yet sought to anchor their analysis in the richness of social policy.

Finally, we need to return our gaze closer to home and to something we repeat as a mantra but rarely explore the meaning of. If social policy is a 'field of study', what does this actually indicate? In welfare's early skirmishes with the postmodern it could be suggested that it has come to denote a process of fencing off and excluding – an intellectual *non paserán*. However, this need not be so, though we do need to update our cartographical self-image (particularly in the light of Baudrillard's vision of the map preceding the actual territory). In such an atlas, social policy would be shown as a specific but none the less localised relief detail in a wider projection of the social sciences. The contour lines connecting welfare to the surrounding terrain would thus become more apparent and new vantage points arise.

Ultimately, then, this has been an extended plea for mutual common sense and open-mindedness in social policy's dealings with the postmodern. For those active in the study of welfare, this most of all requires a shift from a 'subject-bounded' approach to an intellectual strategy driven by concepts. Concepts defy subject boundaries and can be found in different disciplinary settings. Moreover, a positive reaction to new formulations need not threaten the integrity of academic subjects and indeed can enrich and enliven them. In this fashion then there may yet be a postmodern social policy.

ACKNOWLEDGEMENT

I am grateful to colleagues Karen Morse and Mary Rayner for their helpful comments on this chapter and for ongoing conversations.

BIBLIOGRAPHY

Baker, J. (1979) 'Social conscience and social policy', *Journal of Social Policy* 8, 2: 177–206.
Barthes, R. (1977) *Image–Music–Text*, New York: Hill & Wang.
Berman, M. (1982) *All that is Solid Melts into Air*, London: Verso.
Bertens, H. (1995) *The Idea of the Postmodern: A History*, London: Routledge.
Burrows, R. and Loader, B. (eds) (1994) *Towards a Post-Fordist Welfare State?*, London: Routledge.
Cahill, M. (1994) *The New Social Policy*, Oxford: Blackwell.
Carter, J. (1997) 'Post-Fordism and the theorisation of educational change: what's in a name?', *British Journal of Sociology of Education* 18, 1: 45–61.
Carter, J. and Rayner, M. (1996) 'The curious case of post-Fordism and welfare', *Journal of Social Policy* 25, 3: 347–67.
CNAA (Council for National Academic Awards) (1990) *Social Policy and Administration in Polytechnics and Colleges*, London: CNAA.
Derrida, J. (1967) *Of Grammatology*, Baltimore: Johns Hopkins University Press.
Derrida, J. (1970) 'Structure, sign and play in the discourse of the human sciences', in R. Macksey and E. Donato (eds) *The Structuralist Controversy: The Language of Criticism and the Sciences of Man*, Baltimore: Johns Hopkins University Press.
Erskine, A. (1996) 'The burden of risk – who dies because of cars', *Social Policy and Administration* 30, 2: 143–57.
Fitzpatrick, T. (1996) 'Postmodernism, welfare and radical politics', *Journal of Social Policy* 25, 3: 303–20.
Foucault, M. (1977) *Discipline and Punish: The Birth of the Prison*, London: Allen Lane.
Foucault, M. (1980) *Power/Knowledge: Selected Interviews*, Brighton: Harvester Press.

Glennerster, H. (1988) 'A requiem for the Social Administration Association', *Journal of Social Policy* 17, 1: 83–4.

Hall, S. and Jacques, M. (eds) (1989) *New Times*, London: Lawrence & Wishart.

Hillyard, P. and Watson, S. (1996) 'Postmodern social policy: a contradiction in terms?', *Journal of Social Policy* 25, 3: 321–46.

Huby, M. (1995) 'Water poverty and social policy: a review of issues for research', *Journal of Social Policy* 24, 2: 219–36.

Kemeny, J. (1992) *Housing and Social Theory*, London: Routledge.

Lynton, N. (1989) *The Story of Modern Art*, London: Phaidon.

Lyotard, J.-F. (1979) *The Postmodern Condition: A Report on Knowledge*, Manchester: Manchester University Press.

Marshall, T.H. (1970) *Social Policy in the Twentieth Century*, London: Hutchinson.

Penna, S. and O'Brien, M. (1996) 'Postmodernism and social policy: a small leap forwards?', *Journal of Social Policy* 25, 1: 39–61.

Spicker, P. (1995) *Social Policy: Themes and Approaches*, Hemel Hempstead: Prentice Hall/Harvester Wheatsheaf.

Taylor-Gooby, P. (1994) 'Postmodernism and social policy: a great leap backwards?', *Journal of Social Policy* 23, 3: 385–404.

Taylor-Gooby, P. (1997) 'In defence of second best theory: state, class and capital in social policy', *Journal of Social Policy* 26, 2: 171–92.

Titmuss, R.M. (1958) *Essays on the Welfare State*, London: Allen & Unwin.

Titmuss, R.M. (1974) *Social Policy: An Introduction*, London: Allen & Unwin.

Turner, B. (1990) 'The interdisciplinary curriculum: from social medicine to postmodernism', *Sociology of Health and Illness* 12, 1: 1–23.

Wilding, P. (1992) 'Social policy in the 1980s: an essay in academic evolution', *Social Policy and Administration* 26, 2: 107–16.

Williams, F. (1989) *Social Policy: A Critical Introduction*, Cambridge: Polity Press.

Chapter 3

Postmodernism, poststructuralism and social policy

John R. Gibbins

INTRODUCTION

Debates about postmodernity have entered disciplines and fields of study at different times in different ways and with different effects. As late as the 1980s books on postmodern sociology and politics were still considered avant-garde. While various voices have entered the debate on the value and relevance of postmodernism for social policy, it is only now being felt to have a serious impact. Poststructuralism is an approach of longer lineage and greater impact upon sociology, but again its voice in social policy has been mute and its impact almost non-existent. My aim here is fourfold: first to make a contribution to the current highly critical debate about the relevance of postmodernism to social policy; second, to show that the relevance of postmodernism for social policy becomes more evident when considered alongside poststructuralism; third, to argue that an eclectic and culturalist postmodernism, built upon the study of language, knowledge and reproduction, may provide a significant perspective and resource for policy analysts and practitioners; and finally, to explore some resulting implications of this approach for social policy. I can here neither make a critical judgement on the adequacy of either postmodernism or poststructuralism, nor move to the detail of effects and implications in specific areas of social policy. My study remains at the theoretical level of exposition, analysis and connection of theory to the field of study called social policy.

POSTMODERNISM AND SOCIAL POLICY

Of the many reasons given by critics of the claims for a postmodern perspective on social policy, two are most generally produced and entertained. One is that the perspective's various textual embodiments are too diverse, disparate, incoherent and inconsistent to be of value. The second is that it lacks a political and pragmatic application, providing a mystification, a gloss of terminology, to cover a paucity of practical critique, understanding of real inequalities and solutions to social problems (Taylor-Gooby 1994). In response to the first point, Penna and O'Brien have presented a neat reply to the charge that postmodernists conflate a number of separate theoretical positions and paradigms, stressing both differences between them (postindustrialism, post-Fordism, poststructuralism and postmodernism) and the points of conjunction (Hillyard and Watson 1996: 322–3; Penna and O'Brien 1996; Rose 1991). While agreeing with this response it is possible to go beyond the pragmatism that it invokes, namely that postmodernism provides 'the discipline of social policy with alternative theoretical perspectives and political agenda [sic] with which to address the complexity of current restructuring' (Penna and O'Brien 1996: 60). I also reject the charge of lack of relevance, and argue that, in the current practical and theoretical situation, postmodernism provides one of the best available resources on 'important questions' and not just a 'small step forwards' (Rosenau 1992: ix).

A claim for the relevance of postmodernism to social policy has two strands. First, it alone seems to account for the strange situation in the world that social scientists seek to understand and define; and second, postmodernism is both more persuasive and coherent (though synchronic rather than synthetic) than its critics believe. Too much has been written on the former to need extensive elaboration here, but we can argue with Bauman that the setting – economic, political, social, cultural and intellectual – which accompanied the emergence of the modern field and disciplines of social policy, has changed beyond a point where the proposed agendas, paradigms and language utilised are appropriate (Bauman 1991, 1992).

The feelings that a familiar world has melted before them – feelings of dissonance, insecurity, strangeness and loss – have, some critics argued, been experienced mainly by middle-class professionals whose occupations were undergoing radical restructuring, such as journalists, academics, architects and artists. But the phenomenon is reflected widely in popular cultural forms, such as dystopias, and in both phenomenological and empirical studies of other people's perceptions, feelings and attitudes (Kaase and Newton 1995; Kroker and Kroker 1988; van Deth and Scarbrough 1995). Another source of critique, namely the notion that this shift was only one of perception and had no correlates in practices, behaviour and action, has also been demonstrated to be inaccurate, as Helen Wilkinson's *No Turning Back: Generations and Genderquake* illustrates (Wilkinson 1996).

What the changes were in the world that postmodernists identify we sought to explain in 'Postmodernism' (Gibbins and Reimer 1995), but this should be read alongside and contrasted with similar, competitive accounts of the transformation of modernity by Ulrich Beck on 'reflexive modernization and modernity' and Anthony Giddens on 'high and late modernity' (Beck 1992: 1–15, 87–90, 104–6, 1996: 3–7; Giddens 1991a: 4–5, 10–32, 1991b: 1–10, 149–50, 163–73; Giddens et al. 1994: 1–55, 174–7, 210–13). Our claim is that 'many of the practices and preconditions of politics in the modern world are being undermined by technological, informational, organisational, social and

above all cultural changes which create discontinuities, incongruity, dissonance, fragmentation and dis-sensus' (Gibbins and Reimer 1995: 303–4), and,
one may add, a new apprehension about unpredictability, uncertainty and the
growing awareness of risks (Beck 1992).

Like most postmodernists, we see these as associated (though not causally
determined) by the transition to a postindustrial, information and consumer
society; the disorganisation of capitalism, socialism and bureaucracy;
transnationalism and globalisation processes; the decline of an international
order brokered by the US; the restructuring of employment, unemployment
and leisure discussed in the post-Fordist debate; the restructuring of the
social categories, classes, gender, race and sexuality; and the dissolution of
old and the emergence of new knowledges and discourses.

We disagree with structuralist opponents in the refusal to have a
base/superstructure model of determination. Our model is more horizontal,
multicausal and interdeterminant, placing knowledge, culture and reproduction on a level plane with economy, class and production. Postmodernist
research is as yet inconclusive on determination and the agencies of change,
but researchers do not all buy shares in the reflexive modernisation thesis promoted by Fitzpatrick, in which science and technology are the agents which
are undermining the logic, relationships and identities that sustained first-
stage modernity (Fitzpatrick 1996: 308–12). Mediaisation (the process in and
by which the media, rather than the family and class, take over the role of
socialisation), knowledge creation and identity construction may be at least as
important in the postmodernisation process as technology and post-Fordist
organisational change. Consumerism and the logic of reproduction may be
coming more significant in effecting change than the logic and practice of
production.

That postmodernists do not agree on a narrative or an explanatory paradigm to link all of these levels and effects together should not, however, be
used as an argument for rejecting the hypothesised argument. First, in no
other theoretical position or paradigm is there unity amongst its adherents on
fundamentals. A peripheral analysis of the history of disciplines, schools of
thought, theories and methods, including Marxism, feminism and positivism,
reveals similar tensions, incongruities and irreconcilables. Postmodernism
should and can expect to develop by, through and because of these debates
into a more mature academic perspective, but paradox, irony and ambivalence are accepted as features by its adherents.

Postmodernism, as an academic paradigm and perspective, is undergoing
a process of formation, deconstruction, argument and debate not dissimilar
to that of its predecessors, except in two major regards. First, most paradigms
are driven by the urge for sovereign supremacy and a total coherence. Second,
they base their legitimacy upon claims about foundations and methods that
can produce universal truths of general application, as with Marxism.

Postmodernism develops without such modernist presuppositions. It refuses to accept the supremacy of any metanarrative or perspective, rather seeing the conflict of models, the deconstruction of the dominant, and the reworking of suppressed elements of the canon as preconditions for advance. Next, like poststructuralists, postmodernists are suspicious of claims for coherence, both as a feature of the world and as a feature of argument. Calls for coherence are often reflections of internal crisis (Bourdieu 1988: 174–81). The 'myth of coherence' was first coined in the history of ideas by Quentin Skinner, but postmodernists may see it as of wider application (Tully and Skinner 1988: 39–41). It is unjustifiable to claim that all actors in a category, or all the actions of one actor in his/her life, or all the statements of an author in a text, are driven by the demand for coherence. It is as grave an error to assume all authors act on a coherent life plan as it is to assume that all drug takers do. Multiple selved identities rarely manage a consistent narrative, and when they do, it is usually a fiction, in which 'we impose some narrative form onto our lives, each of us in the ordinary process of living is a fitful novelist, and the biographer is a literary critic' (Rose 1985: 14).

Postmodernists are people who share little, except a refusal to subscribe to universal truths or even a commitment to foundational beliefs, facts or methods. All truths to them are relative to something, most centrally languages or discourses, and all foundations double as conclusions to prior discourses. Foundations are always the contingent products of previous thought and practice, never absolute prehistorical axioms. The origins of this lie not in old-style epistemology, but in the discoveries about the axial place of language and discourse in the creation and maintenance of meanings and forms of life that we find in Saussure and Wittgenstein, and that are echoed in Oakeshott, Rorty and Bernstein, and more potently in French poststructuralism. If, as Wittgenstein argues, all meaning is constructed in language systems; and if all words and phrase mean what they are used to mean in the context of the vocabulary of a practice, its underlying form of life, conventions of usage, the intentions of authors and understanding of the audience; then universalism, absolutism and essentialism are unjustified aspirations (Winch 1958). For universalists and structuralists, research has moved to the question of whether language has universal forms, syntactical rules and physiological foundations. The jury is out on this question.

Postmodern social policy is learning, with difficulty, to live with these considerations, and some recent contributions are encouraging (Penna and O'Brien 1996; Fitzpatrick 1996; Hillyard and Watson 1996). Broadly, the postmodern academic project may be defined as the attempt to understand and respond to a world being transformed, without the supports found in modernism, namely a confidence in absolutes and foundational structures, truths, knowledge, meanings and methods. Postmodernists, in turn, have to live with the effects of their own understandings, with ambivalence and uncertainty, a plurality of postmodernisms, truths, knowledges and disciplines.

They do so by elevating the idea of political practice, and the practice of conversation, into a metaphor and exemplar for good practice.

Social policy, for generations, has been erected upon understanding and solving problems that arise from the operation and antagonism of agreed foundational structures and a largely agreed vocabulary. What is the effect of problematising these structures and vocabularies, and how can a new social policy operate in the void created? Social policy has also been tied to the idea of the expert, knowledge-propelled progress via welfare, and to universalism, indeed to the whole gamut of assumptions inherited from the Enlightenment (Hillyard and Watson 1996: 324–5). What is the effect for social policy of abandoning such groundings?

STRUCTURALISM, POSTSTRUCTURALISM AND SOCIAL POLICY

Structuralism is a collective label for a variety of loosely related philosophical positions that emerged in France in the middle decades of the twentieth century. While diverging on the source and identity of the underlying structures that shaped reality, they all subscribed to the idea of their existence and constructive power. Whether (for Saussure) the foundational structures were sign systems, or (for Lévi-Strauss) they were the binaries implicit in myths, or (for Althusser) they were classes implicit in ideologies, structuralism celebrated and reworked the claims of Marx, Durkheim and Freud, namely that humans were made and operated by structures and forces beyond their personal or collective control (Hewitt 1992: 133–50; Kurzweil 1980; Sturrock 1979). Taylor-Gooby's earlier text on social policy exemplifies this approach (Taylor-Gooby and Dale 1981).

Enshrined within many social science paradigms, methods and theories, this claim was elaborated and deconstructed by the poststructuralists, a diverse group associated with Jacques Derrida, Gilles Deleuze, Emmanuel Levinas and, most famously, Michel Foucault (Foucault 1970, 1972, 1977, 1979). Disagreeing on methods, practices and politics, these thinkers shared the desire to challenge and to destroy the tyranny of structures, both in theory and practice, that had held western intellectuals and citizens in chains for decades. They denounced the search for foundational structures as fruitless; they ransacked languages, discourses and categories for the multiple meanings, metaphorical release, irony and paradox that revealed the simplification of semiotic relationships and binary opposites. They took the liberty made evident in the deconstruction of language as an invitation to uncover and explore the differences, distinctions and diversities that structuralist discourses, language and theory had repressed.

While American anti-foundationalism was different in form and approach, similar conclusions and practices were being developed by Richard Rorty and Richard Bernstein (Bernstein 1976, 1985; Rorty 1979, 1989). In Britain, several broadly hermeneutic researches, by Oakeshott, Skinner and Bauman, were concluding that texts have no essential meaning, that unstable meanings reflect contested interpretations from audiences, producers, reproducers and authors; that meaning was never more than a temporary contingent agreement, often little more than adherence to a tradition (Bauman 1987, 1992, 1997; Oakeshott 1975; Skinner 1985). All concluded that knowledge was produced in language, and that languages, and hence knowledges, were plural, relative and incommensurable.

The implications of poststructuralism were rapidly worked out by western intellectuals first in linguistics, literature, art history, cultural studies and media studies, and later in history, political theory and sociology, but rarely in social policy. There, the normal science paradigm was structuralist, though being restructured, with gender and race added to class as foundational categories in the new critical social policy agenda. I wish here to focus on only three of the many profound insights of poststructuralists which may have implications for social policy, namely the method of deconstruction; the rejection of binaries; and the acceptance that social policy analysts construct their own subjects and objects and their disciplinary and repressive regimes and practices.

Deconstruction

As exemplified in the work of Derrida, deconstruction is a method for attacking the traditional laws of thought and logic in western philosophy and thinking, which provide the grids, categories and structures for life as well as thinking (Norris 1982). Involving the search for exceptions to the rule, paradox, irony and the search for difference, deconstruction was used originally to undermine such binaries as appearance and reality, ideal and actual, inside and outside, fiction and non-fiction. But in the writings of Foucault the whole structuralist edifice of the law, state and the regulatory practices of medicine, social work, sexology, penology and psychology came under scrutiny, and with devastating effect (Boyne 1990; Cousins and Hussain 1984; Dreyfus and Rabinow 1982; Gane and Johnson 1993). Not only were literary and actual cases of exceptions and exclusions unearthed from the past, but contemporary discourses in the social sciences, understood within the framework of power/knowledge, came under scrutiny, and their exclusory and repressive potential was realised (Derrida 1967, 1982; Foucault 1973, 1980). With Foucault's writings and the work of Jacques Donzelot on social workers and health visitors, deconstruction had come to the gates of social policy, only to be given limited entry (Donzelot 1979).

The rejection of binaries

The deconstuction of binaries, as prelude for creativity in thinking and inventiveness in practice, was, however, made effective in social policy by feminism.

Its exposure of the fabricated nature and repressive effect of the binaries natural/artificial, man/woman, reason/emotion, active/passive, independent/dependent were models of what poststructuralism can do for social policy. Rulers/ruled, exploiters/exploited, white/black, abled/disabled, heterosexual/homosexual, healthy/sick, educated/ignorant, housed/homeless, employed/unemployed are just some of the common binaries that structure and define social policy research and practice and are awaiting serious, but avoided, attention (Hillyard and Watson 1996: 324, 327–8).

The construction of subjects and objects

Welfare discourse, we can learn from poststructuralists like Donzelot, is part of a modern system and apparatus for regulating and controlling mass populations in confined spaces. Social policy constructs its subjects, such as the needy, disabled and homeless, onto whom bodies, minds, values, interests and behaviours are inscribed. It constructs regulatory and disciplinary regimes through which power is inscribed upon individuals and groups, and circulated through the social body, mostly for its own interests (Hewitt 1983, 1990, 1992: 159–63; Squires 1990). This problem of mass populations, created by the new health, sanitation and housing discourses and practices of the nineteenth century, requires the state to fund policy analysis and formation by recognised professional experts (Baron 1988; Cohen and Scull 1983; Hewitt 1992: 151–73). The power and status of social research, social science and social administration were premised upon promises by generations of scholars to provide workable solutions to the problem of governance (Burchell *et al.* 1991). In particular, power lies with those able to invent and impose their categories, the taxonomies that control everyday life. Social policy has been one of the most prolific generators of such taxonomies, of desert, need, want and quality of life, the effects of which have been dubious (Forder 1974: 39–57).

Further links with poststructuralism

One other major source of opposition to the postmodernist project, which poststructuralism may help us to transcend, lies in the disputed nature of the binaries involved: modern/postmodern, modernity/postmodernity, modernisation/postmodernisation. That clear-cut division and distinctions have proved impossible to sustain, that many features invoked in one can be found in areas of the other, that modern and postmodern often coincide in one place or person are features of the contemporary debate that it is unnecessary to dispute. The ideas that postmodernity is a uniform thing or time period, that postmodernisation is a linear process, that the postmodern depicts something essential, are false and rejected by postmodernists.

While some postmodernists see postmodernity as a thing, they do not see it as a period with definite beginnings and ends; rather it is an unfinished project, whose directions are both uncharted, unknown and disorganised. From Kant through Lévi-Strauss to the deconstructionists, binaries have been understood as human impositions, grids and categories to make the world more navigable. Postmodernists, learning from deconstructionists, treat binaries as historical, contingent artefacts, and not realities.

The strong linkage in context, mutual influence and effects of postmodernism and poststructuralism has been argued elsewhere (Lemert 1992: 28–42; Sarup 1988). The linking themes and concepts are anti-foundationalism, deconstruction, irony, difference, plurality, diversity, relativism, methodological and political pragmatism. The main impact of these points for social policy must be the rejection of any idea of itself being a unitary discipline, with agreement on aims, methods and field of study. However, social policy's experience of combining disciplines, in multidisciplinary or interdisciplinary research on a field of study, has at least protected it from the necessity of wholly reinventing itself. Its multiparadigmed tradition is proving to be an asset and not a liability.

POSTMODERNISM

Most analysts in the field of social policy treat postmodernism from within structuralism rather than poststructuralism; that is, they treat postmodernism as an epiphenomenon of the restructuring of the global economy, society and polity, treating the economy as foundational, often as little more than an ideology. When it comes to social policy, they look at the effects of capitalist globalisation and post-Fordist management processes upon work and employment, central and local government. In turn, these processes are seen to impact upon social classes, families and communities, producing dealignment, breakdown and restructuring of the familiar to accommodate the new demands. In turn again, the restructuring of society is seen to impact upon the political level, not only upon parties that decline as social movements rise, but in the state, local government and welfare, and in their impacts upon social service delivery and policy formation. Within this structuralist model, postmodernism is understood as the cultural and ideological (including academic) epiphenomenon of late capitalist modifications, in which citizens are told they are being given choice, options and power when in fact these are legitimations of restriction, regulation and disciplining.

Such an interpretation is plausible and in some ways persuasive. It is certainly well researched and argued in the Marxist forms of postmodernism, such as those elaborated by Jameson, Harvey and Smart (Harvey 1989; Jameson 1984, 1989, 1991; Smart 1993). But in this section, I wish to deal with my third aim: to reorientate the debate and to focus another account of postmodernity upon social policy; that is, one informed by the arguments of poststructuralism. In particular, I wish to intensify the gaze of social policy analysts on the cultural level, for instance upon the changes taking place in the postmodern self, in the identities of individuals and groups, and in the postmodern lifestyles they create and share. I argue that social policy can benefit from exploring the implication of poststructuralism and postmodern cultural studies, and that while not ignoring the structuralist and restructuring models, we should add the new focus to our endeavours.

What threads or voices are there in the postmodern debate other than the neo-Marxist variant? While historians argue the genealogy of the term 'postmodernism', there is some agreement that it was first coined by Frederic de Onis in 1934 to refer to the anti-modernist current in Spanish and Latin American poetry between 1905 and 1914 (Rose 1991: 13–15). This usage, mainly limited to the field of literary studies, refers to a style of writing. Recent research has trumped this claim, identifying a German philosopher, Rudolf Pannwitz, as using it in 1917, to refer to the growing nihilism in western culture, traced to the musings of Friedrich Nietzsche (Rose 1991: 190). A religious adaptation was coined by Bernard Iddings Bell in 1939; he used the term to refer to the cultural phenomenon in which secular thought was unable to replace or make good the void left by the decline in religious thinking.

Also in 1939 we had the usage by Arnold Toynbee referring to a new epoch, the one typified by the triumph of mass society (Rose 1991: 9). So by 1945, four valid usages were available, none at this stage being economistic and structuralist, and all referring to the cultural level and to cultural change in particular. None agreed on the 'modernism' that the 'post' referred to, in terms of either dates, features or effects; and none agreed on how 'post' is to be used. In 1945 two unrelated authors writing on architecture, Bernard Smith and Joseph Hudnut, adopted the term to refer to a reaction to modernist abstract aesthetics, a usage later adopted by Charles Jenks. The first clear sociological and structuralist usage appeared in 1959 from Daniel Bell (Turner 1989). He combined an epochal usage with a sociological model of the transformation towards a new type of social order. The next development in this field was that of Jameson in 1984, mentioned above (Bertens 1995: 160–84). Since then almost all of the usages above have been revived and reworked, with the addition of the French poststructuralist usage and the culturalist poststructuralist adaptation most closely associated with Mike Featherstone and Bryan Turner (Featherstone 1988, 1991; Turner 1990). More recently, the term has been used to refer to a cultural movement rather than a process, one expressing avant-garde and radical political and aesthetic change (Heller and Feher 1989).

A new taxonomy of postmodernism is neither needed nor necessary for us to see that other usages than that depending upon structuralist and economistic underpinnings were, and are, available. These agree on focusing debate upon something called modernism, and not capitalism. While postindustrialists critique industrialism, and post-Fordism transforms Fordism, postmodernism is contrasted with modernism. They all seem to suggest by

'post' that their position is a 'break' from, something 'different' and, sometimes 'after'. What that looked like is disputed, but it has many dimensions,
only some of which are economic and technological. While there is no agreement, most authors see modernity as multidimensional, featuring such
diverse elements as industrial production; priority given to production and
technology; a class-based social division of labour; the modern state; rationalism; materialism; faith in education, science and progress; and the growth
of individualism and mass culture, plus a regimented division of the private
and public worlds. Not all have binary opposites in postmodernity; some
continue and others have been transformed.

The agents of change differ, but we can note three especially prevalent theories in dispute: Marxist structuralism, poststructuralism and culturalism.
Poststructuralist postmodernism is happy to be eclectic and accept a plurality of ever-changing agents of change. The culturalist approach has several
dimensions which stress the capacity of knowledge, disciplines, the media,
consumerism and the reproduction system, especially the mass media, to
alter the world. Lyotard can be located between the two approaches. Having
concluded that Marxist structuralist analysis no longer has explanatory or
emancipatory potential, he addressed the reasons why.

Three interrelated factors have combined together, according to Lyotard, in
a complex way to undermine the modern order: the mercantilisation of
knowledge; the transmission of knowledge; and the attendant decline in legitimacy and legitimation principles for knowledge (Lyotard 1984: 39; Sarup
1988: 117–25). Yet underpinning knowledge is language, and Sarup and
others argue, correctly, that Lyotard saw the revolution in language and in
discourse philosophy as driving the knowledge level (Sarup 1988: 118–20).
Computers, as a form of technology, may be identified as major agents in the
process. The collapse of traditional language games, the circulation of new
narratives and the collapse of metanarratives are given political and social
significance.

Jean Baudrillard identifies the triumph of reproduction over production,
and the detachment of image from object, of simulation from the simulated,
and of signs from what they signify as the key agent (Baudrillard 1983a,
1983b). In his third order of simulacra, talk of reality is empty; we can only
know and operate at the level of signs. Baudrillard is hence identifying reproduction, and especially the mass media, as the core agent. Bo Reimer and I
argue an extension of this in our theory of mediaisation, which looks more
closely at the impact of various media on everyday life (Gibbins and Reimer
1995: 309; Reimer 1994). Several processes in the media are identified as for-
mative: the immediacy of contact made possible by electronic forms; the
transnationality of penetration; the concentration of reproduction in ever
fewer hands; and the self-referential nature of the media. The media are
replacing traditional forms of socialisation in providing the structure, meaning and calendar of everyday life. Consumerism, the practice of prioritising

consumption of goods and services over all other reason for being, is related (Featherstone 1983, 1991).

To conclude this section, I propose two other entry points into postmodern social policy: lifestyles and the self. Recent lifestyles research has usually been sociological and concentrated upon the particular, usually rare and exotic lifestyles – looking at various youth cultures, for instance. But there are good reasons to believe that the notion could be applied with benefit to social policy and to the more general, the more common and mundane. Bourdieu has described the class habitus, and we could go on to develop race and gender habitus as well as researching the newer and stranger lifestyles practised by the youth groups, gays and lesbians, travellers, greens, healers, foodies and new mystics (Bourdieu 1984). We also hypothesised that lifestyles are becoming not only more important as centres of identity and for relationships, but more pluralised (Gibbins and Reimer 1995: 11). People are exploring alternative lifestyles, moving beyond a base where vocation, class or a sport may dominate, towards an exploration of other practices and lifeworlds. So a married mother shares a life with work friends and another at a health and sports club, and may gender bend while exploring on the Internet. A redundant male miner from south Wales may have a life with young mothers around the school and may study art with the Open University, while maintaining a 'drinking-and-rugby' culture with old friends. The implications of this for social policy are enormous in range and significance. We might have to look beyond the current canon of groups to study and look at new lifestyle groupings, such as drug takers, travellers, gays and lesbians, lesbian mothers. Next we might have to look at the different groups within large groupings, such as black mothers or professional black mothers. Third, we might see that inequalities may follow lifestyle as well as class and gender lines, as with travellers and gays.

If postmodernists reject metanarratives and replace them with multiple narrative disciplines, and reject methodological foundationalism and essentialism, so they also reject the ideas of an essential human nature or self; structured lifestyles based on social categorisation; and the ideas that values are merely ideological epiphenomena of these primary structures. Rather postmodernists assert that the subject should be seen as essentially decentred or without fixed content; that s/he has few if any fixed, universal or essential characteristics. The self is a multiple personality, with plural, distinct and often conflicting facets and needs, finding expression in ever-changing and highly personalised, eclectic lifestyles, now more usually held together by particular patterns of personalised preferences and values than by the imposition of the dull routine of everyday life or of social-structural and functional necessities. Giddens, Connolly, Taylor and we ourselves have hypothesised that accompanying the 'disembedding' of the self from its traditional social location is a process of the 'reinvention' of the self (Connolly 1991; Giddens 1991a; Taylor 1989). We hypothesise the emergence of new structures of feeling and new patterns of values and preferences amongst western citizens that have an impact on behaviour, practices and institutions, including areas considered in social policy (Gibbins and Reimer 1995). We can explore usefully the impact of values on social policy, such as feminist, green, postmaterialist and postmodern values (Inglehart 1977; Squires 1993; van Deth and Scarbrough 1995; Weeks 1995). We could, however, consider as one connection between these factors the extension of the neo-Marxist idea that capitalism has destroyed its own logic and sources in its search for profit. Having seen the necessity of bringing the worker to the market as consumer, the market has now destroyed the deferential consumer and created the postmodern expressive subject. Restructured consumers, like reconstructed workers and their unemployed counterparts, have come to terms with their situation by constructing narratives of their own from the diverse and disjointed outputs of the media available (Burrows and Marsh 1992; Shields 1992; Warde 1990). The postmodern self could be one response to the challenges of late capitalism, as Jameson originally hypothesised (Jameson 1984).

POSTMODERNISM, POSTSTRUCTURALISM AND SOCIAL POLICY

This summary and conclusion is organised into four sections. The first looks at the effect of poststructuralism; the second is on the impacts of the broader academic enterprise of postmodernism on the social policy theory; third, I will summarise the changing world that postmodernisation has delivered and to which social policy must respond; and finally, suggest some agenda items for a future postmodern social policy.

The effects of poststructuralism

Poststructural debates suggest that academics in the field need to enter a phase of deconstruction: deconstruction of the canon, the dominant language, the conceptual glossary and discourses. Social policy has constructed its own truths and legitimations for its own normalisation processes. Deconstruction of the dominant binaries constructed and deployed over recent decades can make way for the invention of alternative, non-binary schemes. Poststructuralism suggests that, in social policy discourse and practice, we should encourage and be prepared to accept more the self-made categories and subjective classifications of individuals and groups, such as the practice of 'sexing the self', as a response to the deconstruction and collapse of gender and sex binaries (Probyn 1993; Weeks 1994, 1995). Deconstruction of essentialist notions in theory and discipline areas can, however, be supported by the confidence that language is fluid, flexible and adaptable, so allowing transformation. Slavish subscription to foundationalism – the orientation to find and ground all behaviour on single or dual structures, and especially gender and class structures – can be abandoned, freeing up social policy to explore modifications of the old and inventions of the new. Finally, from poststructuralism we may learn to abandon the deep-seated and mistaken belief in the unconscious determination of the surface by deep structures, in favour of a horizontal model in which the complex interplay of a variety of factors and processes is imagined and explored.

The impacts on social policy theory

From a postmodern perspective the impacts on social policy as a discourse are profound. We accept that the objects of study are constituted in social policy itself. We abandon essentialism, foundationalism and structuralism at all levels and proceed to explore the diversity, difference and distinctions that are at the heart of all language, discourse and taxonomies. The drive to find a new conceptual, theoretical and methodological consensus around a grand theory should be abandoned in favour of a new pluralism and pragmatism. As its criteria of validity, social policy can therefore abandon its subscriptions to the courts of Enlightenment reason, in empirical correspondence, theoretical coherence and absolutist synthesis, in favour of a pragmatic conception of truth and an eclectic notion of synchrony, in which discrete parts make up a broader picture, like instruments in an orchestra. Similarly, the notion that the subject must progress on the principle of theoretical exclusion, ejecting cuckoos or sparrows from the nest, would be better replaced by a notion of inclusion, welcoming resources that may be of help. Two fallacious notions within social policy need abandonment or reformulation: the notion of unilinear change through time beloved of most modernisation theorists, and the comparative notion of a universal pattern across space. We should accept the guidance of Bauman that the character, forces and effects of postmodernisation over time and space are disorganised, ambiguous and ambivalent (Bauman 1992, 1997).

The changing world

Having rethought its own enterprise, postmodernist social theory should respond to the changing world that theorists of the postmodernisation of the world identify. Three features of change in the world should especially attract our attention. Firstly, there is the disruptive and yet inventive potential of changes in individual and collective identities. If social policy has to deal with new selves and groups who are more self-authored, autonomous and assertive, it will need to change its assumptions, aims and practices (see the chapters by Croft and Beresford and by Smaje in this volume). Disputes over identities and between identities will be expected to grow, and ways to maintain peace and well-being to be explored. At issue is the solution to the riddle of how we can allow a plurality of ever-diverging individuals and groups to share a common space, and to negotiate ways of living and proceeding that give expression to the legitimate but incommensurable interests and values of others. How to reconcile the results of the processes of disembedding, pluralisation and empowerment is the problem inherited by postmodern social policy, with which every police force, prison, school, hospital and community must grapple. Changing needs, desires, problems, uncertainties and risks, emerging from the new situations and relationships, also pose immediate challenges.

John Clarke and Norman Ginsburg (in this volume) describe the range of particular effects of postmodernisation on the welfare system: the fragmentation of welfare delivery; the retreat from universalism in provision; the decline and challenge to the experts and professions; the loss of faith in the very idea (metanarrative) of welfare and security provided from cradle to grave; the tide going out on the idea that government or European Union can provide social cohesion; the privatisation of public problems; the prioritisation of desire over need; and the recognition that risk can only be managed and not eradicated or successfully insured against. Whether all are responses to postmodernisation as advocated by postmodernists is doubtful. Many seem better explained within the context of more materialist, structural clashes, involved in old economic, class and party political rivalries about the role of the state and its relations in capitalism as understood in crisis theory (Offe 1984). All of these items are attributable to postmodernism only if you accept the Jameson Marxist structuralist variant.

Similarly, Allan Cochrane's justified scepticism (in this volume) about the much-vaunted subsidiarity and the devolution of power, and about the rise of individual, group, local and institutional autonomy and participation in welfare services, cannot be laid at the door of postmodernism and the postmodernisation process, but at the door of academics, politicians and managers who operate late capitalism by offering post-Fordist solutions.

Some agenda items

Affirmative postmodernism and its agenda setting is in its infancy. As yet few politicians and managers are responding to its analysis and problematics. Before agreeing to its strangulation at birth, the academic community may be better advised to turn to the task of addressing and reconstructing the political agenda in response to the postmodernist analysis of social policy. The outlines of this can be found in various recent texts, which advocate for the future (rather than celebrate the arrival of) the empowerment of citizens; the encouragement of autonomy, self-actualisation and expressivism at the individual level; the development of new politics, and new political structures and organisations, such as new social movements, at the group level; the recognition legitimation and support of new types of family, network and lifestyle; the search to craft particular packages of service for particular cases; the prioritising of particularism (not selectivism) over universalism; the addressing of welfare risks, issues and solution at the global, local and transnational levels; the pluralising of services; the recognition that a new set of welfare values and principles is needed to deal with a more cosmopolitan and differentiated society; and the exploration of solutions to welfare problems at other levels than and in additional agencies to those of the central and local state (Beck 1996; Bernstein 1991; Betz 1991; Brown 1988; Cooper 1994; Evans 1993; Gibbins 1989; Giddens 1994; Heckman 1990; Laclau and Mouffe 1985; Mouffe 1988; Nicholson 1990; Reimer 1989; Rosenau 1992: 144–55; Squires 1993; Weeks 1994, 1995; Yeatman 1994).

BIBLIOGRAPHY

Baron, C. (1988) *Asylum to Anarchy*, London: Free Association Books.
Baudrillard, J. (1983a) *Simulations*, New York: Semiotext(e).
Baudrillard, J. (1983b) *In the Shadow of the Silent Majorities: Or the End of the Social and Other Essays*, New York: Semiotext(e).
Bauman, Z. (1987) *Legislators and Interpreters: On Modernity, Postmodernity and Intellectuals*, Cambridge: Polity Press.
Bauman, Z. (1991) *Modernity and Ambivalence*, Cambridge: Polity Press.
Bauman, Z. (1992) *Intimations of Postmodernity*, London: Routledge.
Bauman, Z. (1997) *Postmodernity and its Discontents*, Cambridge: Polity Press.
Beck, U. (1992) *The Risk Society: Towards a New Modernity*, London: Sage.
Beck, U. (1996) *The Reinvention of Politics*, Cambridge: Polity Press.
Bernstein, R. (1976) *The Restructuring of Social and Political Theory*, Philadelphia PA: University of Pennsylvania Press.
Bernstein, R. (1985) *Philosophical Profiles: Essays in a Pragmatic Mode*, Cambridge: Cambridge University Press.
Bernstein, R. (1991) *The New Constellation: The Ethical–Political Horizons of Modernity/ Postmodernity*, Cambridge: Polity Press.
Bertens, H. (1995) *The Idea of the Postmodern: A History*, London: Routledge.
Betz, H.-G. (1991) *Postmodern Politics in Germany: The Politics of Resentment*, Basingstoke: Macmillan.
Bourdieu, P. (1984) *Distinctions*, London: Routledge.
Bourdieu, P. (1988) *Homo Academicus*, London: Polity Press.
Boyne, R. (1990) *Foucault and Derrida: The Other Side of Reason*, London: Unwin Hyman.
Boyne, R. and Rattansi, A. (eds) (1990) *Postmodernism and Society*, Basingstoke: Macmillan.
Brown, S. (1988) *New Forces, Old Forces and the Future of World Politics*, Glenview IL: Scott, Foresman.
Burchell, G., Gordon, C. and Miller, P. (eds) (1991) *The Foucault Effect: Studies in Governability*, Hemel Hempstead: Harvester Wheatsheaf.
Burrows, R. and Loader, B. (eds) (1994) *Towards a Post-Fordist Welfare State?*, London: Routledge.
Burrows, R. and Marsh, C. (1992) *Consumption and Class: Divisions and Change*, London: Macmillan.
Cohen, S. and Scull, E. (eds) (1983) *Social Control and the State*, Oxford: Martin Robertson.
Connolly, W. (1991) *Identity/Difference: Democratic Negotiations of Political Paradox*, Ithaca NY: Cornell University Press.

Cooper, D. (ed.) (1994) *Sexing the City: Lesbian and Gay Politics within the Activist State*, London: River Oram Press.

Cousins, M. and Hussain, A. (1984) *Michael Foucault*, London: Macmillan.

Derrida, J. (1967) *Of Grammatology*, Baltimore: Johns Hopkins University Press.

Derrida, J. (1982) *Margins of Philosophy*, Brighton: Harvester Press.

Donzelot, J. (1979) *The Policing of Families*, London: Hutchinson.

Dreyfus, H.L. and Rabinow, P. (1982) *Michel Foucault: Beyond Structuralism and Hermeneutics*, Brighton: Harvester Wheatsheaf.

Evans, D. (1993) *Sexual Citizenship: The Material Construction of Sexualities*, London: Routledge.

Featherstone, M. (1983) 'Consumer culture', *Theory, Culture and Society*, 1, 3: 4–9.

Featherstone, M. (1987) 'Lifestyle and consumer culture', *Theory, Culture and Society*, 4, 1: 55–70.

Featherstone, M. (1988) 'Postmodernism', *Theory, Culture and Society*, 5: 2–3.

Featherstone, M. (1991) *Postmodern Sociology*, London: Sage.

Fitzpatrick, T. (1996) 'Postmodernism, welfare and radical politics', *Journal of Social Policy*, 25, 3: 303–20.

Forder, A. (1974) *Concepts in Social Administration: A Framework for Analysis*, London: Routledge and Kegan Paul.

Foucault, M. (1970) *The Order of Things: An Archaeology of the Human Sciences*, London: Tavistock.

Foucault, M. (1972) *The Archaeology of Knowledge*, London: Tavistock.

Foucault, M. (1973) *The Birth of the Clinic: An Archaeology of Medical Perception*, London: Tavistock.

Foucault, M. (1977) *Discipline and Punish: The Birth of the Prison*, London: Allen Lane.

Foucault, M. (1979) *The History of Sexuality. Vol. 1: An Introduction*, London: Allen Lane.

Foucault, M. (1980) *Power/Knowledge: Selected Interviews*, Brighton: Harvester Press.

Gane, M. and Johnson, T. (1993) *Foucault's New Domains*, London: Routledge.

Gibbins, J. (ed.) (1989) *Contemporary Political Culture: Politics in a Postmodern Age*, London: Sage.

Gibbins, J. (1990) 'The new state and the impact of values', unpublished paper, European Science Foundation.

Gibbins, J. (1995) 'Lifestyles', unpublished paper, European Science Foundation.

Gibbins, J. and Reimer, B. (1995) 'Postmodernism', in J.W. van Deth and E. Scarbrough (eds) *The Impact of Values. Vol. 4: Beliefs in Government*, Oxford: Oxford University Press.

Giddens, A. (1991a) *Modernity and Self-Identity: Self and Society in the Late Modern Age*, Cambridge: Polity Press.

Giddens, A. (1991b) *The Consequences of Modernity*, Cambridge: Polity Press.

Giddens, A. (1992) *The Transformation of Intimacy: Sexuality, Love and Eroticism in Modern Society*, Cambridge: Polity Press.

Giddens, A. (1994) *Beyond Left and Right: The Future of Radical Politics*, Cambridge: Polity Press.

Giddens, A., Lash, S. and Beck, U., (1994) *Reflexive Modernisation: Politics, Tradition, and Aesthetics in Modern Society*, Cambridge: Polity Press.

Harvey, D. (1989) *The Condition of Postmodernity*, Oxford: Blackwell.

Hekman, S.J. (1990) *Gender and Knowledge: Elements of a Postmodern Feminism*, Boston: Northeastern University Press.

Heller, A. and Feher, F. (1989) *The Postmodern Political Condition*, Oxford: Blackwell.

Hewitt, M. (1983) 'Bio-politics and social policy: Foucault's account of welfare', *Theory, Culture and Society*, 2, 1: 67–85.

Hewitt, M. (1990) 'Bio-politics and social policy', in M. Featherstone, M. Hepworth and B.S. Turner (eds) *The Body: Social Process and Cultural Theory*, London: Sage.
Hewitt, M. (1992) *Welfare, Ideology and Need*, Hemel Hempstead: Harvester.
Hillyard, P. and Watson, S. (1996) 'Postmodern social policy: a contradiction in terms?', *Journal of Social Policy*, 25, 3: 321–46.
Inglehart, R. (1977) *The Silent Revolution: Changing Values and Political Styles among Western Democracies*, Princeton NJ: Princeton University Press.
Jameson, F. (1984) 'Postmodernism, or the cultural logic of late capitalism', *New Left Review* 146: 53–92.
Jameson, F. (1989) 'Marxism and postmodernism', *New Left Review*, 176: 31–45.
Jameson, F. (1991) *Postmodernism, or the Cultural Logic of Late Capitalism*, London: Verso.
Kaase, M. and Newton, K. (1995) *Beliefs in Government*, Oxford: Oxford University Press.
Kroker, A. and Kroker, D. (1988) *The Postmodern Scene: Excremental Culture and Hyper-Aesthetics*, London: Macmillan.
Kurzweil, E. (1980) *The Age of Structuralism: Lévi-Strauss to Foucault*, New York: Columbia University Press.
Laclau, E. and Mouffe, C. (1985) *Hegemony and Socialist Strategy*, London: Verso.
Lemert, C. (1992) 'General social theory, irony, postmodernism', in S. Seidman and D.G. Wagner (eds) *Postmodernism and Social Theory*, Oxford: Blackwell.
Lyotard, J.-F. (1984) *The Postmodern Condition: A Report on Knowledge*, Manchester: Manchester University Press.
Mouffe, C. (1988) 'Radical democracy: modern or postmodern?', in A. Ross (ed.) *Universalism Abandoned? The Politics of Postmodernism*, Minneapolis MN: University of Minnesota Press.
Nicholson, L.J. (ed.) (1990) *Feminism/Postmodernism*, London: Routledge.
Norris, C. (1982) *Deconstruction: Theory and Practice*, London: Methuen.
Oakeshott, M. (1975) *On Human Conduct*, Oxford: Clarendon Press.
Offe, C. (1984) *Contradictions of the Welfare State*, London: Hutchinson.
Penna, S. and O'Brien, M. (1996) 'Postmodernism and social policy: a small step forwards?', *Journal of Social Policy*, 25, 1: 39–61.
Probyn, E. (1993) *Sexing the Self: Gendered Positions in Cultural Studies*, London: Routledge.
Reimer, B. (1989) 'Postmodern structures of feeling: values and lifestyles in the postmodern age', in J. Gibbins (ed.) *Contemporary Political Culture: Politics in a Postmodern Age*, London: Sage.
Reimer, B. (1994) *The Most Common of Practices: On Mass Media Use in Late Modernity*, Stockholm: Almquist and Wiksell.
Rorty, R. (1979) *Philosophy and the Mirror of Nature*, Oxford: Blackwell.
Rorty, R. (1989) *Contingency, Irony and Solidarity*, Cambridge: Cambridge University Press.
Rose, M. (1991) *The Postmodern and the Postindustrial*, Cambridge: Cambridge University Press.
Rose, P. (1985) *Parallel Lives: Five Victorian Marriages*, Harmondsworth: Penguin.
Rosenau, P.R. (1992) *Postmodernism and the Social Sciences: Insights, Inroads, and Intrusions*, Princeton NJ: Princeton University Press.
Sarup, M. (1988) *Poststructuralism and Postmodernism*, London: Harvester.
Shields, R. (1992) *Lifestyle Shopping: The Subject of Consumption*, London: Routledge.
Skinner, Q. (1985) *The Return of Grand Theory in the Human Sciences*, Cambridge: Cambridge University Press.
Smart, B. (1993) *Postmodernity*, London: Routledge.

Squires, J. (ed.) (1993) *Principled Positions: Postmodernism and the Rediscovery of Values*, London: Lawrence & Wishart.

Squires, P. (1990) *Anti-Social Welfare: Welfare Ideology and the Disciplinary State*, Hemel Hempstead: Harvester Wheatsheaf.

Sturrock, J. (1979) *Structuralism and Since: From Lévi-Strauss to Derrida*, Oxford: Oxford University Press.

Taylor, C. (1989) *Sources of the Self: The Making of the Modern Identity*, Cambridge MA: Harvard University Press.

Taylor-Gooby, P. (1994) 'Postmodernism and social policy: a great leap backwards?', *Journal of Social Policy*, 23, 3: 385–404.

Taylor-Gooby, P. and Dale, J. (1981) *Social Theory and Social Welfare*, London: Edward Arnold.

Tully, J. and Skinner, Q. (eds) (1988) *Meaning and Context: Quentin Skinner and his Critics*, Cambridge: Polity Press.

Turner, B. (1989) 'From postindustrial society to postmodern politics: the political sociology of Daniel Bell', in J. Gibbins (ed.) *Contemporary Political Culture: Politics in a Postmodern Age*, London: Sage.

Turner, B. (1990) *Theories of Modernity and Postmodernity*, London: Sage.

Van Deth, J.W. and Scarbrough, E. (eds) (1995) *The Impact of Values. Vol. 4: Beliefs in Government*, Oxford: Oxford University Press.

Warde, A. (ed.) (1990) 'Sociology of consumption', *British Journal of Sociology*, Special Issue, 24, 1.

Weeks, J. (ed.) (1994) *The Lesser Evil and the Greater Good: The Theory and Politics of Diversity*, London: Rivers Oram Press.

Weeks, J. (1995) *Invented Moralities: Sexual Values in an Age of Uncertainty*, Cambridge: Polity Press.

Wilkinson, H. (1996) *No Turning Back: Generations and Genderquake*, London: Demos.

Winch, P. (1958) *The Idea of a Social Science*, London: Routledge and Kegan Paul.

Yeatman, A. (1994) *Postmodern Revisionings of the Political*, London: Routledge.

Chapter 4

Oppositional postmodern theory and welfare analysis

Anti-oppressive practice in a postmodern frame

Martin O'Brien and Sue Penna

INTRODUCTION: POSTMODERNISM AND POSTMODERNITY

To explore questions of the 'postmodern' is to engage in a highly complex and disputed theoretical field. 'Postmodern' is a label that has been used to refer to a bewildering array of cultural, political, economic, social and philosophical shifts in contemporary societies. For example, when we compiled our notes for this chapter we were able, from just two sources (Morley and Chen 1996; Lyotard 1992), to identify the following list of meanings and definitions of postmodernity/ism:

- the end of a history of white males and the beginning of 'other' histories;
- the end of western cultural dominance;
- a new cultural age in the west;
- a new historical era;
- an expression of thought or the rethinking of sets of established intellectual problems;
- a field of cultural struggle;
- a movement in architecture and the arts;
- a loss of confidence in the idea of progress and modernisation;
- a trend in poststructuralist philosophy;
- the end of Enlightenment rationalism.

The term 'postmodernism' is also frequently used to refer to the (over-) intellectualisation of relatively straightforward problems by bourgeois academics (Ebert 1995; Norris 1990) or 'robots' (Inglis 1996; Penna and O'Brien 1997). In some mainstream social theory, the very term 'postmodern' engenders convulsive fits of vilificatory rage combined with more or less explicit accusations that anyone who values anything done in its name has sacrificed her/his political and intellectual soul on the altar of commercialised modishness. Even if there were no other good reasons for thinking through postmodern perspectives (of which there are, in fact, many such reactions indicate that they have touched some raw theoretical nerves worthy of closer inspection. In this chapter, we outline some of the characteristics of postmodern social theory in order to contest the prevalent view that postmodernism is nothing but a bourgeois abstraction from reality. We then go on to provide a critique of the competency requirements for 'anti-oppressive practice' in contemporary social work education and training, based on our exposition of postmodern theory.

The multiplicity of meanings that is attached to postmodernity and postmodernism suggests that these terms are circulating in a number of contested fields or arenas. They indicate, at least, some of the theoretical dynamism that characterises these fields. The struggle around their meanings, and its confrontational character, however, similarly suggest that the dynamism is not only theoretical, but also political. We have addressed these terminological differences and their relationships to concepts of modernity in some detail elsewhere (O'Brien and Penna, forthcoming). In this chapter, we focus on the distinction between 'postmodern*ism*' and 'postmodern*ity*'. Postmodern*ism*, here, comprises an 'elective affinity', described by Hall (1996: 289, after Weber) as 'certain theoretical shifts which occur at about the same time in a number of different but related fields of work'. Thus, there are postmodern approaches in art, architecture, geography, sociology, literary criticism, philosophy, pedagogy, dance, cinema and many other technologies of cultural and social production, each of which pays attention to certain analytical themes, but each of which also generates somewhat different consequences. These differences are rooted partially in the substantive concerns of the organising social fields and partly in the conceptual looseness of the 'postmodern' itself. 'Postmodernism', in short, describes a number of stylistic and focal convergences between fields of knowledge and power. This conception of postmodernism draws attention to, for example, the 'linguistic turn' in social and cultural theory (the concern with discourse, meaning, symbolic and syntactic processes), the 'aestheticisation' of politics through the disruption of binary categories (public/private, high/low culture, sign/signifier, and so on) or the rejection of 'metanarratives' (of science, politics and reason) as empirical cases of the convergence of postmodern thematics across social locations (West 1990).

This approach to postmodernism draws attention to the partiality of the themes, styles and foci that comprise the contents of the 'affinities' or 'convergences'. 'Partiality' is used here in its active sense, of inclining or tending towards certain positions, viewpoints or conclusions. Postmodern*ity*, or 'the postmodern', can be construed as the social and political relationships through which such inclinings or tendings are sustained. We do not, in this chapter, adjudicate on which of the many interpretations or descriptions of these relationships is correct. We note that they have been described through the agonism of language games (Lyotard), the cultural logic of late capitalism (Jameson) and the hyperdifferentiation of a simulated social (Baudrillard), for example. We discuss social and political issues in postmodern theory later in the chapter. Our point is that the formal concept of postmodern*ism* (the affinity or convergence) makes sense only in the context of the substantive

concept of postmodern*ity* (the relationships that sustain the former's partiality, or what makes it into an affinity or convergence). This approach to
postmodernity proposes that all 'modern' institutions and discourses, all of
the categories and metanarratives, are partial, upheld and voiced by someone,
somewhere, in some circumstance. Indeed, in these terms, the Enlightenment
itself should be described as an 'elective affinity', a tendency or inclination,
that has been sustained through sets of social and political relationships. In
postmodern perspectives 'Enlightenment' and 'modern society' do not represent a once-and-for-all split with the past, but processes in the present whose
partiality is contested and defended through political action.

LUDIC AND OPPOSITIONAL POSTMODERN THEORY

These observations lead to the issue of 'postmodern theory', specifically,
what is 'theoretical' about postmodern perspectives or, alternatively, in what
ways do such perspectives provide ways of theorising. In our view, postmodern perspectives provide two related critiques that are useful for theorising
social welfare. These are, first, the focus on the materiality and dynamism of
discourse and, second, the deconstruction of the Cartesian subject. We deal
with each in turn.

In relation to the first point, postmodern perspectives propose that 'knowledge' about the world cannot be separated from its telling or 'voicing'.
Theoretically, what is at stake in the emergence and application of organised
knowledges – such as science or medicine and their validation in programmes
of environmental or social policy, for example – is the way that experiences,
perspectives, languages and symbols are centralised and marginalised in the
canons of legitimate discourse. Here, postmodern philosophy insists that *how*
the world is known – as well as *what* is known about it – comprises a politics
of voice: a political arrangement of included and excluded knowledges, narratives and his/herstories.

In relation to the second point, postmodern critiques reject the ontological
distinction between the knower and the known, or between subject and
object. Under the influence of poststructuralism, postmodern perspectives
examine how it is that specific constructions of the 'knowing subject' have
been (and are) developed and maintained: is the Cartesian subject of
Enlightenment thought an abstract, 'knowing' entity, devoid of any social,
cultural, political or economic contents? Or is this subject itself a *fiction*
through which the progress and power of 'modern' knowledge has been/is
narrated? Theoretically, the emergence of an abstract human subject ('man'
in general) who bears rights and responsibilities and is endowed with capacities, needs and desires is treated as an historical event – as something that has
been invented and amplified historically – rather than as the universal realisation of 'man's' inherent nature. Analytically, contemporary institutions –
including welfare institutions – are construed as maintaining the fiction of

this universal subject through social practices that are inflected by political differences: although there are no limits to the divisions and distinctions that cut across human populations and their experiences, modern social institutions maintain and co-ordinate hierarchies of difference through which certain identities, knowledges and histories – of gender, 'race', age, sexuality, class, embodiment, for example – are privileged in relation to others that are subordinated or suppressed.

Through these two sets of critiques it is possible to elaborate a postmodern theoretical framework that situates the social process of *narration* (the telling of history and 'truth') in the cultural validation of *voice* (in the identity of the teller) through a politics of *location* (situating the narrative and the teller in relation to specific struggles). The concepts of narration, voice and location are widely used in postmodern analyses of cultural and political struggles. They draw attention not only to who is doing what to whom in what circumstances but also, more importantly from our point of view, to who gets to voice the doing and in what ways, with what consequences. In these respects, postmodern theory can be said to be 'critical' – in that it exposes the axes around which valid and legitimate knowledges revolve, challenging conventional wisdoms and accepted theories. At this level, all postmodern perspectives are critical, but not at all in the same way. To clarify this point, it is useful to make a distinction between 'ludic' postmodernism and 'oppositional' postmodernism or, more accurately, between what is 'ludic' and what is 'oppositional' about postmodern perspectives. 'Ludic' or 'spectral' postmodernism (often associated with Lyotard and Baudrillard) construes politics as the interplay of signs and meanings in a heterogeneous world of (incommensurable) differences. Here there is an insistence on the impossibility of grounding theoretical concepts in any essential or foundational reality, a move that poses problems for important traditions in left theory. In Marxist theory, for example, it is argued that the reality of the world – including its exploitations, oppressions and discriminations – is distorted through the ideological dominance of false ideas. The spread of these ideas throughout society comprises a false consciousness or, at least, a misapprehension of the ways that social and political systems operate to maintain the economic dominance of capital.

Rather than focusing on the (distorted) representation of the 'real', ludic postmodernism asserts that all representations, all meanings, are unstable, varying from context to context, entangled in chains of signs and symbols. The meaning or significance of the real can never be categorically or conceptually fixed, in either sense of this term: the real cannot be 'pinned down' in theory and it cannot be 'repaired' in theory. Since there is not a fixed system of true representations and false representations, then theory cannot be conceived as a mental construct serving to guide emancipatory or utopian action more or less 'correctly'. It has been a central claim of both reformist and revolutionary traditions that specific forms of knowledge – whether positivist social science (in the liberal tradition) or historical materialism (in the Marxist tradition) – provide a common representational space where differences or discriminations (of class, primarily, but also of embodiment, sexuality, 'race' and so on) can be apprehended in their basic or raw reality. A correct or true theory, in this account, will overturn the system of false ideas and lead to the elimination of exploitation, oppression and domination.

This construction is opposed in postmodern theory. It can be understood as 'oppositional' in its resistance to the conventional linkages between 'false' knowledge and domination, on the one hand, and 'true' knowledge and emancipation, on the other. Such conceptual linkages are fictions (they are narrated by particular voices in particular locations) that generate their own violence: when theory is constructed as 'representing' the truth of the real, it leads to the conceptual obliteration of alternative realities (it commits an act of conceptual violence); at the same time, the construction is itself an attempt to *implement* the truth, in the face of opposition, resistance and rejection, in programmes of political, not merely conceptual or theoretical, action (it commits an act of political violence). The relationships between these two violences saturate European historical and political theory. For example, an exclusive club of enlightened nineteenth-century liberals fought for decades to prevent mass access to any kind of political influence on the theoretical basis that with power came a responsibility that only the enlightened few were able to carry. Alternatively, the proletarianisation of the working classes was simultaneously condemned and celebrated by Marxism at the same time as its destruction of alternative economic, social and political arrangements was seen as a necessary effect of the passage into communism. The liberal project entailed that different groups of people (European men, European women, African men, African women, Asian men, Asian women and so on) all represented different stages of 'enlightened' development and thus 'fitness' to take part in their own governance. The Marxist project entailed that opponents of mass proletarianisation were 'deviationists' or 'alien elements' who needed re-educating. The point is that the claim to a universally 'true' representation of reality, particularly in normative theories of emancipation or progress, requires that the worlds of experiential and sensuous life be construed as homogeneous in some or all respects and that the homogeneity itself is the basis for practical action. The homogenisation, as we noted, denies or obliterates the subjective realities, the divergences and heterogeneity of the peoples in whose name the representation is applied.

In postmodern theory, the linkage between the 'conceptual' and the 'sensible' through the logic of representation is a linkage maintained in violence. This is why Lyotard upholds the figure of incommensurable language games, why Baudrillard emphasises the symbolism of consumer culture, and why postmodernism more generally focuses on the movement of signifiers rather than on the signifier/signified relationship (Sarup 1993). Each of these theoretical positions is an attempt to disturb the representational logic of traditional social theory. Postmodern theory focuses not on the representations themselves (on whether a Marxist perspective is 'truer' than a liberal perspective, for example) but on the discourses and practices that reiterate them in the social world. Discourses and practices – of the body, deviance, the nation or health, for example – are not distinct phenomena (where one is representative of the other). Instead, they comprise a configuration of differences – sexual, racial, regional, communal, for example – which is politically dynamic.

The attempt to circumvent, or at least to take seriously, the violence of the conceptual–sensible dyad is the basis of 'oppositional' postmodern theory. To write, to speak or, in this context, to theorise in full awareness of this violence – in awareness of the ways that representational discourses deny and destroy the many conceptual (and sensible) realities of heterogeneous groups – is not a simple matter of choosing politically correct words to describe identities and experiences. Nor is it the adoption of the right sets of 'values' that give respect and autonomy to individuals on a case-by-case basis. Theorising in a postmodern frame requires a shift in the political linkage between theorist and theorised – the 'subject' and 'object' of theory.

This is why postmodern theory pays particular attention to processes of identity-construction and the politics of subjectivity, to the ways that meanings, cultural codes and knowledge production are entangled in the construction and maintenance of power relations. Whilst they may not be privileged in this regard, postmodern perspectives have contributed to the development of a field of writings that recover – or renarrate – the histories and voices of those excluded from knowledge production, analyse the historical locations and relations of marginality and theorise the cultural politics of marginalisation (Julien and Mercer 1996; Richard 1993). The latter focus has exposed the extent to which particular identities and voices have occupied a pivotal role in cultural constructions of progress, rationality and truth. These identities and voices define a 'centre' – a unique and superior position – whose masculine, racialised and gendered outlines uphold a 'fiction of universality' (Law 1996: 15; Richard 1993: 463–4) that suppresses and delegitimises any deviations from its 'normality'. The decentring of this subjective centre of authority through the focus on narrative, location and voicing is one of the main features of oppositional postmodern theories.

POSTMODERN DECENTRINGS

A number of different approaches to this decentring have been put forward in an attempt to define an 'oppositional' postmodern theory. These include the critical pedagogy of McLaren (1994, 1995) and Giroux and McLaren (1994), amongst others; the 'engaged' postmodernism put forward by, for example,

Mohanty (1992); and the social postmodernism or postmodern critical theory developed by Fraser (1994, 1995), for example. Below, we make brief comment on each of these approaches in order to provide a framework for thinking through the emergence of anti-oppressive practice in social work in postmodern terms.

'Critical pedagogy' is based on Freire's work on education for empowerment in Latin America. Its political character is summed up neatly by McLaren:

> Critical pedagogy is more than a de-sacralization of the grand narratives of modernity, but seeks to establish new moral and political frontiers of emancipatory and collective struggle, where both subjugated narratives and new narratives can be written and voiced in the arena of democracy.
>
> (McLaren 1995: 83)

This approach is concerned with resisting forms of social and cultural oppression and developing a transformative politics. The precondition for human emancipation is seen to be the recovery of the voices of the oppressed (Macedo 1994: xviii). Oppression, occurring in myriad tangible forms, is understood as an effect of different configurations of power and of discursive regulation. It is seen as the outcome of both exploitative economic relations and cultural practices which construct oppressive subject positions and identities (McLaren and Lankshear 1994a). The emphasis on subjectivity, discourse and meaning is considered to be essential in order both to recover the voices and histories of oppressed peoples and to identify conditions for empowerment and the cultural struggle it entails. In order to establish these 'moral and political frontiers', McLaren (1994: 194–5) argues that the cultural and critical focus of postmodern theorising needs to be guided by a 'substantive political project' supported by 'utopian' thinking.

A different 'oppositional' focus in postmodern theorising is exemplified by Mohanty (1992) and Martin and Mohanty (1988). The concern here is with questions of feminist and anti-racist theory and struggle, with shifts as well as continuities over time. The crucial issue for Mohanty (1992) is the ways that difference has become institutionalised within feminist discourse – the ways that 'difference' is foregrounded in theoretical investigation. Mohanty proposes that feminism and feminist theory have developed through encounters with postcolonialism, anti-racism, peasant struggles, gay and lesbian movements and, equally importantly, poststructuralist and postmodern discourses. These various political and intellectual movements demonstrate the impossibility of a 'universal subject' and the importance of historicising and locating political agency, leading Mohanty to pose the following question:

> How does the politics of location in the contemporary United States determine and produce experience and difference as analytical and political categories in feminist 'cross-cultural' work? By the term 'politics of location'

I refer to the historical, geographical, cultural, psychic, and imaginative boundaries which provide the grounds for political definition and self-definition for contemporary US feminists.

(Mohanty 1992: 74)

According to Mohanty, a theory that takes the experience of struggle (and not just its 'form' or underlying 'values') seriously implies that the theorist is always *engaged* with specific social, cultural and political locations. The theorist is not abstracted from the experience of struggle, even if the latter does not affect all of the different contestants in the same ways. There is no escape out of the experience of discursive and material location in contested political projects: to struggle is to engage in a politics of location. Mohanty's postmodern emphasis on the locatedness of struggle refutes the possibility of a transcendental politics, and furnishes a critique of the 'value' emphasis in the critical pedagogy literature. It provides a concept of located agency whose efficacy is rooted in the engagement with specific material and discursive relations, rather than transcending these in a utopian dreamscape of universal emancipation. It does not, however, provide a theory of how the locations come to be structured or configured as they are (whether, in the absence of any specific agent, the political location would still exist). In short, there is the beginning of a postmodern *social* theory but the interactions of the struggles and locations is not addressed in any detail.

A useful contribution to this theoretical task is provided by Fraser (1994, 1995), who develops a postmodern perspective on 'publicity' or the 'becoming public' of social and political struggles and claims. Fraser argues that, historically, members of subordinate social groups have formed alternative publics – *subaltern counterpublics* – which allow the formulation of oppositional interpretations of identities, interests and needs. These counterpublics emerge in response to exclusions from dominant publics, and expand discursive space, so that the proliferation of subaltern counterpublics means an increase of discursive contestation (Fraser 1995: 291). Modern societies, here, are characterised not by a single public sphere of rights-granting authorities, but by a multiplicity of public spaces in which different struggles are conducted and through which different inclusions/exclusions and centralisations/marginalisations are organised. Entry into a public sphere is no guarantee of political 'inclusion' in any wider sense and, indeed, may result in intensified or reconfigured exclusions, because participatory parity is not fully realisable where systematic inequalities exist (Fraser 1995: 292). Fraser exemplifies this issue in her analysis of the American Senate Judiciary Committee hearings around Anita Hill's claim of sexual harassment against Supreme Court nominee Clarence Thomas. The episode indicated that different gender, 'race' and class interests were mobilised by factions in the struggle and that the claims contest was part of an inherently broader range of public political conflicts than the 'private' issue of sexual conduct.

Contestation around the Thomas/Hill hearings, writes Fraser, 'became the condensation point for a host of anxieties, resentments and hopes about who gets what and who deserves what in the United States' (Fraser, 1995: 305).

Specific claims and counterclaims, the acquisition or loss of particular rights and duties – that is, the 'public sphere's' substantive contents – are 'condensed' through a wider range of (intra- and inter-) sexual, gender, regional, racial and class conflicts. They represent unequal, often discriminatory and sometimes exploitative relations between marginalised groups. There can be no guarantee of ethical universality in a democratic public sphere: the political ideals embedded in particular claims and counterclaims are necessarily fractured in the contestatory social organisation of different public spaces (O'Brien and Penna 1996: 199–200).

Our brief discussion of postmodern theoretical approaches suggests that it is disingenuous to suggest that postmodernism *tout court* delegitimises political struggles or sweeps away the possibility of radical action to counter oppression, exploitation and domination. This proposition is now a well-rehearsed feature of the critique of postmodernism (Ebert 1995; Hewitt 1996; Jameson 1991; Norris 1990). Yet, it seems to us that the criticism is wide of the mark by some distance: it refuses to address what is specifically theoretical about postmodern perspectives, and instead rearticulates precisely those normative assumptions that are contested in postmodern work (that a utopian vision is the only coherence that matters in political struggle, that differences can be structured away under the rubric of a transcendental revolutionary schema, that the incapacity of any of the social agents of Enlightenment theories to achieve emancipation is merely a contingent matter disconnected from the philosophical and theoretical categories that uphold the agent's purported transformative role, and so on). We contend that through the concepts of narration (the telling or recounting of the nature and experience of struggle and change), voice (the identity and authority of the teller) and location (the engagement with contested political relations in diverse struggles), postmodern writings have provided a more sophisticated theoretical framework for the analysis of social change than has been acknowledged in much of the mainstream sociological and social policy literature. Viewed through the lenses of postmodern theory, discourses and practices in the social world reveal the political dynamism of contemporary struggles around difference and culture. The dynamism both exposes and compounds the fragmented relationships between institutions and groups in modern social (welfare or otherwise) programmes and projects. Below, we explore the emergence and propagation of 'anti-oppressive practice' in social work education and training through the concepts of voice and location, in particular, in order to illustrate this element of political dynamism.

POSTMODERN ANTI-OPPRESSION?

In recent years, there has been a shift in professional social work education to an emphasis on competency- and skills-based training. The various 'competencies' that have to be demonstrated during training are underpinned by a central requirement that they derive from, and concretely display the operation of, anti-discriminatory and anti-oppressive values. Social workers in training, educational and practice locations are required to exhibit their understandings of the 'structural oppressions' of class, 'race', gender, disability, age and sexuality, which understandings provide a basis for interventions that oppose the former's 'effects' on service users. We do not have the space here to address the contradictory nature of these requirements in detail. Instead, we wish to focus on the locatedness of anti-oppressive practice (AOP) in specific struggles that have cut across the social welfare field.

In political and ideological terms, AOP owes much to the radical social work movement of the 1960s and 1970s, which itself expressed a number of competing claims and perspectives. These include Marxism and radical sociology, especially deviancy and labelling theory, feminism and anti-racism. In the effort to grasp the characteristics of and solutions to social inequality, both the academic debates and social movement strategies broadened their intellectual horizons beyond issues of economic inequality and class oppression to address the experiences and perspectives of gay and lesbian people, disabled people and older people, for example. The incorporation or translation of the different oppositional movement politics and their associated critiques into radical social work philosophy involved a reconfiguration of the discourses of inequality and discrimination. We do not suggest that such politics and critiques are simply absorbed and then applied by practitioners in any mechanical sense. Instead, we propose that their emergence and propagation is a feature of the political locating of claims and counterclaims by different publics in struggle. These latter include professional or expert publics, producer, consumer, client and carer publics, for example, intersecting politically through racialised, gendered, embodied, sexualised and stratified publics. In our view, it is the intersection of these many different publics in struggle that has made social work, as Clarke (1996: 50) comments, 'a particularly clear focal point for cultural politics and equality campaigns from a range of sources'. In postmodern theoretical terms, social work discourse and practice comprises a 'condensation' (Fraser 1995) of counterpublic struggles through which the normative and meliorative dimensions of social work interventions are persistently fragmented and decentred. The fragmentation arises because the processes by which issues become or are made public (their 'publicity') are agonistic – they push and pull, challenge and contest the centred identities, values and discourses of reform and melioration.

An example of the fragmentation of publicity is the contest around the construction of 'race' in social work. In giving voice to the racial discriminations that pervade all areas of social life, anti-racist movements have politicised the racial 'complexion' or configuration of public services: their 'whiteness' has been located politically in the context of racialised practice. Whereas 'race relations' and 'multiculturalism' in the UK in practice constructed non-whiteness as 'race' (as 'other' races), the anti-discrimination and anti-oppression perspectives construct 'race' as including, not excluding, 'whiteness' (Ahmad 1993: 2–3; Dalrymple and Burke 1995: 16–18). Law makes a similar point in relation to the legal configuration of equal rights policies in the UK:

> The deconstruction, or analysis of the underlying meanings and assumptions, of the gender and culture neutral legal subject against whom comparisons of equal treatment are made reveals a subject which is white and male. Here, the racialised and ethnocentric values and assumptions built into legal forms, rules and principles become a focus of attention.
>
> (Law 1996: 15)

In a similar way, the whiteness of social services is not simply an issue about numbers of people from different ethnic groups providing or receiving them. It refers to the conventions, assumptions, norms, rules and resources that predominate – culturally and institutionally – and their public whitening of the claims and counterclaims of marginalised groups.

Ahmad (1993), for example, in an analysis of social work interventions with black families, observes differences in approach between black and white social work practitioners. Through a number of case studies, Ahmad examined social work assessments, working practices and interpersonal dynamics and argued that black social workers provided more 'user-centred, sensitive services'. White assumptions and norms about black people's needs, characteristics and lifestyles provide the foundation for a 'disadvantage' perspective which retains a focus on black families as problem families. A persistent focus on 'racial disadvantage' – in relation to poverty, employment, health, housing, education, command of English, generational conflict and immigration problems – results in a discursive and cultural construction of black 'victims'. This general pathologising of black people is rooted in the centrality of whiteness in the perspectives, methods and dynamics of social work. Arguing for a distinctive black perspective in social work, Ahmad challenges white scholars and practitioners to define their own theoretical position:

> It is often asked what is a Black perspective. Interestingly enough, the same question is hardly ever, if at all, directed towards White academics, writing books and articles on Black people, or for that matter on any other issues ... Yet, they must have a perspective that relates to them being White. I suggest that White writers have not had to define White perspective, as

'White' is accepted as the 'norm'... For Black perspective is much more than a string of words. It is more a statement against 'White norms': it is an expression of assertion that cannot be bound by semantic definition.

(Ahmad 1993: 3)

A 'black perspective' in social work is, thus, a counterperspective: it exists, at least partially, in and through the unreflexive centrality of a 'white perspective' in social work. Thus, Ahmad observes, the Eurocentric focus of social work theory and practice obscures the historical and contemporary consequences of colonialism, the legacy of slavery and the relations of subordination and domination that underpin the white encounter with 'other' races. This 'voicing' of whiteness and white racism as a missing link in social work discourse and practice shifts the focus from 'black' as 'other', inferior in relation to whiteness. It constructs 'white' as a political issue and decentres whiteness from its unarticulated superiority. In this sense, to issue a claim, to contest a norm, to disobey a rule or demand a resource is to engage in the public location of 'whiteness': in how and where it will be located politically in struggles over services and resources (see de Gale 1991).

We are not proposing that a white or a black perspective in social work comprises a unified idea (a 'representation') or value held by different 'races'. Rather, we suggest that anti-racist struggles are dynamics of change in the cultures of racism where those ideas or values conflict. Social work and social welfare institutions and discourses are sites of historical and contemporary struggle, not only over resources and entitlements but also over the meaning and experience of Britishness, nationality, professional and institutional life and, importantly, over what is and is not to count as legitimate knowledge about these experiences (Ahmad 1993: 63; Gus 1991: 91). In this regard, anti-racist struggles are precisely that: struggles. They are not the foundation stones of a moral or ideological consensus on the nature of oppression and disadvantage. Rather than 'summing' to an emancipatory politics, struggles around class, 'race', gender, age or embodiment *generate* divisions and publicise different forms of inclusion and exclusion.

For example, the development of feminist social work practice has involved a commitment to validating the complex patterns of women's experiences. The validation represents a struggle for recognition of women's nurturing and caring experiences as well as their political and economic contributions to modern social life. Feminist social work, reinterpreting and rewriting women's experiences, has situated these within the context of patriarchal social relations, where men's power to define the parameters of women's lives is construed as the central problem requiring attention. In this way it has provided a political space in which women's histories can be examined in relation to the pathological inadequacies of patriarchal structures, rather than the pathological inadequacies of individual women.

Such experiences, however, are not enveloped only in patriarchal structures and processes: women's locations are criss-crossed also by racist, homophobic, disabling and ageist structures and processes. Indeed, women's experiences and struggles are, in Fraser's terms, 'condensations' of the conflicts and relationships between and within the political, cultural and economic dimensions of these social fields. The condensations render the experiences of womanhood as complex, not simple, patterns of inequality and difference. For example, as Langan observes:

> Race does not simply make the experience of women's subordination greater, it qualitatively changes the nature of that subordination. However, while different oppressions interact and reinforce one another, emphasising 'difference' *per se* may lead to division and conflict.

> (Langan 1992: 5)

Langan intended her observation as a warning not to go 'too far' along the postmodern path. Yet the point of the postmodern emphasis on difference in the first place is to draw attention to and theorise division and conflict. Nor does postmodern theory emphasise 'difference *per se*'. Rather, postmodern theory emphasises the importance of specific differences in challenging the binary categories of dominant identity structures – 'man'/'woman', 'black'/'white', 'citizen'/'alien', for example. The challenge to such binary categories involves rejecting any assumption that the categories are inclusive and subverting the hierarchies of identity and subjectivity sustained by contemporary social institutions. We have offered examples from anti-racist and feminist discourses on social policy and social work but the challenges are issued by many diverse groups simultaneously. 'Queer theory' has highlighted the heterosexuality embedded in legal, taxation and other cultural and regulatory systems; disability theory has exposed the ways that some forms of embodiment are validated by modern economic and political systems whilst others are subject to systematic and institutionally entrenched discriminations and marginalisations (Oliver 1990; Seidman 1994).

The general theoretical point we wish to make is that the translation of 'anti-' philosophy into the discourses and practices of organised social work illuminates the logic of 'supplementarity': the production of 'excessive' semiotic and political spaces through the definition and control of appropriate, permissible and 'realistic' competencies and commitments. The use of the 'anti-' phrase to depict contemporary social work competencies itself is a curious choice, since, on the one hand, it is used to pit social work 'against' or 'counter' to a number of specific cultural and political currents in contemporary society whilst, on the other hand, it is used to reaffirm specific sets of values that are entrenched in the professional and institutional structures of social work (notably, individual autonomy and self-determination and the necessity of a balance between care and control) (CCETSW 1995). 'Anti-' practice is situated firmly and only as a value preference that potential social workers must exhibit during training. In other words, it is not, in concrete terms, 'anti-' anything as such – it is not against the state, capitalism and the accumulation of private wealth, nuclear families, imperialism, colonialism and nationalism, economic globalisation, fundamentalism, rationalisation, modernisation, privatisation, pit-closures, MTV, genetic manipulation, Rupert Murdoch, the car-dependency culture, excessive product packaging, swearing in public or fox-hunting, for example. More problematically, it assumes (and in its training programmes, attempts to impose) a monolithic notion of 'racism', 'sexism', 'ageism' and so on as 'structural oppressions' that individual social workers are expected to 'counter ... using strategies that are appropriate to role and context' (CCETSW 1995: 2). For reasons of space we comment on only two aspects of this problematic construction.

First, in the publicity material for the CCETSW (1995) guidelines on competencies and training (*New Requirements for the Diploma in Social Work*), the approval of Des Kelly, deputy general secretary of the Social Care Association, is quoted: 'the new paper [on DipSW skills and requirements] will help standardize training so someone from a course in Sunderland will have the same core skills to offer as someone from one in Portsmouth'.

It is of note, here, that Des Kelly could not 'appropriately' counterpose 'Toxteth' and 'Mayfair' or any other similar pairing. It is of note not because social workers are not trained in Toxteth or Mayfair but because it is difficult to envisage what 'core' social work skills might transfer between work with the bottom-income decile (who are found in Toxteth) and work with the top-income decile (who own Mayfair). Yet how, by working only on the bottom decile, is social work to 'counter' structural oppression – in our example in its social class manifestation – other than by training the poor in the use of sophisticated assault weapons in order to 'disadvantage' the top decile? This question draws attention to the contestatory logics of public action, on which we commented above. Here, we would note that 'anti-practice' philosophy obscures its own institutional and political location or, phrased positively, 'supplements' that location with an imaginary unity of experience and value. Social work's contradictory political location (*in* Sunderland and Portsmouth but *between* Toxteth and Mayfair) sustains specific geographies of inclusion and exclusion and at the same time denies the very specificity of those discriminations that the 'anti-practice' philosophy is meant to address: why is it that social work's 'core skills' so easily traverse the cultural distance between Sunderland and Portsmouth but not the cultural distance between Toxteth and Mayfair? Is it because such skills are applicable to the poor en masse – that is, in spite of their uniqueness, autonomy and diversity – whereas the rich are 'too unique' and 'too diverse' to have their place in the 'structural oppressions' countered by social work's values? What we can see here is precisely the *trace* of diversity and uniqueness, that which must, in practice, be excluded in order for the integration of social work's values to occur. 'Diversity' and 'uniqueness' are discursive supplements that enable the institutions of social work to ignore, in their formal training and enskilling programmes, what it is that unites Sunderland and Portsmouth yet differentiates Toxteth and Mayfair.

The second aspect we wish to comment on is that CCETSW's professional construction of AOP – mirroring a model derived from the National Vocational Qualification (NVQ) approach to learning and education – emphasises, as we have noted, the acquisition of practice competencies that reflect core social work values. In social work training courses, students are required to provide evidence of AOP competencies in written and placement work. What such competencies look like in practice, however, remains mysterious. How do anti-sexist and anti-racist competencies connect with each other in different circumstances – in Muslim, Catholic or Hindu communities, for example? What anti-racist and/or anti-sexist strategies should be followed? Competencies, supposedly, are derived from a theory of AOP, yet there is not a unified AOP theory from which strategies can be so derived. Debates and disputes around anti-racism or anti-sexism, for example, express different analyses of the causes, experiences and consequences of oppression and generate different 'anti-' strategies: which analysis should provide the general theory for the development of specific social work competencies? Who is to decide which analysis is the appropriate one? Anti-racist, feminist, disability and other movements do not provide single, unified theories of oppression. Instead, they are characterised by theoretical and political divisions that mark such movements as publics in struggle. AOP demands that the diversity and multifaceted character of oppressed publics are acknowledged, yet its competency requirements can only be achieved by disregarding the political and intellectual struggles within which it is situated. Competencies are discursive constructions of professional knowledge that decouple such knowledge from the political struggle of which it is a part. Yet, in practice, AOP competencies remain situated within uncertain, unstable and shifting cultural and political arenas where the right or correct values are intrinsically problematic. Counterpublics do not share the same values either with each other or with social work professionals; rather, these are the site of intense dispute.

Contemporary cultural and political conflicts around difference, identity and inequality are dynamics of social change. They shift the parameters in and through which social welfare practitioners encounter the everyday and institutional processes of exploitation, oppression and discrimination. No professionally imposed value-base or competency accreditation system can generate interventions with predictable effects that offset or ameliorate the ways that these processes are worked out. Today's professional competencies and values will be tomorrow's professional closures and ideologies because they will be challenged and transformed in the conflicts and compacts between different publics in struggle.

Voicing inequality, locating its dimensions, experiences and consequences, and retelling or renarrating the relationships between 'race', gender, class, age, disability and region, for example, involve challenging the codes, conventions and symbolic hierarchies of contemporary professional and institutional orders. These processes also involve contesting and disputing with the voices, locations and narratives of multiple publics in struggle. Exploitation and oppression are not the aggregate products of individual characteristics: a third-generation-immigrant, Irish, working-class male with a bad chest is not by definition more or less oppressed than a second-generation-immigrant, Chinese, middle-class female with poor eyesight. The social work competencies that apply in relation to these two 'identities' (and the relationships between them) derive not from the voices, narratives and locations through which the latter are sustained and challenged, but from the reconfiguration of social work's own professional and institutional value-base and the embedded logic of its continuous displacement and decoupling from the experiences, motivations and goals of politically dynamic groups in struggle.

CONCLUSION

In this chapter we have tried to clarify some of the important theoretical issues in postmodern writing and apply these to the discourses and practices of contemporary social work. Our purpose has been to indicate some of the ways that postmodern perspectives contribute to theorising the disputes, divisions, fragmentations and differences that social workers encounter in the institutional and everyday locations where they are called upon to do social work: to make decisions, write reports, assess needs, negotiate and co-ordinate resources, manage case loads or care for and control the lives of individuals and groups. These activities comprise not only the 'social' work of distribution or melioration, but also the political work of location and identification (or voice) and the cultural work of interpretation and definition (or narration).

The political and cultural constructs through which claims and counterclaims are organised and processed are not the coherent products of theoretically accurate value systems. They are the partial outcomes, the uncertain expressions of specific discourses and practices. We have argued that such discourses and practices are intrinsically unstable and that the instability is a feature of the contested 'publicity' through which politically dynamic groups struggle for social change. The 'anti-oppressive practice' focus of social work education and training, for example, itself comprises a political moment in the production and regulation of discrimination and inequality. There is not a value-base, a competency, a theoretical perspective or professional code that enables the translation of social work's anti-oppressive values into anti-oppressive practice because 'anti'-oppression is precisely a *struggle* within and against a multiplicity of divergent projects and programmes: it is 'anti-' in substance as well as in form.

ACKNOWLEDGEMENT

We would like to thank Hilary Graham and Chris Smaje for comments on (and debates about) earlier drafts of this chapter.

BIBLIOGRAPHY

Ahmad, B. (1993) *Black Perspectives in Social Work*, London: Venture Press/BASW.

Barrett, M. and Phillipps, A. (eds) (1992) *Destabilizing Theory: Contemporary Feminist Debates*, Cambridge: Polity Press.

CCETSW (Central Council for Education and Training in Social Work) (1995) *New Requirements for the Diploma in Social Work*, London: CCETSW.

Clarke, J. (1996) 'After social work?', in N. Parton (ed.) *Social Theory, Social Change and Social Work*, London: Routledge.

Dalrymple, J. and Burke, B. (1995) *Anti-Oppressive Practice: Social Care and the Law*, Buckingham: Open University Press.

de Gale, H. (1991) 'Black students' views of existing CQSW courses and CSS schemes 2', in Northern Curriculum Development Project (ed.) *Setting the Context for Change*, vol. 1 of the Anti-Racist Social Work Education Series, London: CCETSW.

Ebert, T.L. (1995) 'The knowable good: post-al politics, ethics, and red feminism', *Rethinking Marxism* 8, 2: 39–59.

Fraser, N. (1994) 'Rethinking the public sphere: a contribution to the critique of actually existing democracy', in H.A. Giroux and P.L. McLaren (eds) *Between Borders: Pedagogy and the Politics of Cultural Studies*, London: Routledge.

Fraser, N. (1995) 'Politics, culture and the public sphere: toward a postmodern conception', in L. Nicholson and S. Seidman (eds) *Social Postmodernism: Beyond Identity Politics*, Cambridge: Cambridge University Press.

Giroux, H.A. and McLaren, P. (eds) (1994) *Between Borders: Pedagogy and the Politics of Cultural Studies*, London: Routledge.

Gus, J. (1991) '"Taking sides": objectives and strategies in the development of anti-racist work in Britain', in Northern Curriculum Development Project (ed.) *Setting the Context for Change*, vol. 1 of the Anti-Racist Social Work Education Series, London: CCETSW.

Hall, S. (1996) 'For Allon White: metaphors of transformation', in D. Morley and K.-H. Chen (eds) *Stuart Hall: Critical Dialogues in Cultural Studies*, London: Routledge.

Hewitt, M. (1996) 'Social movements and social need: problems with postmodern political theory', in D. Taylor (ed.) *Critical Social Policy: A Reader*, London: Sage.

Inglis, F. (1996) 'Review of *Media Matters: Everyday Culture and Political Change*, by John Fiske, London: University of Minnesota Press, 1994', *Sociological Review* 44, 1: 154–6.

Jameson, F. (1991) *Postmodernism, or the Cultural Logic of Late Capitalism*, London: Verso.

Julien, I. and Mercer, K. (1996) 'De margin and de centre', in D. Morley and K.-H. Chen (eds) *Stuart Hall: Critical Dialogues in Cultural Studies*, London: Routledge.

Langan, M. (1992) 'Introduction: women and social work in the 1990s', in M. Langan and L. Day (eds) *Women, Oppression and Social Work: Issues in Anti-Discriminatory Practice*, London: Routledge.

Langan, M. and Day, L. (eds) (1992) *Women, Oppression and Social Work: Issues in Anti-Discriminatory Practice*, London: Routledge.

Law, I. (1996) *Racism, Ethnicity and Social Policy*, Hemel Hempstead: Prentice Hall.

Lyotard, J.-F. (1992) 'Note on the meaning of "post-"', in *The Postmodern Explained: Correspondence 1982–1985*, Minneapolis MN: University of Minnesota Press.

McLaren, P.L. (1994) 'Postmodernism and the death of politics: a Brazilian reprieve', in P.L. McLaren and C. Lankshear (eds) *Paths from Freire*, London: Routledge.

McLaren, P.L. (1995) *Critical Pedagogy and Predatory Culture: Oppositional Politics in a Postmodern Era*, London: Routledge.

McLaren, P.L. and Lankshear, C. (1994a) 'Introduction', in P.L. McLaren and C. Lankshear (eds) *Paths from Freire*, London: Routledge.

McLaren, P.L. and Lankshear, C. (eds) (1994b) *Paths from Freire*, London: Routledge.

Macedo, D. (1994) 'Preface', in P.L. McLaren and C. Lankshear (eds) *Paths from Freire*, London: Routledge.

Martin, B. and Mohanty, C.T. (1988) 'Feminist politics: what's home got to do with it?', in T. de Lauretis (ed.) *Feminist Studies/Critical Studies*, Basingstoke: Macmillan.

Mohanty, C.T. (1992) 'Feminist encounters: locating the politics of experience', in M. Barrett and A. Phillipps (eds) *Destabilizing Theory: Contemporary Feminist Debates*, Cambridge: Polity Press.

Morley, D. and Chen, K.-H. (eds) (1996) *Stuart Hall: Critical Dialogues in Cultural Studies*, London: Routledge.

Norris, C. (1990) *What's Wrong With Postmodernism? Critical Theory and The Ends of Philosophy*, London: Harvester Wheatsheaf.

Northern Curriculum Development Project (ed.) (1991) *Setting the Context for Change*, vol. 1 of the Anti-Racist Social Work Education Series, London: CCETSW.

O'Brien, M. and Penna, S. (1996) 'Postmodern theory and politics: perspectives on citizenship and social justice', *Innovation: The European Journal of Social Sciences* 9, 2: 185–203.

O'Brien, M. and Penna, S. (forthcoming) *Theorising Welfare: Enlightenment and Modern Society*, London: Sage.

Oliver, M. (1990) *The Politics of Disablement*, Basingstoke: Macmillan.

Penna, S. and O'Brien, M. (1997) 'Inequality, transformation and political agency: reflections on Teresa Ebert's "red feminism"', *Rethinking Marxism* 9, 3: 95–102.

Richard, N. (1993) 'Postmodernism and periphery', in T. Docherty (ed.) *Postmodernism: A Reader*, London: Harvester Wheatsheaf.

Sarup, M. (1993) *An Introductory Guide to Post-structuralism and Postmodernism*, 2nd edn, London: Harvester Wheatsheaf.

Seidman, S. (1994) 'Introduction', in S. Seidman (ed.) *The Postmodern Turn: New Perspectives on Social Theory*, Cambridge: Cambridge University Press.

West, C. (1990) 'The new cultural politics of difference', in R. Ferguson, M. Gever, T.T. Minh-ha and C. West (eds) *Out There: Marginalization and Contemporary Cultures*, New York/Cambridge MA: New Museum of Contemporary Art/MIT Press.

Chapter 5

Quality assurance and evaluation in social work in a postmodern era

Barbara Fawcett and Brid Featherstone

INTRODUCTION

Quality assurance in social work is widely understood as relating to the monitoring of predetermined definitions and standards which are, or should be, built into contracts and services (Payne 1995). This can be seen to be linked to evaluation, a term largely associated with concepts of efficiency and effectiveness and the extent to which services or their component parts match stated or predetermined goals (St Leger *et al.* 1993; Wright *et al.* 1994). We maintain that both quality assurance and evaluation, as currently used within social work, can be regarded as forming part of a modernist project applied to a postmodernist era, where the large certainties of modernism have been translated into 'small certainties'. Other features of these 'small certainties' include rationality, objectivity and managerialism (Howe 1994; Parton 1994). Links can also be made between how evaluation and quality assurance are currently used and Lyotard's emphasis on performativity as being all there is, in terms of knowledge production in a postmodern era.

   In this chapter, we will use a case study to explore the current use and relevance of quality assurance and evaluation for a disabled service user, her partner and her children. We will then explore formulations drawn from feminist, postmodern perspectives, which we argue can be used to critique both the 'small certainties' of modernism applied to a postmodernist era and remaining part of the modernist project, and also notions of performativity found in some postmodernist perspectives. We will then sketch out possible alternatives.

POSTMODERNITY AND POSTMODERNISM

At the outset, it is useful to outline briefly what is being referred to by the term 'postmodern era' and how this links to concepts of postmodernity and postmodernism.[1]

   Concepts such as postmodernity and postmodernism are intricately interconnected and are variously interpreted by different writers (Smart 1993;

Bauman 1992). Some authors use 'postmodernism' and 'postmodernity' to denote the same thing (e.g. Harvey 1989), others make distinctions (e.g. Bauman 1992; Sarup 1993; Smart 1993). In this chapter, distinctions are being made between the terms, and references to a postmodern condition or era draw from concepts of postmodernity. Postmodernism, in turn, is being viewed as a range of theoretical perspectives which can be related in various ways to discussions about postmodernity or the postmodern condition. To rephrase this succinctly, 'postmodernity' is being used to refer to the condition and 'postmodernism' as a way of understanding the condition (Williams 1992).

With regard to the ways in which concepts like postmodernity and postmodernism can be used, there are again differences of orientation. Smart (1993) suggests that there are three main approaches. The first views the culture of postmodernity (and in turn postmodernism) as being broadly continuous with modernity, the second regards postmodernity (and postmodernism) as constituting a distinct break with modernity or the modern, and the third sees postmodernity and postmodernism in relational terms, as a means of relating and responding to modernity and modernism in all their aspects. Cahoone (1996), whilst accepting that it is impossible to capture the diversity of postmodernism fully, attempts a three-part classification system to aid understanding. He refers to historical, methodological and positive orientations. Historical postmodernism suggests that the social and/or political and/or cultural organisation of modernity has/have changed fundamentally and we therefore face a different world. Methodological postmodernism is deconstructive rather than prescriptive, whilst positive postmodernism, in applying general postmodern themes to particular subject matter, offers alternative visions or understandings.

Although the attempts at classification given by Smart (1993) and Cahoone (1996) differ, they can be seen to share a general broad aim, which is to produce groupings which facilitate the assimilation and application of complex material. In this vein, we propose that there is a fourth way in which the term 'postmodernism' can be used which utilises the work of feminist postmodern writers. This perspective will be developed throughout this chapter.

QUALITY ASSURANCE AND EVALUATION: THE CURRENT CONTEXT

A case study

We maintain that quality assurance and evaluation can be unpacked to pose a series of questions. In relation to quality assurance within social work these include: 'what is it and how is it determined?' and 'what constitutes quality?'. With regard to evaluation, questions include 'what and who are being evaluated?', 'by whom?', 'how is this taking place?' and 'what are the implications?'.

There are further questions related to that of 'what are the discourses operating and how are the legitimating processes applied?'. As Lyotard (1994) points out, issues of legitimisation become key, as does 'who decides what knowledge is, and who knows what needs to be decided' (Lyotard 1994: 9).

In order to explore these questions, this chapter focuses on a case study involving a disabled woman, her partner/carer and their children in contact with social services. To elaborate further, Jane is a 21-year-old woman brought up in care, with three children aged 7 months, 3 years and 5 years. Two years ago she discovered she had rheumatoid arthritis and following the birth of her third child she became a wheelchair user. Early in 1996 Jane, her partner Ramzan and their children were living in an unadapted rented house where Jane, no longer able to climb stairs, had to sleep in the kitchen.

Jane was interviewed in February 1996 as part of a research project exploring how disability is constituted within accounts. At the time of the interview, Jane did not receive any home-care support because her partner lived with her. She also attended a day centre for disabled people twice a week so that she could have a bath and a break from her domestic environment. Whilst she attended the centre her partner looked after the children. Extracts from the interview which refer to Jane's contact with formal and informal support networks are given below.

Jane said in relation to the formal support she received:

> I've had support and everything like that, I've got my own social worker, then I've got a social worker from the disability team and I've got a social worker involved with my little boy 'cos he's fascinated with fire at the moment[2] ...
>
> I mean the one that comes in for my little boy, she just comes and chats to him about dangerous fires and helps him try to understand why his mum's in a wheelchair and she watches him play and watches how he behaves and things, and then she says to me what she thinks I'm doing wrong, she'll tell me, this is what you should do or what I could do instead or maybe do it, in a different way and you know she's been quite helpful. The social worker from the disability team ... she actually got involved with me because I got depressed and she gave me some vouchers to go and stay in a nursing home every weekend or something and when she'd done that she said I don't need to have anything more to do with you now ... I asked her to look into getting some help with cleaning and I was told basically that the funding is not there, you know for getting somebody to come and clean round ... My own social worker which I've had since I was 16, because I was in care to start off, she's the after care worker and she doesn't really come any more. If I need something I phone her up and she tries to deal with it and she phones me back, that's about it really.

With regard to informal support networks, Jane has her partner and his parents:

I feel sorry for the carers more than anything else, because he [Ramzan] doesn't have a chance to relax from the moment he wakes up, until the children and myself are asleep. I mean there's been times when he's just walked out and left me alone all day because he couldn't handle it, and I'd be the same I think ... He's got family but he doesn't like asking them, because I mean he's quite a bit older than me and his parents are old you know, so he shouldn't have to be asking them ... Yes, well depression sets in and then things just get impossible don't they? I mean he's already halfway there, he's not coping very well. I've asked for the help and they've said there's no money available. If I had enough money I'd pay for somebody to come and look after me, I'd pay for somebody to come and take over for a while.

... Well I actually called the social worker and I said I need to see you. I need you to come and see me and when she came I said he's had enough, I said look at the state [of the house] I mean it were disgusting, it were really horrible you know because I were depressed, he were depressed, nothing were getting done, and she said there's no money available. Well I said to her you know we're desperate, if we don't get some help he's going to end up losing his temper or getting violent or something, he doesn't want to do that and I don't want to face that. I said we need some help and she's not been in touch, says there's no money available and she'll keep looking into it but that's about it. I told her, it's urgent, we need help you know, and then he lost his temper, got violent and we had to leave, had to move away and stay in a hotel, but we asked for help. I said you can't blame him because we asked you for help. I mean luckily it's not often that he flips like that, he's learned to control himself a bit ... it's like elastic stretching too far and, but his can go a bit further than some people's.

The excerpts from the interview with Jane have been included to facilitate an examination of the meanings and implications that terms like 'quality assurance' and 'evaluation' could have in this particular situation. However, before looking at applications, it is useful to look at these terms in relation to the questions posed earlier.

Quality assurance and evaluation within social services departments and other organisations are often viewed in a non-problematic and straightforward fashion, typical of modernist projects which ascribe single, transparent, universalist meanings to words and terms. Objectivity is striven for and questions related to the knowledge frameworks applied, while the questions of how projects in the fields of quality assurance and evaluation are both constituted and legitimated, how decisions are made, and what the implications are and for whom are often obscured. Smart maintains that: 'The idea of order as a task, as a practice, as a condition to be reflected upon, preserved and nurtured is intrinsic to modernity' (Smart 1993: 41). In a postmodern era the search for order continues, but the grand designs of modernism can be seen to have given way to, as we indicated earlier, the search for 'small certainties'.

Accordingly, quality assurance and evaluation, as tasks, can often be seen to be about making things fit, polishing over rough and fragmented patches (such as extreme service-user distress, contradictions and uncertainty) and ascribing fixed, ordered subject positions. Performativity and market forces are accepted as the way to proceed, and alternative discourses and a critical consideration of the legitimising processes applied tend not to feature.

With regard to quality assurance in the fields of social services and health, Hudson (1990) points to its association with one-dimensional, commercial and industrial models and to the insistence on precise measurability and efficiency. Pfeffer and Coote (1991) maintain that the current emphasis on quality and total quality management have become inextricably connected with an overriding concern for value for money and economic efficiency. Quality is open to numerous definitions, but the model predominantly adopted in social services and health tends to be that which draws from industry, where services conform to standards decided by experts, designers, professionals or managers, who in the process are expected to take the consumer view into account (e.g. Cassam and Gupta 1992; DoH/SSI 1991). There are exhortations to make service-user needs the focus of professional and managerial standards (e.g. Flynn and Miller 1991), but as Payne (1995) states: 'It is easy to forget in devising evaluative systems to make arrangements for maintaining accountability to the service user, by building their responses into checks on service attainments' (Payne 1995: 210).

Those who have focused on evaluation in social work (e.g. Cheetham et al. 1992; Everitt and Hardiker 1996; Powell and Goddard 1996) highlight the fact that the approach used does not have to be unilinear and one-directional. Cheetham et al. (1992), for example, consider how pluralistic evaluations can demonstrate an appreciation that a unified consensus cannot be assumed and that multiple and conflicting outcome criteria can be used (Cheetham et al. 1992: 33–4). Powell and Goddard (1996) describe how evaluative approaches can seek to incorporate the perspectives of the various stakeholders and emphasise multiplicity and plurality in terms of interests, concerns and success criteria. Arguably, however, these approaches draw predominantly from modernist scenarios and, although there are elements of deconstructive critique involved, stakeholders views tend to be accepted at face value and the location of the various subjects within the discourses operating remains unchallenged. Subjects are regarded as having experiences and occupying identities which are unified, essential, fixed and coherent, and, as a result, contradiction, change, discontinuity and the possibility of occupying different subject positions simultaneously are ignored. Pluralistic evaluations also seek to obtain the views of various categorised groupings such as 'the disabled' or 'women'. This can serve to obscure differences within groups and promote an emphasis on homogeneous rather than heterogeneous features, which are then taken to be representative of that particular group.

Everitt and Hardiker (1996) develop an approach which they term 'critical evaluation', which focuses on mechanisms of oppression and on locating evaluative initiatives within varying frames of reference. They utilise post-modernist perspectives to reject truth claims and acknowledge that knowledge and power are inextricably linked. They see evaluation as a 'dia-logical process' (Everitt and Hardiker 1996: 151) which facilitates the ability of all involved to consider the meaning of experiences and their relationship to the discourses operating. This approach moves away from one-dimensional 'normative' perspectives and acknowledges how power and knowledge are interwoven within discourses. However, Everitt and Hardiker can be seen to privilege certain perspectives uncritically over others (for example, those of service users) and to continue to operate at times within frameworks which position certain kinds of knowledge outside power relations. Such knowledge is then viewed as automatically emancipatory. Their approach has also been critiqued by Trinder, who regards their primary task as being to make 'eman-cipatory truth claims rather than explore the question of why people are saying what they say' (Trinder 1996: 28).

In relation to the case study, it is important to acknowledge that in a system where resources take precedence over 'needs', quality assurance and evalua-tion, even in relation to the 'small certainties' of the modernist project, are found wanting. Jane had three social workers (hardly an efficient arrange-ment), none of whom was working with her to review and assess her total situation and none of whom seemed to have adopted a 'needs-led' approach. Jane found the social worker who worked with the child helpful, but her effectiveness, in concentrating on a single family member and not addressing the total family situation, is questionable. With regard to services received, Jane, in order to have a bath and 'socialise', was merely allocated a two-day-a-week placement at a day centre for disabled people. As it happened, Jane was full of praise for this centre, but nobody reviewed and evaluated her progress in relation to predetermined objectives, or even monitored and appraised the suitability of this placement for Jane and her family in terms of specified outcome criteria. There were no contracts in operation, either between any of the social workers and Jane or between Jane and the centre, and so quality and standards could not be monitored. With regard to service-user involvement, Jane's self-assessed needs relating to cleaning were not met, on the grounds of resource constraints and because they did not fit into a pri-ority category, and her cry for psychological help and support went unheeded. It is also interesting to note that the social worker from the dis-abilities team eschewed a pre-community care role of acting as an advocate for her client and merely reiterated a gate-keeping response to requests for assistance. Jane was not offered, and was even unaware of, the possibility of having an advocate to argue her case on her behalf.

However, it is also questionable whether quality assurance and evaluation applied as 'small certainties' would have significantly improved the situa-tion. The setting of predetermined objectives and outcome criteria would have streamlined the process and facilitated measurability, but the key question to ask here is whether it would have significantly improved Jane's situation from the perspective of Jane and her family. Their involvement in the overall evaluative process, the setting of standards and the monitoring of quality would have helped, but the questions posed earlier relating to who decides what quality is and how is it determined and constituted still apply. The questions raised with regard to evaluation, in terms of who and what are being evaluated, by whom, how this is taking place and what the implications are, also remain pertinent, as do issues related to power and knowledge production.

POSTMODERN CRITIQUES OF THE CURRENT CONTEXT

Quality assurance and evaluation have been subject to postmodern critiques. In relation to evaluation, Fox (1991) rejects claims from economists and others that evaluation can ever be rational and objective, and views such claims as merely representing an unacknowledged subjective value system which privileges managerially defined criteria such as efficiency and effectiveness. He critiques the idea of 'neutral' process and outcome evaluations and single resolutions, on the basis that these do not take into account all the differing views present in any one situation of what constitutes 'outcome' success. Fox maintains that rationality as the 'keystone' of evaluation has to be rejected. Instead of focusing on one rationality and regarding it as a means of accessing the 'truth' of any situation, he argues that it is important to recognise a whole variety of rationalities which reveal not 'the truth' but 'versions of reality constituted by interests' (Fox 1991: 742).

Trinder (1996), in her discussion of dominant research perspectives within social work, points to the re-emergence of the positivistically orientated empirical practice movement. She suggests, given postmodern critiques of modernist scientific projects, that such an emphasis initially appears perverse but, located within the context of wider social and political trends, it makes sense. Trinder maintains, like Parton (1994) and Howe (1996), that: 'what we have is a re-framed modernist back to the future project tied to neo-liberalism' (Trinder 1996: 241–2). In such a framework, individual accounts, attention to causes and context are lost and an overriding, rigid and narrow focus on measurement, control, intervention, outputs and surface explanation, which are regarded as neutral and objective, prevails. Trinder (1996) associates empirical research practice with being tied to the ongoing shift in social work towards managerialism, quality assurance, consumerism and audits.

Howe (1996), taking a definition of postmodernism as 'unrestricted liberal modernism' and in an argument reminiscent of Lyotard, points to the emphasis in current social work practice on performativity. The social worker is not required to think and act independently and use his/her own knowledge, skills and experience, rather s/he is required to be competent, according to a prescribed set of competency criteria. As Howe says, there has been a move from 'reason to rote' (Howe 1996: 92), from professionals to technicians. Such technicians operate within managerially or organisationally defined situations and are subject to related evaluation and quality assurance mechanisms. They are not trained to think independently, to deal with out-of-the-ordinary situations, or to cope with complexity, uncertainty and creativity. This can lead, as Howe points out, to meanings being imposed upon service users in relation to the organisational and competency parameters set. Welfare services become commodified and defined in economic terms and the development of social relationships between social workers and service users becomes irrelevant.

Clarke, although voicing reservations about 'postmodernist tales' (Clarke 1996: 41), offers an effective critique of the current situation in relation to social welfare and social work. His contribution, despite not specifically focusing on quality assurance and evaluation, can be seen to be relevant because of its emphasis on managerialism and top-down determinants. Clarke (1996) reviews welfare restructuring in relation to four broad areas. These are marketisation, mixed economies of welfare, the continuing transfer of responsibilities from formal to informal provision, and the process of managerialisation. He sees bureaucracy and professionalism, with all their tensions and contradictions, as comprising the organisational and individual tenets of social work. These he maintains have been undercut and rendered untenable as a result of political, organic and conjunctional factors.[3] Clarke asserts that this crisis and the shifting field of organisational power have 'created the space for management' to emerge 'as a new force' with its development being 'intimately linked to the expansion of managerial authority' (Clarke 1996: 59).

Clarke highlights the likely consequences of 'the managerial mode' being 'the chosen agent of public sector re-structuring'. He sees managerial organisational changes and managerial authority in social work as likely to exacerbate the tendency away from general public service initiatives and issues such as anti-oppressive practice, and towards managerially specified 'core' areas of concentration and 'top-down' definitions of 'need' and 'danger'. Greater targeting and concentration on areas regarded as 'key' will, he asserts, lead to increased levels of stigmatisation for users of services. Managerial 'ownership' of resources, missions and objectives, a source of supposed strength for the new system, he views as a means of giving managers and organisations perverse incentives to reduce or remove claims on their resources and to engage in 'buck passing'. He also points to significant changes in relation to features such as social worker autonomy and discretion, with professional judgement being subject to 'managerial imperatives and resource control' (Clarke 1996: 59). Professional autonomy is also likely to be further constrained by the devolution of resources and budgets, with workers internalising budgeting disciplines and gate-keeper roles. Accordingly, managerial categories of cost, efficiency and risk will come to dominate operational policies, and discordant perspectives emanating from service users or social workers will be dismissed or responded to only at a rhetorical level. In addition, narrow corporate loyalty and identity are likely to replace a professional culture and value-base, with workers operating in a narrow-focused and bounded manner.

FEMINIST POSTMODERN PERSPECTIVES AND APPLICATIONS

In relation to the effects of postmodernism, Smart refers to a 'postmodernism of reaction', which promotes a culture of eclecticism and affirms the status quo, and a 'postmodernism of resistance', which is about deconstructive critique and resisting the status quo (Smart 1993: 20). Lyotard, largely as a result of his focus on performativity as being all there is in terms of knowledge production in a postmodern era, and also of his interpretation of postmodern social criticism as having to be 'local, ad hoc and non theoretical' (Sarup 1993: 54), has been regarded as a postmodern writer who embraces the former stance (e.g. Sarup 1993).[4] Lather (1994) has critiqued such a differentiation as merely instituting more binaries, and, although the danger of reinstituting modernist oppositional frameworks has to be considered, Smart's analysis remains useful in highlighting differences in applications, especially in relation to areas like quality assurance and evaluation.

Feminists who have embraced postmodern perspectives, such as Fraser and Nicholson (1993), are indeed critical of Lyotard's orientation, but have avoided creating an alternative binary by offering a reformulated postmodern perspective. They argue that the retention of non-universalist, temporally, historically and culturally situated, large-scale theoretical perspectives, which reject standpoint positions and which view the social, subjectivity and identity as diverse, interrelational and complexly constructed, remains possible. There is also space for local, context-specific perspectives. Fraser (1995) asserts that large- and small-scale narratives are important so that the distorting tendencies present in both can be counteracted.

Drawing on Fraser and Nicholson (1993), we maintain that by using specifically feminist appropriations of postmodernism which contribute to the 'fourth way' referred to earlier, it is possible to view postmodern social criticism as grounded, yet anti-foundationalist, so that recognition of social differences and divisions and the weighting of criteria in relation to concepts of justice, equity and fairness maintain viability. Accordingly links can be maintained between the theoretical and the political, and the 'de-politicising agnoticism' of some postmodern perspectives is avoided (Clarke 1996: 42). The 'fourth approach' also effectively moves beyond performativity and utilises critique, making it feasible to develop theoretical tools which can be employed to

CORNWALL COLLEGE
LEARNING CENTRE

analyse and appraise aspects of postmodernism and also modernist projects, including the 'small certainties' of quality assurance and evaluation.

The utility of the 'fourth approach' will now be examined in relation to three areas which can be regarded as key. These are knowledge production, notions of self or subjectivity, and questions of difference.

Knowledge production

With regard to knowledge production, feminist postmodern perspectives can be seen to offer a means of moving away from fixed truth claims, which include modernist notions of objectivity and also feminist validations of experiences achieved through struggle against oppression, towards the historical, social and cultural location of knowledge. Accordingly all knowledge and related positionings, including those of feminists and service users, are viewed as non-innocent and partial. To give an example here, the 'fourth approach' can be used constructively to deconstruct accepted 'facts' related to social welfare and other areas, and at the same time, taking on board the reformulation alluded to above, continue to focus in a non-essentialist and non-fixed manner on feminist concerns such as the bringing of private matters into the public arena and/or (in relation to Jane) the social barriers model of disability (see also Fraser 1993).

In relation to the case study and issues of quality assurance and evaluation, it is possible to use the feminist appropriations of postmodernism to emphasise flexibility and inclusivity rather than rigidity and exclusivity, and to highlight the fact that all knowledge produces its own gaps, omissions, contradictions and regulatory possibilities. In Jane's case, this points to the importance of not regarding particular positions, experiences or knowledge bases, whether they belong to Jane, the social worker/care manager or agency, as normatively privileged, and of always recognising the plethora of options available. It is also about not focusing on one problem or person to the exclusion of others, and not treating specific statements and meanings as constituting the full statement of the position. With regard to Jane, attendance at the day centre was the only service offered and actioned in response to Jane's admission that she felt depressed and required assistance bathing. This might have been the only course of action resources would allow, but her 'story', in terms of how she related past, present and future events, how she made sense of situations at different points in time and how possible courses of action might link into these, was ignored. The emphasis in relation to Jane was also on problem areas and on negative aspects of her life. Feminist postmodern perspectives direct attention towards positive areas where things are currently working well.

Subjectivity and the social

Flax (1992) explores a notion of justice as a way of constructively applying a postmodern orientation and of responding to issues of subjectivity, difference and diversity in a way that goes beyond mere pragmatism. In this project, she reformulates the liberal view of justice to take account of 'self' and citizenship and unhinges it from its universalistic, essentialist roots. She regards discourses about justice as being inextricably linked to concepts of 'self' or subjectivity and active notions of citizenship. With regard to notions of 'self', she argues that a feminist view of an interconnected, integrated and social 'self' differs from the Enlightenment view of 'self' as unified, essential and rational, where individuality is sovereign and inviolate. She maintains that a feminist view of 'self' is not incompatible with a non-objective, non-rational, yet historically grounded 'self'. In relation to postmodern orientations, she takes issue with concepts of 'self' as a position in language propounded by Derrida (1978). Similarly, she contests Foucault's view of 'self' as an effect of discourse and maintains that a feminist postmodern self would have to be 'differentiated, local and ahistorical' but that it could be a social 'self' (Flax 1992: 201).

By 'active citizenship', Flax means the importance of ongoing processes of negotiation and (as does Fraser 1993) the viewing of need as publicly actionable – the making public of private miseries (Flax 1992: 206). She asserts that justice, understood as a process, could be utilised as a means of positively valuing and responding to difference via a focus on key aspects such as reconciliation, reciprocity, recognition and judgement. Here, 'reconciliation' refers to an ongoing 'unity of differences' which feature mutuality and incorporation rather than the annihilation of opposites and distinctions. 'Reciprocity' relates to an emphasis on the sharing of authority and a mutuality in decision-making processes in the absence of dominating perspectives of 'objective standards' or 'normative practices' (Flax 1992: 206). 'Recognition' is about accepting and positively regarding difference whilst simultaneously recognising sameness in terms of how the other is like oneself. 'Judgement', in turn, highlights our connectedness and obligation to others and the quality of care that arises out of this.

Feminist postmodern perspectives reintroduce notions of 'self' and subjectivity in ways that do not privilege experience but that decentre subjects, pointing to non-essentialist features which are always in process and which regard the self or subject as a predominantly social entity. Subjectivity is seen as changing, complex and contradictory, always influenced by relational and biographical forces, and as an area ripe for interrogation about the realising of potential rather than the deciphering of 'truth' (Hekman 1995). Subjects are also not regarded as merely occupying discursive positions, but can be seen as both constructed and capable of critique.

Identities are not unitary, but, borrowing from Flax (1992), the notion of a core self does not have to be rejected, merely reformulated. Accordingly we can be seen as having a shifting core that continually changes in relation to others. We therefore can be seen to relate differently to different people in different situations using varying aspects of our fluid 'core' self. This highlights the ways in which we differentially relate to others – in Jane's case, as disabled service user, mother, partner, carer, centre user, care leaver, young woman and so on – and the ways in which we continually develop relational, interconnected, integrated and social selves which are yet not essential, rational and unified (Flax 1992). In Jane's case, social factors in terms of her relationship with her children, partner, other disabled women and men, relatives and friends are of great importance and continually form and reform her sense of self so that, in accordance with feminist postmodern perspectives, she is more than a position in language or an effect of discourse. This social notion of self, linked to non-essentialist versions of citizenship and justice, further flags up the positive part that Jane can play in all her interactions and interconnections. It also gives social workers and care managers other positions to occupy and explore.

Questions of difference

Feminist postmodern applications have also grappled with issues of difference, and there is an emphasis on moving away from valorising difference and towards regarding it as a resource rather than an obstacle, especially in relation to political change (Sawicki 1991). There is also an understanding that notions of difference are always unstable and that categories are actually constituted through exclusion.

It can often appear that contemporary masculinity derives impetus from fear and anxiety of relatedness and the exaggeration of difference. In contrast, contemporary femininity can seem to be founded on fear of difference and on desires to foster illusions of relatedness. Interconnectedness, intersubjectivity and emphasis on the 'we' rather than the 'I' are significant features of postmodern feminist orientations. In terms of postmodern feminist perspectives and the 'fourth approach', there can be seen to be a move away from either/or scenarios, and a focus on exploring the developmental conditions that foster selves which are able to appreciate differences and not exaggerate relatedness, but which do not need to annihilate or destroy.

Postmodern feminist applications deconstruct and interrogate taken-for-granted categorisation processes built on difference, such as 'men', 'women' and 'disability'. These approaches examine the ways in which such categories are constructed and linked within social work discourses. With regard to Jane, her difficulties are categorised and compartmentalised, with different social workers or care managers responding to different problematised areas. Aspects such as the difference and sameness between herself, her mother, the social worker/care manager and others remain unexplored, as do areas related to connectedness and obligation. This fosters a unidimensional approach which in relation to evaluation and quality assurance emphasises rigidity, inflexibility, the fixing of positions, and privileged standpoints being uncritically imposed. In contrast, the fourth approach put forward here creatively interprets difference, with differences being explored, appreciated and, to cite Williams (1996), temporarily fixed to challenge oppressive scenarios or to campaign for change.

FEMINISM, POSTMODERNISM, QUALITY ASSURANCE AND EVALUATION

In relation to quality assurance and evaluation, the orientations presented by Fox (1991), Trinder (1996), Howe (1996) and Clarke (1996) are well within the frame of reference of feminist postmodern perspectives and are generally endorsed. However, as mentioned earlier, the 'fourth way' of interpreting and applying postmodernism has something additional to offer. Suggestions have already been made in relation to knowledge production, notions of self or subjectivity and questions of difference. At this stage it is useful to return to the questions posed earlier relating to the knowledge frameworks used to define quality assurance and evaluation, to see if there are further pointers that can be made as to how social workers can use such concepts and practices in their work.

With regard to the knowledge frameworks utilised and the control of knowledge, it is pertinent to restate how all knowledge claims (including those made by Jane), managerial 'small certainties' and postmodern performativity criteria are continually open to deconstruction and critical interrogation. Focusing on managerial 'small certainties', rigid, 'top-down' procedures might appear to produce clear, fixed positions and separate the thinkers, planners and organisers from the doers, facilitating control, but they are unlikely to be sustainable in an era where features such as flexibility, fluidity and diversity predominate. In addition, an exclusive focus on modernist 'small certainties' or postmodernist performativity, which lack integrating, non-essentialist yet located narratives, is likely to lead to the complete disintegration of social work, as these areas are unable to provide the coherence required for social work to retain viability.

In contrast, the 'fourth way' propounded highlights practices that accord with the multiplicity and diversity of postmodernity or a postmodern era, and that can also be combined and temporarily fixed to form, depending on the situation, both large-scale and small-scale narratives. These practices emphasise participation, interaction, negotiation and a focus on 'what works' for all concerned. This includes Jane being given the space to tell her story within understandings which see needs as constructed. There is also a focus on process as well as outcome in social worker–service user relationships and the opening up of space for change, with regard to Jane's story, in the responses of the workers and the services offered.

CONCLUSION

Social work, with its emphasis on reason and rationality, social and economic progress, expert knowledge, a core self and professionalism (Clarke
1996; Philp 1979; Williams 1996), can be seen as constituting part of the
modernist project. In a postmodern era change is inevitable, but the form that
that change is to take is not fixed or immutable. There is, drawing on feminist
postmodern perspectives and the 'fourth approach', a range of critical and
creative possibilities that can be explored and applied, and some of these have
been looked at with regard to Jane. Evaluation, quality assurance and managerialism applied as modernist 'small certainties' to a postmodern era, and
postmodern notions of performativity, are not the only options. This is not to
dismiss evaluation, quality assurance and managerialism out of hand, but to
use the 'fourth approach' to question and critique how they are currently
being interpreted, defined and applied.

Finally, it is argued that the 'fourth approach' counters the fragmentation
and superficiality of some postmodern accounts by retaining the possibility
to weight criteria, maintain a critical perspective, develop an interrelational
view of a social self, and creatively address questions of difference. In addition it is contended that this approach, although incorporating considerable
diversity and variation, makes it possible to develop theoretical tools that can
be used to analyse and critique aspects of modernist and also postmodernist
projects, and to open up possibilities in a manner which can be regarded as
productive.

NOTES

1 It is also important to emphasise at this point that, for the purposes of this chapter, we are incorporating poststructuralist orientations within our interpretation of
   modernism. We acknowledge that there are authors who would broadly agree
   with us on this (e.g. Barrett 1992; Best and Kellner 1991; Sarup 1993) and also
   those who would disagree (e.g. Huyssen 1990).
2 The interview was undertaken as part of a research project entitled 'Researching
   into disability from feminist postmodernist perspectives'. Excerpts from different
   points in the interview have been included. '...' denotes the transition to a different excerpt. Every attempt has been made in the use of different excerpts not to
   detract from the overall coherence of the account.
3 Political factors relate to the political emphasis placed by the Conservative government of the 1980s and early-to-mid-1990s on privatisation and marketisation.
   Organic factors refer to the instability in social democratic forms of the welfare
   state, the limited universality of social work due to its focus on normative family
   forms, and the historically contradictory and unstable nature of bureaucratic professional regimes such as social work. Conjunctional factors focus on how
   political and organic tensions are manifested and intersect at particular points
   (Clarke 1996).
4 Lyotard (1994) tends as well to regard performativity as being linked to two elements of didactics. These are simple transmission reproduction (technical,
   how-to-do-it information) and extended imaginative reproduction (imaginative

and strategic thinking and problem solving). Although Lyotard laments the separation in academic institutions of simple transmission reproduction from extended imaginative reproduction, he does not see both as necessarily needing to be made accessible to everybody. Instead, to aid performativity, extended imaginative reproduction only needs to be accessible to the few who direct and lead.

BIBLIOGRAPHY

Barrett, M. (1992) 'Words and things: materialism and method in contemporary feminist analysis', in M. Barrett and A. Phillips (eds) *Destabilising Theory: Contemporary Feminist Debates*, Cambridge: Polity Press.
Bauman, Z. (1992) *Intimations of Postmodernity*, London: Routledge.
Best, S. and Kellner, D. (1991) *Postmodern Theory: Critical Interrogations*, Basingstoke: Macmillan.
Cahoone, L. (1996) 'Introduction', in L. Cahoone (ed.) *From Modernism to Postmodernism: An Anthology*, Oxford: Blackwell.
Cassam, E. and Gupta, H. (1992) *Quality Assurance for Social Care Agencies*, Harlow: Longman.
Cheetham, J., Fuller, R., McIvor, G. and Petch, A. (1992) *Evaluating Social Work Effectiveness*, Buckingham: Open University.
Clarke, J. (1996) 'After social work', in N. Parton (ed.) *Social Theory, Social Change and Social Work*, London: Routledge.
Derrida, J. (1978) *Writing and Difference*, trans. A. Bass, Chicago: University of Chicago Press.
DoH/SSI (Department of Health/Social Services Inspectorate) (1991) *Training for Community Care: A Joint Approach*, London: HMSO.
Everitt, A. and Hardiker, P. (1996) *Evaluating for Good Practice*, Basingstoke: BASW/Macmillan.
Fawcett, B. (in progress) 'The constitution of disability within accounts', research project, University of Bradford.
Flax, J. (1990) *Thinking Fragments: Psychoanalysis, Feminism and Postmodernism in the Contemporary West*, Berkeley CA: University of California Press.
Flax, J. (1992) 'The end of innocence', in J. Butler and J. Scott (eds) *Feminists Theorise the Political*, London: Routledge.
Flynn, N. and Miller, C. (1991) *Caring in Our Communities: The Management Agenda*, London: NISW.
Fox, N.J. (1991) 'Postmodernism, rationality and the evaluation of health care', *Sociological Review* 39: 709–44.
Fraser, N. (1993) *Unruly Practices: Power, Discourse and Gender in Contemporary Social Theory*, Cambridge: Polity Press.
Fraser, N. (1995) 'False antithesis', in L. Nicholson (ed.) *Feminist Contentions: A Philosophical Exchange*, London: Routledge.
Fraser, N. and Nicholson, L. (1993) 'Social criticism without philosophy: an encounter between feminism and postmodernism', in M. Docherty (ed.) *Postmodernism: A Reader*, Hemel Hempstead: Harvester Wheatsheaf.
Giddens, A. (1990) *The Consequences of Modernity*, Cambridge: Polity Press.
Harvey, D. (1989) *The Condition of Postmodernity*, Oxford: Blackwell.
Hekman, S.J. (1990) *Gender and Knowledge: Elements of a Postmodern Feminism*, Boston: Northeastern University Press.
Hekman, S. (1995) *Moral Voices Moral Selves: Carol Gilligan and Feminist Moral Theory*, Cambridge: Polity Press.
Hollway, W. (1996) 'Gender and power in organisations', in B. Fawcett, B.

Featherstone, J. Hearn and C. Toft (eds) *Violence and Gender Relations: Theories and Interventions*, London: Sage.

Howe, D. (1994) 'Modernity, postmodernity and social work', *British Journal of Social Work* 24: 513–32.

Howe, D. (1996) 'Surface and depth in social work practice', in N. Parton (ed.) *Social Theory, Social Change and Social Work*, London: Routledge.

Hudson, B. (1990) 'Quality Street snarl up', *Health Services Journal* April 1990: 636–7.

Huyssen, A. (1990) 'Mapping the postmodern', in L. Nicholson (ed.) *Feminism/Postmodernism*, London: Routledge.

Jackson, S. (1992) 'The amazing deconstructing woman', *Trouble and Strife* 25: 25–31.

Lather, P. (1994) 'Staying dumb? Feminist research and pedagogy with/in the postmodern', in H. Simons and M. Billig (eds) *After Postmodernism: Reconstructing Ideology Critique*, London: Sage.

Lyotard, J.-F. (1988) *The Differend: Phases in Dispute*, Manchester: Manchester University Press.

Lyotard, J.-F. (1994) *The Postmodern Condition: A Report on Knowledge*, Manchester: Manchester University Press.

Parton, N. (1994) 'Problematics of government, (post)modernity and social work', *British Journal of Social Work* 24, 1: 9–32.

Payne, M. (1995) *Social Work and Community Care*, Basingstoke: Macmillan.

Pfeffer, N. and Coote, A. (1991) *Is Quality Good for You?*, London: IPPR.

Philp, M. (1979) 'Notes on the form of knowledge in social work', *Sociological Review* 21, 1: 83–111.

Powell, J. and Goddard, A. (1996) 'Cost and stakeholder views: a combined approach to evaluating services', *British Journal of Social Work* 26: 93–108.

Sarup, M. (1993) *Poststructuralism and Postmodernism*, Hemel Hempstead: Harvester Wheatsheaf.

Saussure, F. de (1974) *Course in General Linguistics*, London: Fontana.

Sawicki, J. (1991) *Disciplining Foucault: Feminism, Power and the Body*, London: Routledge.

Smart, B. (1993) *Postmodernity*, London: Routledge.

St Leger, A.S., Schnieden, H. and Walsworth-Bell, J.P. (1993) *Evaluating Health Service Effectiveness*, Milton Keynes: Open University.

Trinder, L. (1996) 'Social work research: the state of the art (or science)', *Child and Family Social Work* 1: 233–42.

Weedon, C. (1987), *Feminist Practice and Poststructuralist Theory*, Oxford: Blackwell.

Williams, F. (1992) 'Somewhere over the rainbow: universality and diversity in social policy', in N. Manning and R. Page (eds) *Social Policy Review 4*, Nottingham: Social Policy Association.

Williams, F. (1996) 'Postmodernism, feminism and the question of difference', in N. Parton (ed.) *Social Theory, Social Change and Social Work*, London: Routledge.

Wright, K., Haycox, A. and Leedham, I. (1994) *Evaluating Community Care*, Buckingham: Open University.

Part II

Critical social policy
and postmodernity

Chapter 6

'One step beyond'

Critical social policy in a 'postmodern' Britain?

Kirk Mann

INTRODUCTION

In this chapter I want to try and engage with some of the recent sociological literature on postmodernity/post-traditional society and the accounts of welfare that it provides. Despite some interesting observations, a central flaw in these accounts is the narrow definition of welfare that is used. Thus the concern here is not what social policy might glean from postmodernism (Hillyard and Watson 1996; Taylor-Gooby 1993) but what critics of modernity can learn from social policy. This may be a rather shocking suggestion; after all, social policy is part of the 'empiricist tradition' and is not noted for its contributions to theory (Taylor-Gooby 1981). It will be suggested that any attempt to go 'beyond left and right' (Giddens 1994) could usefully begin with Titmuss's account of the 'social division of welfare' (Titmuss 1958b). However, in highlighting the diverse and different meanings that social policy and welfare can have, the chapter also poses the question of what it is that now distinguishes a 'critical' social policy from 'orthodox' perspectives. The uncertainty which supposedly characterises postmodernity, along with the erosion of the traditional ideologies and constituencies for grand social engineering projects, poses some difficult questions for the future. A measure of scepticism, something that typifies postmodernist accounts, may be a healthy response and may serve to distinguish a 'critical social policy' from 'orthodox' accounts; particularly if New Labour form the next government.[1]

POSTMODERNISM AND SOCIAL POLICY

It is not the intention of this chapter to provide the definitive account of what is, or is not, postmodernism (see the introductory chapter in this volume by Carter). Rather the focus is firmly on a few of the key contributors to the debate on postmodernity who have specifically drawn attention to welfare issues. In many accounts by postmodernists, welfare and social policy are not explicitly discussed or are treated as part of the more general failure of social engineering. There are also so many versions of postmodernism that it is tempting to place the term in quote marks, 'registering reservations about its distinctiveness and indicating a provisionality about its use' (Rattansi 1994:16). However, since it is possible to query the distinctiveness of so many sociological terms, I have not done so as it would be rather clumsy. Nevertheless, and again in line with Rattansi, it is important to acknowledge that the label 'postmodernist' should not be too readily attached to all commentators on modernity.

The focus here is on two scholars that have been to the forefront of British sociology, Bauman and Giddens, who have commented on postmodernism and post-traditional society respectively. Giddens is engaging with postmodernists and is concerned with many of the central concerns of postmodernism, but it would be misleading to suggest he is a postmodernist (Giddens 1990, 1994). Bauman could be described as fully engaging with postmodernist accounts but he too stands a little to one side (Bauman 1988a, 1988b, 1993, 1995). In part it is because both commentators retain their commitments to certain ethical, social and political concerns that they wish to comment on welfare and are not, almost as a consequence, 'real' postmodernists. Like so much else the definition of postmodernity is, it seems, ambiguous and it is therefore not surprising that a host of other labels – late modernity, post-traditional society, postscarcity society – compete to explain similar phenomena (Bauman 1995; Giddens 1994; Harvey 1994).

The rather belated discovery of postmodernism by scholars whose main interests remain within social policy should be no great surprise. Taylor-Gooby (1981) was berating social administration for its arthritic 'empiricism' some considerable time ago, although he was not advocating the adoption of any theory. Indeed, more recently it is clear he feels that postmodernity is the wrong theory (Taylor-Gooby 1993). His critique subsequently prompted Hillyard and Watson (1996) to highlight those aspects of postmodernism/poststructuralism that they felt added to our understanding of social policy. They highlight the work of Foucault, in particular, to demonstrate the way that social policy can benefit from an engagement with postmodernism. This is interesting, and has a certain postmodern irony to it, since Dean and Taylor-Gooby (1992) appear to use Foucault's concept of discourse to account for the perception of those who rely on public welfare. Did Taylor-Gooby forget that some consider Foucault a postmodernist or Hillyard and Watson forget that others do not?

Memory loss seems to be one of the few aspects of postmodernity that afflict everyone, since according to Baudrillard (1987) we should remember to 'forget Foucault', whilst the selective amnesia virus has led Rojek and Turner (1993) to 'forget Baudrillard' and Rattansi (1995) to ask if we should simply 'forget postmodernism' or whether we might all enlist in Billig's (1994) campaign of 'sod Baudrillard'. In the circumstances anyone interested in social policy might be forgiven for not remembering to take postmodernism seriously. However, whilst postmodernists are usually happy to debunk any other 'position', the one position they will not tolerate is that of the debunker of postmodernity. O'Neill perceives this as arrogance (1995:1) but it is surely just another of the great 'ironies' that postmodernists are so fond of highlighting.

Mocking postmodernism, however, is easier than dismissing it, since those who identify with the phenomenon persist with some tricky questions. Most obviously, questions that might (if they could be persuaded to take social policy seriously) spring to the postmodernists minds is 'What exactly is a critical social policy?' and 'How does this differ from uncritical social policy?'. Thus, social policy finds itself engaged in a debate that is distinctly postmodern: the search for identity. But, and again in true postmodernist fashion, we (in social policy) should not simply answer the questions that occur to them (the postmodernists) but might usefully pose questions of our own. At this point, assuming they are prepared to engage with the lackeys of social engineering, we have dialogue and debate. Before embarking on my sombre polemic I must confess that to a certain degree I am 'just gaming', as O'Neill (1995:192) suggests Lyotard and Derrida are with their opponents. This may be too playful but hopefully those who are attached to aspects of the postmodernists critique are as content with being playfully teased as they are with teasing others (Rattansi 1995; Soper 1993; Williams 1996).

There is, however, a very serious point that needs to be made. The welfare of millions of people cannot be treated lightly. If there is a general sense of scepticism, a feeling that social policy has failed, or a belief that there is very little that can be done to resolve social divisions, it is crucially important to be clear about the reasons for such analyses. Consequently one of the tasks here is to demonstrate the misunderstandings that permeate accounts of *the* British welfare state by some sociological observers. For citing Giddens (1994) and Bauman (1993, 1995) most frequently and for challenging their accounts there is no apology, but, despite the flaws in those accounts, it would be a mistake to dismiss their contributions. Indeed, it is because both scholars are so influential and have been so significant in the development of sociological theory in Britain that their work merits careful consideration. Most importantly, their work raises questions about how to mobilise support for welfare services that address the needs of the poorest. Their scepticism about the reliability of the traditional pillars of welfare support – which include both the political constituencies that have been mobilised in the past and the moral and political arguments that have been called upon to enthuse supporters – deserves to be taken seriously. Thus the doubts and scepticism of observers of 'postmodernity' brings them and sociology closer to a critical social policy, which has always been sceptical. Moreover, many of the central concerns of a critical social policy are now shared by (so-called) orthodox commentators on social policy, which has itself been more critical for some time. Nevertheless, dialogue and debate need to be promoted: there can be no such thing as a critical social policy that refuses to listen to other critical voices, any more than 'postmodernists' can continue to neglect a social policy that, across the political spectrum, has been critical and sceptical. It is worth noting that, to date, critical commentators on social policy have been more prepared to consider writings on postmodernity than vice versa (Fitzpatrick 1996; Hillyard and Watson 1996; Taylor-Gooby 1993; Thompson and Hoggett 1996; Williams 1992, 1996).

Without wishing to push this claim too far, it is important to acknowledge similarities between the 'postmodernists' and 'critical' social policy. Although it is difficult to see how Nietzsche, Bourdieu or Baudrillard might be reconciled with a critical approach to social policy – unless that is to include *any* criticisms – there are others who clearly want to establish some sort of dialogue with a wider constituency. Within the broad church looking for some postmodern morality there exists a tendency that tries hard to maintain a hold on some of the traditional concerns of British sociology; for example, social justice, poverty and social divisions. For scholars such as Giddens (1994), Bauman (1993) and Harvey (1994) it is still possible to engage with these traditional concerns but not in the traditional – modernist – manner. A postmodern society is, certainly for Giddens and Bauman, also a post-traditional society. Rather than suggesting that postmodernity marks the end of politics, ethics and the aim of a 'good society', it is the manner in which these are to be conducted that is seen to have changed. Appeals to tradition, from both left and right, may be voiced but as fewer people subscribe to tradition, such appeals cannot anticipate a traditional response. Thus to assert, as Prime Minister John Major did, that we need to go 'back to basics' was rather naive and simplistic. There simply is no consensus – if there ever was – over what these basics might be. Just issuing an appeal to tradition is unlikely to pay the political dividends that it might previously have done. Unless such appeals are presented as 'new' and in a non-traditional fashion, as Tony Blair seems intent on doing, they will be greeted with scorn.

Nor has the 'orthodox' approach to social policy been immune to the doubts and queries about public welfare regimes. If the *Journal of Social Policy* is a reliable guide it is clear that many of the criticisms have been taken on board. Moreover, a number of those previously associated with a critical approach have found a receptive audience for their work within a more broadly defined 'orthodoxy'. Some of the older critics were always closely associated with the orthodox school and many of the critical school have since become part of an increasingly broad church that is well established, if no longer so clearly 'orthodox'. Trying to maintain a strict division between two clearly distinguishable schools of thought, or of the contents of the journals *Critical Social Policy* (*CSP*) and *Journal of Social Policy* (*JSP*), is not as easy today as it was fifteen years ago. Of course there are still significant differences of opinion, intense disagreements over how to proceed, and profoundly important contrasts in relation to politics and ethics. But there are very few commentators on social policy who suggest that the welfare status quo is satisfactory, and even fewer who appear to advocate some sort of return to the Keynes/Beveridge model of *the* welfare state. In some senses at least anyone concerned with social policy has become 'critical' and could perhaps be classed as part of the growing critique of modernity.

GOOD INTENTIONS GONE WRONG?

As Williams (1996) points out, there are grounds for seeing welfare states and social policy as essentially modern and diametrically opposed to all things postmodern. Instead, criticism of public welfare by postmodernists tends to take two forms: first, the social engineers of *the* welfare state got it wrong; and second, current defenders of the welfare state continue to get it wrong. As Taylor-Gooby (1993) demonstrates, the first claim is made by various critics of modernity but the second is most forcibly asserted by Giddens (1994) in his ambitious attempt to redefine radical politics.

First, the principle architects and so-called 'founders' of the welfare state are portrayed as naive and shortsighted, failings which led them to promote well-meaning but mistaken policies. Thus, interviewed for *Intimations of Postmodernity*, Bauman asserted that:

> The idea of welfare state provision really was to engage the state in order to create for the ordinary people, who didn't have freedom, the conditions for it. It was very much like Aneurin Bevan's view of the National Health Service, that it was a 'one off' expenditure. You introduce it, then every-body would become healthy; and then there would be no expenditure on national health any more – at least, it would be going down and down, year by year. That was the idea. And it was the same with the welfare state. The welfare state was thought of as an enabling institution, as a temporary measure to provide a sort of safety cushion for people, so that they know they can dare, they can take risks, they can exert themselves, because there is always this safety provision if they fail.
>
> (Bauman 1992: 219–20)

Bauman does in other respects provide a sensitive and erudite perspective on modernity that offers a number of insights (Bauman 1993, 1995). However, and even allowing for the fact that interviews tend to generate rather shallow and narrow responses, this respondent has a remarkably benign view of both the architects and the intentions of *the* welfare state. This view is reiterated when he discusses the dismantling of the welfare state:

> The welfare state, wisely, institutionalised commonality of fate: its provi-sions were meant for every participant (every citizen) in equal measure, thus balancing everybody's privations with everybody's gains. The slow retreat from that principle into the means-tested 'focused' assistance for 'those who need it' has institutionalised the diversity of fate, and thus

made the unthinkable thinkable. It is now the taxpayer's privations that are
to be balanced against someone else's, the benefit recipient's, gains.

(Bauman 1993: 243, emphasis in original)

Bauman seems to applaud the initial good intentions but implies these were
misplaced and have been overwhelmed by the concerns of the anxious taxpayer. An attractive feature of Bauman's account, highlighted by Rattansi
(1994), is the idea of the architects of welfare as gardeners, weeding out the
defectives. Despite this, however, there are difficulties to do with the picture
of *the* welfare state that is painted. *The* welfare state is portrayed in an unambiguous and simple manner, but more of this later. Similarly the clichéd
dichotomy of benefit recipients versus taxpayers is reproduced uncritically. It
may be that public welfare is more visible and makes the recipients of it more
prone to disciplinary measures, but that is largely a consequence of discourses
that neglect other forms of welfare (Sinfield 1978). Only if the observer's
gaze is fixed upon the poorest and if the discourse is conducted in terms that
problematise the least powerful can such a view be sustained.

Smart (1990: 412) claims: 'It is through the work of Bauman (1988a,
1988b) that the question of postmodernity has been placed firmly on the
sociological agenda', whilst Giddens is cited on the cover of *Postmodern
Ethics* (Bauman 1993) as follows: 'Bauman, for me has become the theorist of
postmodernity. With exceptional brilliance and originality, he has developed
a position with which everyone now has to reckon.' If so, then the possibility
of finding much common ground with a critical social policy looks rather
remote. To be fair *the* welfare state does not occupy as central a position for
Bauman as it does for Giddens (1994) or Harvey (1994). It might also be
claimed in Bauman's defence that he is discussing the ideas behind the welfare
state, not the policies that were introduced. This is a somewhat lame response,
since it suggests a disjuncture between the good intentions of the architects
and the actual construction of the welfare state. Nor can Bauman's suggestion that *the* welfare state was 'meant' to cater for a commonality of fate or
to enable risk taking pass without comment. When was this 'meant' to have
happened? When was *the* welfare state intending to cater 'in equal measure'
for citizens? Perhaps I am too firmly grounded in the empiricism of social
policy, but some evidence in support of these remarkable claims is surely
called for. In fact there is ample evidence that the founders of *the* welfare
state – whichever period and founders we care to choose – held ideas that
were not, even in the eyes of their contemporaries, benign (Orwell 1970;
Shaw 1987; Williams 1989). What is more, such an account completely
neglects one of the insights that postmodernists claim: that there is no unitary
cause and no single 'idea' about the way society is, or should be. The patterns
of consumption in the 1930s, the pressure from various groups representing
women, the TUC, employers' organisations, the notion of a postwar settlement, intraclass divisions, racist and nationalistic ideas, employers' changes to

the labour process, and notions of the deserving/undeserving, among other factors, all had an influence, and this suggests we might be a little more sensitive in the way we account for the establishment of *the* welfare state (Mann 1986, 1992, 1994).

The second major criticism of *the* welfare state, that defenders of it continue to get it wrong, is more closely associated with Giddens (1994). Indeed, Giddens places *the* welfare state at the centre of his account of how we might go 'beyond left and right'. His undoubted influence on sociology over the last twenty years, combined with his ambitious project – establishing a future for radical politics as he sees it – means it is not unreasonable to single Giddens's work out for scrutiny. This is particularly important when it is asserted that 'We should be prepared to *rethink* the welfare state in a fundamental way' (Giddens 1994: 17, emphasis in original). He portrays *the* welfare state as developing in response to 'misfortunes that "happen" to people' (p. 18). Thus Giddens sees welfare policy responding post hoc to mishaps, whereas he proposes a proactive role for welfare that 'mobilises life-political measures, aimed at once more connecting autonomy with personal and collective responsibilities' (p. 18). Social policies are generally acknowledged to have served to maintain traditional gender roles with the myth of the male breadwinner and the female carer at their core, although some (e.g. Dennis and Erdos 1992; Green 1993) might take issue with the claim that social policies have gone too far in promoting the traditional heterosexual family, and others might point to features that have been used to promote a measure of independence (Mann and Roseneil 1994). Giddens takes a distinctly critical perspective on the role of the welfare state, mentioning the close link between social policies and economic policies in the postwar period and the accumulation and legitimation functions attributed to social policy.

Thus far, many who identify with a critical social policy may nod enthusiastically, although some may want to quibble with the peculiar reductionism employed – 'peculiar' because it rests uneasily with a theoretical model that seeks to escape any hint of reductionism, 'reductionism' because the idea of certain key functions is difficult to sustain in the light of various critiques, some of which Giddens goes on to cite. Leaving these quibbles to one side, there are more worrying flaws in Giddens's account of social policy.

If, as Giddens (1994: 17) claims, 'the welfare state was formed as a "class compromise" or "settlement" in social conditions that have now altered very markedly', it might be worth considering who was party to that settlement and who was excluded. I have argued at length elsewhere that the foundations for contemporary social divisions were laid by a sectional, economistic labour movement pursuing a pragmatic strategy of social closure and exclusion (Mann 1992). Although he acknowledges the way *the* welfare state developed as an exclusive range of publicly funded, insurance-based schemes that were never designed for those who most needed assistance, Giddens proceeds as if they had been so designed. That is, he acknowledges the sectional interests that promoted insurance but then turns to discuss why it is that *the* welfare state failed to meet the needs of those who were excluded. In running through a series of failures that *the* welfare state is held to be responsible for, Giddens highlights the failures of postwar social democracy and the Fabian strategy. The left, he accepts, were consistently critical of both the strategy and the normative philosophy that informed the orthodox approach to social policy. However, and in contrast to virtually everyone associated with *CSP*, it is Marshall and Crosland whom Giddens takes as his representatives of this critical socialist tradition. Not surprisingly he is able to show that 'the left', in the form of Marshall and Crosland, mounted a flawed defence of *the* welfare state, which now confronts a formidable list of problems (Giddens 1994: 73–7).

RISKY WELFARE

It is important to note that risk and risk assessment are central features of the contemporary welfare state, according to Giddens. He undertakes a discussion of risk that potentially raises a number of themes that could engage with both critical and more 'orthodox' approaches to social policy. In pointing to pensions he takes a good example, one that illustrates both the exclusionary features of insurance-based notions of risk and the inherent limitations for many such schemes. Insurance-based schemes like those in Britain certainly did rely heavily on actuarial calculations, although it is doubtful whether these are still based on any meaningful sense of 'insurance funds' as was the case before World War II. There is not, for example, a pot of money held by anyone marked 'pensions contributions'. The old Friendly Society principles of collective risk assessment are more likely to be carried on by occupational and insurance company pension fund managers. Giddens is surely correct, though, to point to the actuarial assumptions that underpin welfare regimes. However, he fails to appreciate, or if he appreciates it to address, the part occupational and fiscal welfare play (Mann 1992; Rose 1981; Sinfield 1978; Titmuss 1958b).

This myopic view of the provisions available, and by implication of risk assessment, leads to some serious misrepresentation and misunderstanding of what welfare is and how it developed. Indeed, the history and development of social policy actually illuminate modernity and reveal it to be more complex and ambiguous, than is often thought. It is the bizarre manner in which everything can be presented as complex, diverse and ambiguous except the welfare services associated with the state, that is so frustrating. This is most obvious when Giddens discusses the role of *the* welfare state in addressing risk and need.

Giddens has a fixation with the costs and risks that public welfare recipients incur that obscures other forms of welfare. In contrast to the way he observes the role of risk assessment, actuarial principles and calculations about the behaviour of potential claimants are certainly not confined to public welfare recipients. Indeed, when it comes to pensions (his example), it is remarkable that he can discuss the demographic and funding 'crisis' and consider (confusingly) the potential for intergenerational conflict but make no mention of some of the most significant players in the pensions arena. With all pension funds in January 1992 holding assets in the region of £500 billion, according to Goode (1993:157), and with actuarial calculations so important to their future ability to fulfil the 'pensions promise', we have to ask why the focus is only on public welfare. Giddens also neglects, to paraphrase Sennett and Cobb (1973), the hidden benefits of class. Thus the focus on risk and responsibility in respect of public welfare, often associated with benefit fraud, can neglect other collectively calculated risk provisions, such as insurance for home contents, vehicles and holidays. As Cook (1989) has emphasised, the benefit system favours those that already access the more privileged services. Likewise the actuarial calculations used to assess risk often have regressive clauses. For example, for the poor and anyone living in an area where poverty is prevalent, the risk of burglary is greater but so is the possibility of being refused insurance cover or charged additional premiums. If our notion of welfare includes the idea that it provides some form of protection against accidents, unforeseen circumstances and unwarranted hurt – a fairly narrow and conservative definition, it might be thought – then some form of insurance or protection is vital. Unfortunately, Giddens sets an agenda that does not allow for a discussion of 'risk' in this context because he is fixated on existing public welfare policies.

Only someone unaware of the array of occupational and fiscal welfare measures that exist could write:

> As a result of the way in which the welfare state developed, from a concern to assist (as well as to regulate) the poor, 'welfare' has generally come to be equated with improving the lot of the underprivileged. But why not suppose that welfare programmes should be directed at the affluent as well as those in more deprived circumstances?
>
> (Giddens 1994: 193)

Yet Giddens has previously acknowledged that the better off have often benefited more than the poor from the array of welfare services provided (Giddens 1994: 75). Concern that he is unaware of the welfare policies that the state already provides for the affluent is reinforced by his discussion of welfare dependency. Again the focus is, as in so many of the tiresome discussions of the 'underclass', simply on public welfare recipients (Giddens 1994). There is also a tendency to invert the problems of the poor and claim that these are in some way shared across the social spectrum. Thus he emphasises how the affluent also have welfare needs: 'Security, self-respect, self-actualisation – these are scarce goods for the affluent as well as the poor, and they are compromised by the ethos of productivism, not just distributive inequalities'

(Giddens 1994: 193). Indeed, 'The relief of dependency becomes a *generalised* aim in a post-scarcity society. Overcoming welfare dependency means overcoming the dependencies of productivism, and both can be combated in the same way' (1994:193–4, emphasis in original).

Thus benefits provided by state agencies that reinforce traditional labour-market and gender roles are blamed for promoting public welfare dependency. Nor does *the* welfare state cater for the individual needs of either the poor or the affluent. Everyone, it would seem, is discontented and there is little that can be defended, despite the desperate attempt by 'the left' to do so. The answer lies, Giddens claims, in the affluent accepting that paid work does not have to be at the centre of life; a situation the poor have learnt to accept and from which the affluent can learn (Giddens 1994: 194–5). Thus he makes a virtue out of something that the overwhelming majority of those who are poor regard as an unwarranted necessity.

The cavalier manner in which Giddens treats *the* welfare state and, despite some minor caveats, the poor is tempered by a frank admission that his view of welfare amounts to 'utopian realism'. However, and even allowing for the fact that he accepts that his view of how the welfare state might wither away is utopian, we are not informed about the real benefits provided to the affluent. This oversight means he can also neglect the way that benefits for the better off are fiercely defended by some on the right. Recent cuts in MIRAS (mortgage interest relief at source) produced howls from Tory backbenchers concerned that they would lose the votes of home purchasers. Likewise, when the Securities Investment Board accepted that millions of people had wrongly been persuaded to move from occupational pensions to personal pensions, underwritten by a subsidy of around £5 billion, there was a rapid about face by politicians who had previously been applauding the private welfare provisions that had been taken out. Suddenly there were demands from all quarters that the welfare needs of those who had been ill advised to change had to be acknowledged and compensation provided. Giddens appears at times to be unaware of the political influence of specific consumption sectors and how their 'dependencies' often have a higher priority than those of much poorer groups (Harrison 1986). Instead he advocates a system of 'positive welfare':

Schemes of positive welfare, oriented to manufactured rather than external risk, would be directed to fostering the *autotelic self*. The autotelic self is one with an inner confidence which comes from self respect, and one where a sense of ontological security, originating in basic trust, allows for the positive appreciation of difference. It refers to a person able to translate potential threats into rewarding challenges, someone who is able to turn entropy into a consistent flow of experience. The autotelic self does not seek to neutralise risk or to suppose that 'someone else will take care of the problem'; risk is confronted as the active challenge which generates self-actualisation.

(Giddens 1994: 192, emphasis in original)

Perhaps my sociological imagination needs to be stimulated in some way, but it is very difficult to see the people of Basildon, Billericay and Harlow engaging in a discovery of the autotelic self. Of course 'well-being' consists of more than consumption and perhaps the people of Essex (for example) need to be a little more reflexive and a little less materialistic if they are to 'feel good'. Giddens is also surely right to stress the more vulnerable, more dependent and more fragmented nature of contemporary social life. He may also be correct in highlighting the risks of everyday social and personal life that currently lie beyond the scope of public welfare regimes. The suspicion remains, though, that the discovery of the autotelic self is lower down the agenda of the people of Essex than the restoration of MIRAS.

Leaving aside the autotelic self, Giddens does raise an important and difficult question: how are the interests of the poorest to be represented and how might these engage with other interests to promote the well-being of all? Within an older Marxist account the answer lay with the labour movement, which, it was assumed, had certain shared interests with the poor (Miliband 1974). This was always a rather optimistic view, and the evidence in Britain is that a divided working class pursued sectional interests which in turn promoted divisive social policies (Mann 1992). With the labour movement at its lowest ebb, certainly since the 1930s but arguably this century, this seems to be another tradition that it may not be worth appealing to, if it ever was. Likewise, a number of formerly cohesive localities have been fragmented by economic, social and industrial change (Byrne 1995). Again, an appeal to some idea of the traditional community, to a local or regional coalition of the poor and the affluent, seems unlikely in the near future. It is also important to acknowledge, as Giddens does, that there are significant changes in the way some social groups are more able to negotiate and reflect on their own welfare needs than others. In this context it may be inappropriate to portray all public welfare beneficiaries as victims of forces beyond their control. The poor are active social agents too, even if they operate in highly constrained environments (Mann 1996). If, as Giddens proposes, traditional hopes about the way to represent the interests of the poor appear forlorn, some alternatives need to be considered.

SO WHAT IS CRITICAL SOCIAL POLICY?

There is an initial issue of whether a 'critical social policy' perspective exists in any sense other than as some sort of allegiance to the journal *CSP*. The journal seems to be alive and well but whether there is a clearly defined notion of what a critical social policy would be is debatable. *CSP* defines its own position in a largely negative manner. It is opposed to the radical right and is aware of the inadequacies of the Fabian and other orthodox models. There is an implication that practice, via practitioners and activists, can inform a critical perspective, but this is not intended to exclude theory.

Accessibility by a fairly broad and general audience is encouraged, the implication again being that some wider dialogue should take place. The only standpoint that is set down is that contributors are asked to consider the implications for different social groups. Socialist, feminist, anti-racist and radical perspectives are the preferred approaches to an understanding of welfare policies. Given that within these camps there are some disparate accounts this is a fairly broad platform, although the suspicion remains that certain self-proclaimed socialists, feminists, anti-racists and radicals (e.g. Dennis and Erdos 1992; Paglia 1993) might not be as warmly encouraged as others. The range of contributors has, however, been fairly broad and it certainly does not promote any one position. The great strength of *CSP* has been its diversity and breadth of critique. Thus if postmodernity represents ambiguity and uncertainty, trying to define a critical social policy is a good example. An easy but unsatisfactory definition would be to take all that which finds its way into the journal *CSP* as representative of a critical social policy; in which case we are confronted by a diverse, ambiguous and on occasion contradictory, if not motley, crew.

The crucial point is that despite a rather vague statement of intent *CSP* does not promote a particular standpoint. Numerous standpoints have been expressed in the journal, but these have tended to reflect the contributor's position, and perhaps the views of some of the editorial collective; searching for a single, coherent perspective would be a vain task. *CSP*, like its older, more orthodox companion *JSP*, embraces a fairly broad audience. Only the radical right are excluded from *CSP* and even then one suspects that a carefully crafted libertarian piece on, for example, decriminalisation of drugs or the sex industry could find a place in the journal. Indeed, it would not always be easy to distinguish the position of the radical right from, say, the libertarian left on some social policy issues. Since *CSP* proclaims to be a journal of socialist, feminist, anti-racist and other radical approaches, and these have seen considerable debate over their relationship to the postmodernist critique, it is perhaps surprising that there has not been more doubt and debate within the journal over what precisely a critical social policy would look like (Miles 1993; Rattansi and Westwood 1994; Smart 1993; Thompson and Hoggett 1996).

If we are looking for common ground, it is important to note that a feature of critical approaches to social policy is that they too have been consistently sceptical of those who have claimed that the welfare state is promoting the 'good society'. 'Good for whom?' and 'Good for what?' are the questions that a critical social policy has consistently asked. It has been a theme of many contributions to *CSP* to query welfare measures that seemed to reinforce particular family forms, gender roles, productivism, dependency and ethnic/racial bias. Contributors to *CSP* have also been consistently sceptical of public welfare bureaucracy and practices that failed to engage with the experience, needs and views of the constituents for whom they are nominally intended. Moreover, many of those involved in the new social movements that often feature in the postmodernist literature as indicators of the new direction that politics will take are likely to regard themselves as having a 'critical' perspective. Some will perhaps consider *CSP* as a forum, or even an ally, that addresses their concerns. The women's movement and the host of social and political campaigns that have arisen from it, claimants' unions, anti-racist campaigns, squatters' groups, professionals'/provider groups such as the London to Edinburgh Weekend Return Group (LEWRG 1980), radical teachers and social workers, prisoner and prison reform groups, along with many others, were to the fore in challenging the corporatist welfare state for many years (Rose 1976). Other critical voices within a broadly defined critical social policy stressed the part played by welfare policies in the operation of a capitalist economy (Ginsburg 1979; Gough 1979; O'Connor 1973; Offe 1982). However, even these accounts did not escape scrutiny and critique from within the critical school, with feminist and anti-racist scholars initially wanting to include, subsequently to separate out, additional forms of oppression and division (Mann 1986; Mishra 1986; Williams 1989, 1996). Furthermore, issues of identity, difference, agency and diversity, all now closely associated with the church of postmodernity, have been much debated within social policy circles and for some time (Mann 1986; Williams 1989). Consequently, if, as Bauman (1995) suggests, we now live our lives in 'fragments' that lack the overarching, and overbearing, moral certainties of the recent past, then it is also worth noting that critical voices articulated this in the 1970s (Rowbotham *et al.* 1979). And more recently questions of diversity and difference have crept into welfare policy and practice without any explicit acknowledgement of postmodernity (Williams 1996).

The point is not that postmodernists are echoing earlier discussions – there are always echoes of the past in present debates – but that they have paid scant regard to the extensive debates within social policy. If welfare and social reform are central to an account of modernity's inadequacies, there is a case for paying more attention to those who articulated, and experienced, those inadequacies. It is not unreasonable to argue that *CSP* has in fact articulated many of the concerns associated with postmodernity and for a considerable time. There is, it might seem, a prima facie case for suggesting that there is some measure of agreement between some analysts of postmodernity, some critical social policy accounts, and an increasingly critical 'orthodox' approach to social policy. Before it is thought that a new consensus has been established and in order to promote further dialogue, however, it has to be acknowledged, by some sociologists within the 'postmodern' school, that there are some major obstacles to overcome; not least the view of *the* welfare state that is being propagated.

THE SOCIAL DIVISIONS OF WELFARE

In short, it is simply unreasonable to treat *the* welfare state or social policy as unitary, modernist and unreflexive. In 1955 Titmuss, the first professor of social administration and someone it is probably fair to describe as a representative of the 'orthodox' approach, queried the meaning of *the* welfare state and the purpose of welfare legislation (Titmuss 1958b). His threefold classification of welfare – occupational, fiscal and public – has served as a powerful retort to all those who focus on public welfare alone. Moreover, he was consistently concerned with identifying the social forces that promoted exclusion. He relied on the work of Durkheim (1933) in respect of the division of labour and the concept of anomie to argue that the unrestrained pursuit of sectional interests promoted social divisions and, ultimately, social dislocation. The essay is not without its flaws but it has been revised and revived by successive scholars (Mann 1992; Rose 1981; Sinfield 1978). There can be few social policy undergraduates who are unfamiliar with the idea of a social division of welfare, and it continues to provide a basis for both analysis and substantive research. A good example would be, Ginn and Arber's (1993) work on the way in which pensions – Giddens's exemplar – are gendered by the social division of welfare and its relationship to the social and sexual divisions of labour. If students of social policy are to take seriously the insights offered by contemporary sociological analyses, and the argument here is that they should, it would be helpful if there were some reciprocity.

Interestingly, and lest anyone runs away with the idea that uncertainty is peculiar to the last years of the twentieth century, Titmuss also stated the following in his inaugural lecture at the LSE in 1951, the supposed heyday of the social engineer:

> Uncertainty, then, is part of the price that has to be paid for being interested in the many-sidedness of human needs and behaviour. However, we draw some comfort from Karl Mannheim's thought that it is precisely our uncertainty which brings us closer to reality than is possible for those who have faith in the absolute or faith, I would add, in the pursuit of specialisation.
>
> (Titmuss 1958a: 14)

Of course there have been many within social policy who have neglected this note of caution, and it is not being suggested that social policy has always been postmodern. Nevertheless, the fact that from the first even orthodox accounts of social policy recognised various forms of dependency, that this was closely related to changes in the labour process, demographic, social and familial change, suggests that scepticism is not confined to contemporary critiques.

CONCLUSION

The big problem, which both Giddens and Bauman highlight, is that uncertainty and ambiguity are widespread; and easy answers cannot be found by appealing to some traditional idea or constituency. The contribution of Giddens and Bauman to the debate over the future of welfare is to highlight the problems that confront anyone trying to address the needs of diverse and disparate groups in contemporary Britain. However, and in contrast to Bauman and Giddens, who respectively criticise *the* welfare state for being a well-intentioned but mistaken attempt at social engineering and defenders of *the* welfare state for continuing to get it wrong, it could be argued that neither scholar appreciates the real value of his own perspectives. It is *they* who have a benign but mistaken view of what *the* welfare state intended and *they* who assume critics of the welfare state want to maintain the status quo. In contrast to art, literature and popular culture, social policy is portrayed as definitively and unambiguously 'modern'. Given the lengthy and intense debates within social policy over the meaning and intentions of *the* welfare state, it seems remarkable that anyone should make such assumptions. From the supposed highpoint of consensus in the 1950s to the present day, it is the ambiguity of the welfare state that is noteworthy (Deacon 1982; Gough 1979; Titmuss 1958b; Sinfield 1978).

If we accept that Giddens is setting out an agenda for debate, one that wants to engage with scholars more familiar with the detail of social policy, it is possible to accept his rather narrow account of welfare development and to acknowledge the points he raises about the need for a fundamental rethink. Indeed, there is considerable evidence that the process of reflection and debate over the future of welfare has been under way for some time. There has been a sustained critique of the welfare state from various sources, including feminists, lone parents, disability groups, the left, anti-racist groups, squatters, claimants' unions and many others, for at least twenty years. Trying to find any references to these debates in any of the postmodernist/postscarcity literature is hard work. Failing to acknowledge the challenges that a broadly defined left has mounted is a serious misrepresentation. Likewise, some of the key features that Giddens cites as problematic, most notably acknowledging difference and diversity within the confines of a universalistic welfare state, have also been part of the welfare agenda for a considerable period. The difficulty has often been to find ways of highlighting the dependency and vulnerability of all without suggesting this is the same for all, and without proposing overarching solutions that fail to address specific needs.

ACKNOWLEDGEMENT

I would like to thank Malcolm Harrison, Carol Smart and Fiona Williams for comments on an earlier draft of this chapter.

NOTE

1 This chapter was completed for this collection in January 1997, before the result of the May 1997 general election was known.

BIBLIOGRAPHY

Baudrillard, J. (1987) *Forget Foucault*, New York: Semiotext(e).

Bauman, Z. (1988a) 'Is there a postmodern sociology?', *Theory, Culture and Society* 5: 2–3.

Bauman, Z. (1988b) 'Sociology and postmodernity', *Sociological Review* 36, 4.

Bauman, Z. (1992) *Intimations of Postmodernity*, London: Routledge.

Bauman, Z. (1993) *Postmodern Ethics*, Oxford: Blackwell.

Bauman, Z. (1995) *Life in Fragments: Essays in Postmodern Morality*, Oxford: Blackwell.

Billig, M. (1994) 'Sod Baudrillard! Or ideology critique in Disney World?', in H.W. Simons and M. Billig (eds) *After Postmodernism*, London: Macmillan.

Byrne, D. (1995) 'Deindustrialisation and dispossession: an examination of social division in the industrial city', *Sociology* 29, 1: 95–115.

Cook, D. (1989) *Rich Law, Poor Law*, Milton Keynes: Open University Press.

Deacon, A. (1982) 'An end to the means test? Social security and the Attlee government', *Journal of Social Policy* 2, 3: 289–306.

Dean, H. and Taylor-Gooby, P. (1992) *Dependency Culture*, Hemel Hempstead: Harvester Wheatsheaf.

Dennis, N. and Erdos, G.(1992) *Families without Fatherhood*, IEA Health and Welfare Unit, Choice in Welfare No. 12, London: IEA.

Durkheim, E. (1933) *The Division of Labour in Society*, New York: Free Press.

Fitzpatrick, T. (1996) 'Postmodernism, welfare and radical politics', *Journal of Social Policy*, 25, 3: 303–20.

Giddens, A. (1990) *The Consequences of Modernity*, Cambridge: Polity Press.

Giddens, A. (1994) *Beyond Left and Right: The Future of Radical Politics*, Cambridge: Polity Press.

Ginn, J. and Arber, S. (1993) 'Pension penalties: the gendered division of occupational welfare', *Work Employment and Society* 7, 1: 47–70.

Ginsburg, N. (1979) *Class, Capital and Social Policy*, London: Macmillan.

Goode, R. (1993) *Pension Law Reform: The Report of the Pension Law Review Committee*, chaired by Roy Goode, vol. 1, Cm2342-1, London: HMSO.

Gough, I. (1979) *The Political Economy of the Welfare State*, London: Macmillan.

Green, D.G. (1993) 'Foreword', in J. Davies (ed.) *The Family: Is it Just Another Lifestyle Choice?* IEA Health and Welfare Unit, Choice in Welfare No. 15, London: IEA.

Harrison, M.L. (1986) 'Consumption and urban theory: an alternative approach based on the social division of welfare', *International Journal of Urban and Regional Research* 10, 2: 232–42.

Harvey, D. (1994) 'Flexible accumation through urbanization: reflections on "postmodernism" in the American city', in A. Amin (ed.) *Post Fordism: A Reader*, Oxford: Blackwell.

Hillyard, P. and Watson, S. (1996) 'Postmodern social policy: a contradiction in terms?', *Journal of Social Policy* 25, 3: 321–46.

LEWRG (London to Edinburgh Weekend Return Group) (1980) *In and Against the State: A Working Group of the Conference of Socialist Economists*, London: Pluto Press.

Mann, K. (1986) 'The making of a claiming class – the neglect of agency in analyses of the welfare state', *Critical Social Policy* 15: 62–74.

Mann, K. (1992) *The Making of an English 'Underclass'? The Social Divisions of Welfare and Labour*, Buckingham: Open University Press.

Mann, K. (1994) 'Watching the defectives: observers of the underclass in Britain, Australia and the USA', *Critical Social Policy* 41: 79–98.

Mann, K. (1996) *The Secret Agents Within the 'Underclass': Critical Reflections on some Recent Theories of Poverty*, Copenhagen: CID.

Mann, K. and Roseneil, S. (1994) 'Some mothers do 'ave em: the gender politics of the underclass debate', *Journal of Gender Studies* 3, 3: 317–31.

Miles, R. (1993) *Racism after 'Race Relations'*, London: Routledge.

Miliband, R. (1974) 'Politics and poverty' in D. Wedderburn (ed.) *Poverty, Inequality and Class Structure*, Cambridge: Cambridge University Press.

Mishra, R. (1984) *The Welfare State in Crisis: Social Thought and Social Change*, Brighton: Wheatsheaf.

Mishra, R. (1986) 'The left and the welfare state: a critical analysis', *Critical Social Policy* 15: 4–19.

O'Connor, J. (1973) *The Fiscal Crisis of the State*, New York: St Martin's Press.

Offe, C. (1982) 'Some contradictions of the modern welfare state', *Critical Social Policy* 12, 2: 7–16.

O'Neill, J. (1995) *The Poverty of Postmodernism*, London: Routledge.

Orwell, G. (1970) *Collected Essays, Journalism and Letters*, London: Penguin.

Paglia, C. (1993) *Sex, Art and American Culture*, New York: Viking Press.

Rattansi, A. (1994) '"Western" racisms, ethnicities and identities', in A. Rattansi and S. Westwood (eds) *Racism, Modernity and Identity*, Cambridge: Polity Press.

Rattansi, A. (1995) 'Review essay: forget postmodernism? Notes from de bunker', *Sociology* 29, 2: 339–49.

Rattansi, A. and Westwood, S. (1994) *Racism, Modernity and Identity*, Cambridge: Polity Press.

Rojek, C. and Turner, B. (eds) (1993) *Forget Baudrillard?*, London: Routledge.

Rose, H. (1976) 'Who can de-label the claimant?', in M. Adler and H. Bradley (eds), *Justice, Discretion and Poverty*, Oxon: Professional Books.

Rose, H. (1981) 'Rereading Titmuss: the sexual division of welfare', *Journal of Social Policy* 10, 4: 477–502.

Rowbotham, S., Segal, L. and Wainwright, H. (1979) *Beyond the Fragments: Feminism and the Making of Socialism*, London: Merlin.

Sennett, R. and Cobb, J. (1973) *The Hidden Injuries of Class*, New York: Vintage Books.

Shaw, C. (1987) 'Eliminating the Yahoo: eugenics, social Darwinism, and five Fabians', *History of Political Thought* viii, 3: 521–44.

Sinfield, A. (1978) 'Analyses in the social division of welfare', *Journal of Social Policy* 7, 2:129–56.

Smart, B. (1990) 'On the disorder of things: sociology, postmodernity and the "end of the social"', *Sociology* 24, 3: 397–416.

Smart, C. (1993) 'Proscription, prescription and the desire for certainty?', *Studies in Law and Society* 13: 37–54. (This is reproduced in Smart 1995).

Smart, C. (1995) *Law, Crime and Sexuality: Essays in Feminism*, London: Sage.

Soper, K. (1993) 'Postmodernism, subjectivity and the question of value', in J. Squires (ed.) *Principled Positions: Postmodernism and the Rediscovery of Values*, London: Lawrence & Wishart.

Taylor-Gooby, P. (1981) 'The empiricist tradition in social administration', *Critical Social Policy* 1, 2: 6–21.

Taylor-Gooby, P. (1993) 'Postmodernism and social policy: a great leap backwards?',

University of New South Wales Discussion Article. No. 45, September. Also in *Journal of Social Policy* (1994), 23, 3: 385–404.

Thompson, S. and Hoggett, P. (1996) 'Universalism, selectivism and particularism: towards a postmodern social policy', *Critical Social Policy* 16, 1: 21–43.

Titmuss, R. (1958a) 'Social administration in a changing society'. Also in *Essays on the Welfare State*, London: Allen & Unwin. (First published in *British Journal of Sociology*, (1951), 2, 3.)

Titmuss, R. (1958b) 'The social division of welfare', in *Essays on the Welfare State*, London: Allen & Unwin.

Williams, F. (1989) *Social Policy: A Critical Introduction*, Cambridge: Polity Press.

Williams, F. (1992) 'Somewhere over the rainbow: universality and diversity in social policy', in N. Manning and R. Page (eds) *Social Policy Review 4*, Nottingham: Social Policy Association.

Williams, F. (1996) 'Postmodernism, feminism and the question of difference', in N. Parton (ed.) *Social Work, Social Theory and Social Change*, London: Routledge.

Chapter 7

Postmodernity and the future of welfare
Whose critiques, whose social policy?

Suzy Croft and Peter Beresford

INTRODUCTION

Postmodernist debates highlight difference, diverse subjective realities and the reappraisal of rationalist assumptions about knowledge and understanding. A key development in modern welfare has been the emergence of new movements of the subjects of social policy, including disabled people, people with learning difficulties, psychiatric system survivors and older people. These movements are developing their own critiques, theories, knowledge, objectives, strategies and ways of organising. Ironically, in view of the priorities of postmodernist discussion, they have so far been marginalised by it. While they are sometimes recognised by it as a subject of study, their discourse has so far generally not been included in it.

The broader exclusion which these groups experience has been mirrored in postmodern discussion itself. This chapter examines this exclusion and the implications of the new movements of disabled people and social care service users for social policy, the study of welfare and the themes of postmodernism. It will seek to make connections between emerging postmodernist discussion in welfare and the perspectives of these new movements.

THE EMERGENCE OF DISABLED PEOPLE'S AND SERVICE USERS' MOVEMENTS

During the last fifteen to twenty years, with accelerating strength and authority, groups of people previously conceived of primarily as the subjects of social policy and of other people's discourses have developed their *own* discourses. These groups include disabled people, psychiatric system survivors, older people, people with learning difficulties and people living with HIV and AIDS. The development of their discourses has been related to the emergence of these groups' own movements. They have established their own organisations, action, campaigning, philosophies, developing traditions and cultures, discussions, writings, ideas and knowledge. They have now begun the process of writing up their own histories (Campbell 1996; Campbell and Oliver 1996).

These various movements have similarities but also significant differences. There are overlaps and exchanges between them, as well as separations and distinctions. We would suggest, though, that in general there are fundamental differences between them and traditional approaches to social policy analysis and policy making, of both the political left and right. These are differences in terms of:

- process;
- power and resources;
- aims and objectives;
- philosophy;
- personnel.

Their process is explicitly participatory and democratic, rather than prescriptive and paternalistic, closely linked with other cultural, political, social and self-help activities and a changed social relations of research and theory building. The movements continue to have much less credibility and far fewer financial and other resources than conventional social policy discussions. Their aims and objectives are reflected in the priority which these movements give in their debates and action to safeguarding the civil rights and meeting the needs of their constituencies. This takes precedence over abstracted analysis and description or separate occupational, political or ideological objectives and agendas. Their personnel are generally not dedicated specifically to social policy analysis or theory building, although they do include some academics of their own. Instead, as Jane Campbell has argued of the disabled people's movement:

> The movement is multi-faceted. There is direct action campaigning on the street. There is letter writing and political work in parliament. There is intellectual work and arts. The movement involves all of these and people cross over. People who write the books are also on the picket line. This has given us a much fuller representation because we have a much more holistic approach and understanding.
>
> (Beresford and Campbell 1994: 321)

While the new welfare consumerism, which is particularly developed in the policy of 'community care', where it is framed in terms of 'user involvement' and professional 'empowerment', frequently seeks to frame the interventions and roles of the disabled people's and social care service users' movements and organisations in narrow terms of input to inform and increase the 'efficiency' and 'economy' of existing structures, systems and services, this is certainly not the basis on which such movements and organisations have generally developed. Instead these are essentially independent *political* movements, which are primarily concerned with making both personal and social change and advancing the position of their members (Beresford 1997a). Their key concern has been extending their constituencies' participation, inclusion and autonomy, and they have adopted a range of strategies to achieve this.

MADNESS AND DYING: TWO CASE STUDIES

We want to move next to look briefly at current discussions by and about two such groups of service users. These are discussions by and about psychiatric system survivors, madness and distress; and about dying and people who are dying. There are significant differences between the two. This is not least because while survivors have developed their own distinct movement, the same is not true of people who are dying, although the related movement of people living with HIV/AIDS has been established (see, for example, People Living With AIDS 1996). We also approach these discussions in different ways, bringing different insights; as someone working with people who are dying (including people with cancer, AIDS and motor neurone disease), and as psychiatric system survivors, one of whom is actively involved in the survivors' movement.

We want to consider some central features of discussions by and about these two groups. We also want to highlight some of the key characteristics associated with them. In doing this, we want to make clear that we are not suggesting that there is only one uniform and monolithic expert or experiential discussion. Clearly there is not. There are competing professional perspectives and differences among people with direct experience. But our experience suggests that there are some key characteristics linked with each which can be identified, and we want to headline these.

We will begin with dominant expert discourse on madness and distress. This is a predominantly medical discourse and other disciplines, including social work, have largely adopted its medical model and assumptions uncritically.

- This discourse places an emphasis on the *causation* of devalued behaviour, feelings and perceptions. It emphasises individual physical, biochemical and increasingly genetic explanations.
- It is mainly associated with treatment with mechanical and chemical restraints.
- There is an increasing association of madness and distress with danger and violence in expert, political and media debates.
- The dominant model of madness and distress commands cross-party support from the political left and right and has become a high-profile political and electoral issue.
- This is linked with the community care debate, which has narrowly framed the response to madness and distress in polarised terms of large institution versus medically based maintenance in people's own homes or smaller institutions.

The movement of psychiatric system survivors does not share one agreed view of madness and distress. There is not even any agreement about terminology, some members preferring the term 'survivors', others 'mental health service users'. As Peter Campbell has written:

> The influence of the 'anti-psychiatry movement' on user/survivor action in the 1980s and 1990s is a subject of some interest and uncertainty ... In general, users/survivors will often distance themselves from the 'anti-psychiatric' labelling to gain a decent hearing for their proposals ... The movement's inheritance from 'anti-psychiatry' has been emotional and spiritual rather than programmatic and practical.
>
> (Campbell 1996: 221)

But as Campbell also writes, many survivors do support some of the general propositions put forward by 'anti-psychiatrists' like R.D. Laing and David Cooper:

> The possible intelligibility of madpersons, the possible value of their insights and agonies when in periods usually described as psychosis, are among the respectful declarations that users and survivors warmly welcome and frequently seek to build upon.
>
> (Campbell 1996: 221)

Members of the psychiatric system survivors' movement have challenged dominant psychiatric discourse. They highlight instead:

- survivors' desire for appropriate support rather than medicalised responses, which are often experienced as adding to people's pain, danger and difficulties;
- the need for their feelings, experiences and perceptions and the social relations these have to be acknowledged and understood;
- the demand for respect for their human and civil rights;
- their desire to live an independent life, including access to employment, recreation and social relations (see, for example, Leader 1995; Read and Reynolds 1996).

Now let us turn to the dominant discourse about dying and explore some of its defining features. We include in this both the expert medical and media presentation of death and dying. Bert Keizer, a doctor working in a nursing home for people with terminal illness in Holland, has written:

> The human problem: having a mind, being a body, is nowhere quite so painfully and clearly apparent as in medicine. Painful, because to be a body means you must die. Clear, because to have a mind means that you know this. Though medical training strongly focuses on the body, death is given little attention. An emblem of Death, the skull, can often be found in medical textbooks, but emptied of all symbolism, hidden beneath

anatomical Latin, so that his familiar toothy grin never quite breaks through.

(Keizer 1996: 1)

In contrast, the following seem to be some of the key terms in which we are conventionally encouraged to conceive of death and dying. The two are framed in terms of:

- struggle and competition: the individual winning – fighting, beating cancer, death, illness, morbidity, mortality and not giving up or giving in;
- medical victory: the medical profession and associated medical research overcoming disease through skill, science, knowledge, technology and wisdom. This is linked with the medicalisation and technicisation of death: medical dominance in death and dying. A high percentage of dying takes place in medical institutions, yet this is coupled with the low priority of palliative care in medicine and with the emphasis on cure not support in medical professional values;
- extending life: making it possible for people to have 'more time' (a key concern of oncologists, radiotherapists and related professionals);
- living for ever: the medical and market-led search for immortality, from superfitness and the cult of the body to cryogenics;
- the centrality of faith: spiritual beliefs guiding us in our passage from body to spirit;
- the polarisation of discussion around death as an ideological and rights issue: suffering, the right to life and bad death, versus euthanasia and the right to assisted exit (see, for example Keizer 1996; Kubler-Ross 1986; Nuland 1994; Randall and Downie 1996).

A different picture, reflecting different concerns and priorities, emerges from people who are dying themselves. Their discourse, as one of us (Suzy Croft) has sought to understand it from seven years working as a social worker with people who are dying (and we offer it cautiously), highlights:

- people's desire to live what life there is as best they can;
- being able to make informed judgements, choices and decisions about the possibilities for the rest of their life: exploring treatment and quality of life options;
- being able to deal with their own loss and that of other people;
- pain control (so that life does not have to be so bad as to encourage people's unnecessary desire for death);
- dealing with fear and uncertainty;
- coping with what is happening;
- avoiding impoverishment, through the material changes and losses which are associated in our society with ill health and terminal illness;
- dealing with concerns for those who are close to them, both adults and children (Croft 1996).

COMPETING DISCOURSES

We have only been able to offer brief and initial sketches of some of the salient points of these different dominant expert and subjective discussions. Enquiry into them is still at a relatively early stage. Survivors have only begun to produce their accounts over the last ten to fifteen years. There are still relatively few non-medical discussions of death and dying. For example, it was not until 1995 that the first major study of the sexual politics of death and dying was published (Cline 1995).

But it is clear that dominant and first-hand discussions are not only different, they also compete and are in conflict with each other. Many members of the survivors' movement reject the psychiatric system and its ideology. There is also not much love lost from the other side. Survivors' views are frequently rejected as unsubstantiated and 'unrepresentative' (Beresford and Campbell 1994). While members of the survivors' movement view madness and distress as part of the human condition, both damaging and helpful, frightening and illuminating, the dominant discourse seeks technicist solutions to what is presented as a problem of a distinct and defective group of human beings, either seeking to eradicate it from individuals or starting to explore the possibility of breeding it out of the human species through genetic engineering. The response of the dominant medical discourse on dying is often unsympathetic at individual level to the concerns and approach of its subjects. For example, the focus of some people who are dying on the life they have, rather than on addressing dying, is interpreted in negative terms of people being 'in denial', and not facing or accepting that they are dying.

The two dominant medical discourses on madness and distress and dying are deeply rooted in the scientism and rationalism of the nineteenth century. But the emergence of new discourses from the disabled people's and social care service users' movements has strongly challenged this tradition. Meanings and analysis are now more and more contested. It is increasingly difficult to sustain assumptions that something has one inherent meaning or that there is agreement about meaning. Clear differences in power between different meanings can also be identified. Hierarchies of credibility operate here. The issue of meaning is no longer abstract; it is at the heart of the ideas and activities of these new movements. Just as the survivors' movement has questioned medical diagnostic categories and in some cases the model of mental illness itself, so the disabled people's movement has rejected the medicalised individual model of disability and developed its own sophisticated and dynamic social model of disability, based on drawing a distinction between individual impairment and the disablement resulting from discrimination and social oppression (Crow 1996; Oliver 1996).

Questions of meaning operate at many levels. They change over time. For the Victorians, for instance:

'Good deaths' were rare; the assumption was that 'the manner' of 'dying could provide the final proof of salvation.' The best deaths required either a noble struggle with pain, or its comparative absence, and some last faith-affirming words.

(*Times Higher Education Supplement*, 7 February 1997)

There is no agreement, for example, about the meaning of dying. When, say, is dying dying and when is it chronic illness? Hospices working with terminally ill people, for instance, are much less likely to admit people with chronic heart disease, emphysema and severe strokes, although these illness may be terminal in much the same way as diseases which are admitted, like cancer and motor neurone disease. There are sometimes remissions in the course of cancer which make prediction difficult, even if the assumption of certainty remains. One London social services department has now defined dying in terms of a prognosis of less than six months, because then it is a health authority responsibility and the person will not be assessed by a social worker.

Anne Plumb, a survivor, offers one of the clearest examinations of the gulf between dominant and survivors' meanings of madness and distress:

We may indeed be people who have been diagnosed – labelled – as 'ill' or 'sick'. We have usually been 'treated' with powerful drugs (told sometimes that we will need these drug interventions – these 'medications' – for life) ... We are generally included in disability legislation as 'mentally ill people' ... or as 'mentally disordered' ... Elsewhere we have become people 'with long-term psychiatric disabilities' ... What brings us together ... is our experience of the psychiatric system or 'mental health services' ... This forms the basis of our definition ... rather than a definition of some common personal characteristic or characteristics ... [O]ur difficulties lie in hurt, oppression, a refusal to fulfil prescribed roles ... and society's response to these. This reflects a more widespread shift away from talk of 'illness', 'disorder' or 'defective mechanisms' (chemical imbalances) to talk of *distress* or *dissent*.

(Plumb 1994: 5, 6, 8)

THE RELEVANCE OF POSTMODERNIST DISCUSSION

We now turn to postmodernism. In the debate about the value or otherwise of postmodernism as an idea and development, we remain neutrals, at least until the issue which we are raising regarding the role of service users and their movements in the debate is clarified and resolved. Nor do we see ourselves as experts on the subject. Our increasing realisation has been that we cannot avoid or ignore postmodernism in social policy. It is more and more central in academic debates. There is a growing focus on it and it is also finding its way into supposedly practice-related writings (for example, Parton 1996).

We might expect that the emergence of postmodernism 'as a particular shift in theory and analysis' in social policy, as Fiona Williams describes it (1992: 204), would be helpful and illuminating in a discussion of competing discourses in social policy. The characteristics associated with postmodernity by Nigel Parton, for example – 'a fragmentation of modernity into forms of institutional pluralism, marked by variety, contingency, relativism and ambivalence' (Parton 1994: 27) – reflect the experience of social policy service users. Postmodernist debates highlight difference, diverse subjective realities and the reappraisal of rationalist assumptions about knowledge and understanding. These are issues which service users and their movements raise and highlight too and which would also seem to invite their particular contribution and participation.

We see the emergence of new movements of the subjects of social policy, particularly social care policy, including disabled people, psychiatric system survivors, older people and people with learning difficulties, as a key development affecting modern welfare and its analysis. These movements have developed their own critiques, theories, knowledge, objectives, strategies and ways of organising. While we might expect some problems with postmodern discussion in social policy, for example, because of the nature of its concepts, as Fawcett and Featherstone (1996) discuss, we would also expect it to offer helpful insights for and about service users and their movements. Its emphasis on relativism, subjectivity and diversity all point to this.

THE MARGINALISATION OF SERVICE USERS IN POSTMODERN DISCUSSION

However, ironically, service users and their movements have so far been largely marginalised by postmodernist discussion in social policy. It is this which we want to explore next.

But to begin with, to put this in context, it may be helpful to look at their treatment in other related discussions. Kirk Mann has commented on the failure of broader postmodern debates to address these and related perspectives:

> There has been a sustained critique of the welfare state from various sources, including feminists, lone parents, disability groups, the left, anti-racist groups, squatters, claimants' unions and many others, for at least twenty years. Trying to find any references to these debates in any of the postmodernist/postscarcity literature is hard work.
>
> (Mann, this volume: 99)

Writers from the disabled people's movement argue that mainstream sociology has largely ignored the work of disabled sociologists and the disabled people's movement (Barton 1996).

Another key social policy discussion is that associated with the social care service system. There is now a considerable body of writing, research and analysis following from the practice and policy of 'community care' and 'continuing care'. At the same time, as we have said, service users have developed their own increasingly substantial body of knowledge and canon of writing. Because of the growing numbers and power of service users involved in their own movements, it has been more and more difficult for the dominant service-based discussion on social care to ignore them. The service system, as we have seen, is also increasingly required to 'involve' service users as part of the political commitment to 'consumer choice' in the 'care market'. However, the liberatory objectives of the disabled people's and service users' movements are a poor fit with the market consumerism of the mixed economy of care. As Peter Campbell has said:

> While the growth of consumerist ideology has undoubtedly added to current willingness for service providers and purchasers to consider the views of people with a mental illness diagnosis ... there is a considerable difference between valuing a madperson as a consumer or recipient of mental health services and valuing a madperson as a contributing and insightful member of society.
>
> (Campbell 1996: 220)

The result has largely been a service system which has accepted what service users have to say only so far as it has been required to by legislation and government guidance and the pressure which the movements themselves have been able to bring to bear. It has sought determinedly to tokenise and incorporate service users. While they and their movements are now more powerful than they have ever been, their power and resources are still very restricted. It would be as mistaken to overstate the strength and influence of these movements as it would be to ignore them. As we have suggested elsewhere, although there are some overlaps, two distinct discourses have developed in community care, framed in different terms, with different concerns and objectives (Croft and Beresford 1995). So far, while the viewpoints and knowledge of community care service users appear to be included more in academic and professional community care discussions than in other areas of social policy debate, this involvement is still limited.

Service users and their movements are now beginning to figure in postmodernist social policy discussion. They are identified, described, discussed and analysed within it. In this book, for example, Kirk Mann has addressed these movements, in engaging with recent sociological literature on 'postmodernity', and Barbara Fawcett and Brid Featherstone focus on the experience of a disabled service user to develop a critique of the idea and practice of quality assurance and evaluation in social work in a postmodern era.

But in two key ways service users are still essentially marginalised and tokenised in postmodernist social policy discussion, as they are in the dominant service system discussion. Their marginalisation is reflected first in the limited extent to which their work is as yet included or addressed in post-modernist discussion, and second in the degree to which they are excluded from the process of this discussion. There are some exceptions (notably, Taylor 1996), but this general picture holds.

We will begin with the first of these exclusions: the failure of postmodernist social policy discussion fully to address and include service users' own debates and activities. The enthusiasm with which social policy analysts and commentators have addressed mainstream postmodernist debates has not been matched by a similar enthusiasm for addressing the discourse of the disabled people's and service users' movements. Where efforts have been made to relate service users' and social policy discourses, it has usually come from service users (for example, Barnes and Mercer 1996). Yet the discourse of the disabled people's and social care service users' movements has no less fundamental implications for social policy analysis and discussion, is transformatory in its ramifications, and represents at least as radical a departure in thinking as postmodernist thinking is seen to. This raises the question of why it is that there has not been a comparable focus on and interest in service users' discourse.

Second, service users and their organisations are not included as part of the postmodernist social policy discourse. This mirrors the excluding structures and nature of conventional academic enquiry (Beresford 1997b). It may also be linked with the particular opaqueness of postmodernist discussions. Despite the relevance of service users and their organisations to postmodernist discussion, generally little effort seems to have been made to include or involve them in it. What this means is that most service users, and we are talking here about those who are actively involved in their own organisations and movements, are unlikely to be party to or familiar with postmodernist debates or even to be aware of their existence.

It may be argued that this is not important; that postmodern debates are themselves abstruse and marginal and that they are unlikely to have any real impact on the lives of people on the receiving end of welfare services and social policy. As we have already said, there are many differences within and between social care service users' movements, but the demand which unifies them all is the right to '*speak for themselves*'. Participation – in debates and decisions affecting them, in their own movements, and in mainstream society – is central to the philosophies of these movements. Discussions about them, which do not include them, directly oppose this cornerstone belief.

Sue Penna and Martin O'Brien write in a discussion of postmodernism and social policy which addresses the movements:

Marginalisation/exclusion is inevitably accompanied by resistance and conflict which gives rise to political struggle over the meaning and experience of exclusion. For example, sections of the disability rights movement and the feminist movement challenge the dominant knowledges, procedures and practices of social institutions and their marginality to them.

(Penna and O'Brien 1996: 53)

As we have indicated, postmodernist social policy discussion has not ignored service users and their movements. Instead what it has done is begin to offer its *own* commentary on them. Conventional discussants have developed their own descriptions, analyses and interpretations of these movements, their members and their activities. Those disabled people and service users who have access to their writings and discussions find themselves and their organisations reinterpreted and restructured in them (for example, Rogers and Pilgrim 1991). Instead of challenging the tradition of grand narrative, this discourse replaces one grand narrative with another. Postmodernist commentators are mostly located in conventional academic and policy-making institutions with greater credibility, power and resources than service users and their organisations, so that increasingly they are commanding resources, in the form of research funding, consultancies and academic employment opportunities, to explore the issues and ideas which the users' movements themselves have most forcefully raised – issues around empowerment, collective action, rights and need – and divert them in the direction of their own interests (Barnes and Thompson 1994; Croft and Beresford 1995).

The exclusion of service users and their organisations from postmodern discussion seems to have other negative effects on it. It limits and distorts the discussion's own understanding of such new social movements. For example, David Taylor, discussing the tensions between universalist and particularist approaches to welfare, argues 'they frequently emerge as debates between universalist rights-based arguments in defence of state welfare, and particularist needs-based arguments associated with the self-advocacy of "new social movements"'. (Taylor 1996: 149). Fiona Williams, however, places a different interpretation on these movements:

Some possibilities of the emergence of common and unifying concerns from specific needs can be seen in the development of what could be called the 'New Social Welfare Movements' – those groups that have emerged particularly over the last ten years to push in collective ways for specific needs – self-advocacy groups, survivors' groups, HIV+ groups, women's refuges, black women's refuges, disability groups, women's disability groups, reproductive rights groups, carers' groups. Fragmented, competing and often conflicting as these developments have been, what unites these groups is a concern with the nitty-gritty of empowerment, representation, and ensuring the quality, availability and accountability of user-centred provision ... [they] have the capacity to combine particularist interests with universalist values.

(Williams 1992: 216)

Spicker, writing about empowerment, suggests that by becoming empowered to participate 'People are being empowered to do the kind of things which other people do; and the kinds of things which other people do are often discriminatory' (Spicker 1996: 232).

Some of these arguments do not reflect the reality of the disabled people's, survivors' and service users' movements. They ignore the debates now taking place within these movements addressing and challenging broader discriminations and exclusions which they have mirrored (for example, Morris 1996). One of the key characteristics of the disabled people's and social care service users' movements in the UK is that they challenge the status quo at all levels; they are not concerned only with changing the position of their constituency within the existing order, but believe that there must be change in that order itself if their constituency's rights and needs are to be secured. Peter Campbell has highlighted the dilemma with which this faces the survivors' movements:

> While it may never result in a clear choice between changing services and changing society, the evidence suggests that effective change in future will demand increasingly definite choices and specialisation from local, regional and national organisations.
>
> (Campbell 1996: 224)

The arguments of the movements are more often framed in terms of rights than of needs and there is an increasing concern to challenge the divisiveness of existing public and social policy through building links and alliances (Beresford and Turner 1997; Morris 1996).

If service users are not fully involved in postmodernist welfare discussion, then we have to ask on what basis and how well its commentators will know them and their work. So far, judging from their citations, it appears that most are not even familiar with the published, let alone unpublished, discussions of service users and their movements. They do not generally seem to know the movements on equal terms, and postmodern welfare discussion so far largely appears to have perpetuated rather than challenged the traditional unequal divide between the subjects of social policy and its analysts and researchers. In view of the challenge that postmodern discussion might be expected by its nature to represent to such traditional social relations, this is particularly disappointing. To this extent, we believe that postmodernist discussion mirrors the traditional policy and analysis which it seeks to critique. It is no less excluding and paternalistic. The discourse of the disabled people's and service users' movements offers an alternative to the conventional polarisation of welfare between paternalism and profit, state and market. It is difficult to see how the existing process and product of postmodernist welfare discussion can hold similar promise so long as they maintain their existing pattern of social relations.

Postmodernist welfare discussion and the discourse of the movements of disabled people and social care service users are significantly different. They are different in nature, process, aims and personnel. The reasons they come to their subject are different. The movements are primarily concerned with changing and improving the lives of their members, and their interest in social policy follows from this. Change is not necessarily a central objective of the institutions in which postmodern welfare commentators are located and these institutions are becoming more rather than less constraining (Barnes 1996).

POSTMODERNISM, GRAND THEORY AND THE ROLE OF SERVICE USERS

The nature of the two discussions may also tell us something about their different relations with postmodern debate. While welfare discourse has now engaged with postmodernism with great enthusiasm, it picked up on it late, as welfare tends to do with most things. Before its analysts applied the postmodernist template to social policy, postmodern debates were further developed in other fields.

This still leaves the question of why there is such enthusiasm for postmodernism on the part of social policy analysts, especially since, as we have already noted, the same attachment has not been shown to service users' discourse, despite its strong claim to groundbreaking significance. We do not know what the answer is to this question. We can only offer our own suggestions for discussion. They relate to the weakness and vulnerability of left-of-centre social policy and social policy thinking. Left-of-centre social policy has been undermined and displaced in the UK, Europe and the US. Left-of-centre social policy thinking is weak and uncertain. Both are in retreat and social administration solutions to social issues and problems have come under the most severe and effective attack since their emergence in the late nineteenth and early twentieth centuries. These attacks have come from their recipients and their movements, from citizens' organisations more broadly and from all political quarters. The old left-of-centre grand theory, Fabianism, is in terminal decline, with few political or academic friends.

Faced with this analytical and public policy impasse, postmodernism, with the challenge it makes to traditional assumptions and alignments, comes at a very helpful time for left-of-centre social policy academics and analysts. It offers useful ways of dealing with and rationalising broader political realignments. It highlights issues of difference and social exclusion, which have become increasingly central to social policy from all political quarters (Levitas 1996; Williams 1996). It provides discussants with a new basis and new domains for grand theorising, when others have been lost. This may or may not make it necessary for them to address issues at micro as well as macro level more closely than before, or to work in more equal relationships with the subjects of their policies and prescriptions.

CONCLUSION: MOVING FORWARD

Such grand theorising may or may not be helpful at a time when public policy in the UK and west is becoming more oppressive than it has been in most living memory. We share Kirk Mann's view that 'a very serious point … needs to be made. The welfare of millions of people cannot be treated lightly' (this volume: 87). The key point we want to make here is that if postmodernist welfare discussion does not include and involve the recipients of social policy, drawing on and supporting their ideas, experience and knowledge, then it is unlikely to be an effective or progressive force in social policy. Given the significant differences in approach, understanding and priorities of mainstream social policy discourse and the discourse of disabled people, service users and their organisations, it seems crucial not to continue to incorporate or ignore them. If there is to be a helpful debate about postmodernist welfare and if a postmodernist approach to social policy is to be developed, then it must involve the recipients of policy on full and equal terms.

BIBLIOGRAPHY

Barnes, C. (1996) 'Disability and the myth of the independent researcher' *Disability and Society*, 11, 1: 111–14.

Barnes, C. and Mercer, G. (eds) (1996) *Exploring the Divide: Illness and Disability*, Leeds: Disability Press.

Barnes, C. and Thompson, G. (1994) *Funding for User-led Initiatives*, London: British Council of Organisations of Disabled People/National Council for Voluntary Organisations.

Barton, L. (ed.) (1996) *Disability and Society: Emerging Issues and Insights*, London: Longman.

Beresford, P. (1997a) 'New movements, new politics: making participation possible', in T. Jordan and A. Lent (eds) *Storming the Millennium: The New Politics of Change*, London: Lawrence & Wishart.

Beresford, P. (1997b) 'The last social division?: Revisiting the relationship between social policy, its producers and consumers', in M. May, E. Brunsdon and G. Craig (eds), *Social Policy Review 9*, Sheffield: Social Policy Association.

Beresford, P. and Campbell, J. (1994) 'Disabled people, service users, user involvement and representation', *Disability and Society* 9, 3: 315–25.

Beresford, P. and Turner, M. (1997) *It's Our Welfare: Welfare State Service Users and the Future of Welfare*, London: NISW.

Campbell, J. and Oliver, M. (1996) *Disability Politics: Understanding our Past, Changing our Future*, London: Routledge.

Campbell, P. (1996) 'The history of the user movement in the United Kingdom', in T. Heller, J. Reynolds, R. Gomm, R. Muston and S. Pattison (eds) *Mental Health Matters*, Basingstoke: Macmillan.

Cline, S. (1995) *Lifting the Taboo: Women, Death and Dying*, London: Little, Brown.

Croft, S. (1996) 'How can I leave them?': Towards an empowering social work practice with women who are dying', paper presented at 'Feminism and Social Work in the Year 2000: Conflicts and Controversies' conference, University of Bradford, Bradford, 11 October.

Croft, S. and Beresford, P. (1995) 'Whose empowerment?: Equalising the competing discourses in community care', in Raymond Jack (ed.) *Empowerment in Community Care*, London: Chapman and Hall.

Crow, L. (1996) 'Including all our lives: renewing the social model of disability', in J. Morris (ed.) *Encounters with Strangers: Feminism and Disability*, London: Women's Press.

Fawcett, B. and Featherstone, B. (1996) '"Carers" and "caring": new thoughts on old questions', in B. Humphries (ed.) *Critical Perspectives On Empowerment*, Birmingham: Venture Press.

Keizer, B. (1996) *Dancing with Mr D: Notes on Life and Death*, London: Doubleday.

Kubler-Ross, E. (ed.) (1986) *Death: The Final Stage of Growth*, New York: Touchstone Books.

Leader, A. (1995) *Direct Power: A Resource Pack for People who Want to Develop their Own Care Plans and Support Networks*, Brighton: Community Support Network/Brixton Community Sanctuary/Pavilion Publishing/MIND.

Levitas, R. (1996) 'The concept of social exclusion and the new Durkheimian hegemony', *Critical Social Policy* 16, 1: 5–20.

Morris, J. (1996) *Encouraging User Involvement in Commissioning: A Resource for Commissioners*, Leeds: Department of Health, National Health Service Executive Community Care Branch, West Yorkshire.

Nuland, S.B. (1994) *How We Die*, London: Chatto & Windus.

Oliver, M. (1996) *Understanding Disability: From Theory to Practice*, Basingstoke: Macmillan.

Parton, N. (1994) 'Problematics of government: (post)modernity and social work', *British Journal of Social Work* 24, 1: 9–32.

Parton, N. (ed.) (1996) *Social Theory, Social Change and Social Work*, London: Routledge.

Penna, S. and O'Brien, M. (1996) 'Postmodernism and social policy: a small step forwards?', *Journal of Social Policy* 25, 1: 39–61.

People Living With AIDS (1996) *Living with AIDS*, London: National AIDS Manual Publications.

Plumb, A. (1994) *… Distress or Disability? … A Discussion Document*, occasional paper, Manchester: Greater Manchester Coalition of Disabled People.

Randall, F. and Downie, R.S. (1996) *Palliative Care Ethics: A Good Companion*, Oxford: Oxford Medical Publications/Oxford University Press.

Read, J. and Reynolds, J. (eds) (1996) *Speaking Our Minds: An Anthology of Personal Experiences of Mental Distress and its Consequences*, Basingstoke: Macmillan.

Rogers, A. and Pilgrim, D. (1991) 'Pulling down churches: accounting for the British mental health users' movement', *Sociology of Health and Illness* 13, 2: 129–48.

Spicker, P. (1996) 'Understanding particularism', in D. Taylor (ed.) *Critical Social Policy: A Reader*, London: Sage.

Taylor, D. (ed.) (1996) *Critical Social Policy: A Reader*, London: Sage.

Williams, F. (1992) 'Somewhere over the rainbow: universality and diversity in social policy', in N. Manning and R. Page (eds) *Social Policy Review 4*, Nottingham: Social Policy Association.

Williams, F. (1996) 'Postmodernism, feminism and the question of difference', in N. Parton (ed.) *Social Theory, Social Change and Social Work*, London: Routledge.

Part III

Social divisions and social exclusion

Chapter 8

New horizons? New insights?

Postmodernising social policy and the case of sexuality

Jean Carabine

INTRODUCTION

In recent years sexuality has generated considerable media interest, as evidenced in a multiplicity and range of TV programmes, magazines and books which have taken sexuality as their concern. Similarly, sexuality, specifically its regulation and appropriate expression, has also been the focus of political debates and policy.

I have argued elsewhere (Carabine 1996a, 1996b) that sexuality tends to be ignored in social policy analyses despite the centrality of it in popular discourse, as well as in policy and political debates. Receiving even less attention is the relationship between both sexuality and social policy, which continues to be underresearched and undertheorised. More specifically, heterosexuality is rarely acknowledged or critiqued, and scarcely ever informs social policy analyses. I have also argued for the need to incorporate sexuality centrally in our analyses of social policy both as discipline and as practice (Carabine 1996a, 1996b). One way of doing this is through using aspects of postmodernism, specifically Foucault's work.

The purpose of this chapter (and indeed of my wider project) therefore is first, to argue for sexuality to be included in our analyses of social policy[1] and, second, to suggest ways of doing this. I will suggest that an emergent framework should both account for and recognise the following aspects.

The first is that individuals have multi-identities and so hold both different agendas for welfare and for change, and various positions at the same and different times and in different contexts. Second is difference and the ways in which it is constituted as significant in specific ways and at particular moments. As with identity, difference may be important in some contexts and not in others. Clearly, some differences have become significant enough to have social policies constructed around them.[2] Third is the tendency in much social policy work to reinforce heterosexual norms and relations and taken-for-granted, ahistorical and universalist notions about the sexed body, sex and sexualities. Fourth, developing means by which to examine social policy through the lens of sexuality can tell us how sexuality, and particularly appropriate and acceptable sexualities (heterosexual as well as homosexual), behaviours, relations and contexts at any given moment are constituted in a particular society. It can also inform us about how sexuality discourses interact with and are mediated by a whole range of other discourses which are central to welfare and which are 'played' through social policy. Similarly, using sexuality as a lens can reveal different aspects of social policy processes such as its disciplinary and regulatory functions. In this way we can account not only for the experiences of lesbians and gay men but also critique how social policy, as both discipline and practice, constitutes appropriate and acceptable sexualities in ways which affect heterosexuals, lesbians and gays, albeit differentially, and which are mediated by 'race', class, gender, disability and age. Fifth are the social relations of power and processes of inclusion and exclusion which are constituted through and within social policy and welfare, and, in particular, the ways in which these are operationalised through ideas about acceptable and appropriate sexualities.

WHAT WOULD INCLUDING SEXUALITY IN OUR ANALYSES OF SOCIAL POLICY MEAN?

How might sexuality be included in social policy analyses? Sexuality as an issue for social policy can be explored in a least three main ways. First, it can be included as a topic for consideration within social policy analyses. This might include reference to, for example, reproduction, contraception, abortion, sex education, sexually transmitted diseases, HIV/AIDS, teenage pregnancy, single motherhood, lesbianism and homosexuality. Here the focus might be on needs and the provision of services and benefits for, for example, single and teenage mothers, people with AIDS, or approaches to sex education, and/or on providing data about these categories, and/or on drawing attention to the existence of policies relating to these areas. A second level at which sexuality might be addressed in social policy is through the examination of the power relations which surround sexuality issues. So, for example, social policy writers might analyse or assess the direct and indirect ways in which lesbians and gay men can experience discrimination on the basis of their sexuality. They might also address the ways in which appropriate and acceptable sexuality is the means for establishing access and eligibility to welfare benefits and services, as in critiques of the cohabitation rule. A third and related level is in theorising and critiquing the influence of dominant sexual discourses on social policy. This would require looking beyond sexuality merely in terms of the discrimination of individuals and groups on the basis of their sexualised identities; it would mean going further than seeing sexuality as one means by which eligibility to services and benefits is established. It would mean sexuality would be seen instead as a framework or logic which informs social policy practice and analyses in very particular and real ways rather than as a discrete issue or topic of social policy. What might such a framework look like?

A FRAMEWORK FOR INCORPORATING SEXUALITY INTO
SOCIAL POLICY ANALYSES?

Clearly, as I have outlined briefly above, there are a number of levels at which sexuality might be incorporated into social policy analyses and critiques. However, in this chapter I will focus on integrating sexuality into a framework for informing social policy practice and analyses. Having suggested that sexuality is inextricably linked to gender, 'race', class, disability and age, I want to argue that in order to understand how sexuality works in relation to social policy we have to distinguish it temporarily as a separate logic: heterosexuality. In this way, we can begin to map out the dominant social relations and discourses of sexuality which affect social policy: how do prevalent sexuality discourses inform and constitute social policy, as practice and as a discipline, and what are the social relations involved in this process? Correspondingly, what role does social policy play in constituting what we know to be the 'truths' of sexuality and dominant social relations of sexuality? The aim of the project would be to look at how sexuality affects *all* men as well as *all* women, whilst recognising the differential effects of the power relations involved both between women and men and women and women. Additionally, a focus on heterosexuality reveals that it works in some importantly different ways from, for example, the disciplinary effects of femininity. Unlike femininity, heterosexuality tends to be awarded a privileged status position, and this is mirrored, enacted and constituted through social policy. Whereas femininity is measured against masculinity as the 'norm', heterosexuality is itself the 'norm' by which all – heterosexual or not – are measured, differentiated and categorised.

Next, we can begin to identify the processes of exclusion and inclusion which can result from these dominant social relations and discourses of sexuality when they are 'played' through social policy. This requires that we examine also the various ways that sexuality is mediated by other discourses of social divisions, difference, identity and inequality along with discourses of welfare and social policy, the family and motherhood. In this way, we can begin to identify the ways that social policies treat and affect people differentially and the social relations of power which are involved.

Finally, social policy is also one means through which the 'truths' of sexuality can be challenged and contested. Any framework, therefore, needs to account for the challenges from social movements that have taken issues of sexuality as their concern. Taking on these points, I now want to draw on Foucault's work to actualise a theoretical framework for interpreting social policy.

The aim of this section is to take on board some of the issues raised about an emergent theoretical framework and what it would mean to apply it to an analysis of social policy. In what follows, and because of space constraints, I shall focus on suggesting a framework for integrating questions about regulation, significant differences, differentiating effects, exclusions and inclusions, and questions of eligibility. Other key aspects, such as how sexuality constitutes and is constituted through social policy and the impact of the new social movements (NSMs), are discussed in Carabine (1996a). Foucault's work is central to this project. Indeed, the approach adopted uses a feminist-informed Foucauldian analysis to develop an understanding of the relationship between sexuality and social policy. Foucault has much to offer emergent theorisations of this relationship, particularly through the application of his ideas about sexuality and his concepts of discourse, the body, power/knowledge, disciplinary power, normalisation and biopower (Foucault 1979, 1990).

Of particular importance is the way in which we can use Foucault's work to interrogate, first, sexuality as a discourse which is constituted through, amongst other things, social policy and, second, social policy as practice and discipline as one means by which sexuality itself is constituted. This shows that not only are discourses of sexuality 'played' through social policy as an effect of disciplinary power but also sexuality discourses interact with and traverse other discourses central to welfare and social policy, and in so doing are mediated by those discourses. These other discourses include gender, 'race', disability, age, femininity, masculinity, 'rights', need, citizenship, child care, parenting, motherhood, caring and dependency alongside the professional discourses of welfare.

Drawing on Foucault, I argue that four different aspects – invisibility/ invalidity, normalisation, constitutive and contestation – can be distinguished as being central to the relationship between sexuality and social policy. 'Invisibility' refers, first, to the ways that certain aspects of sexuality are invisible in social policy, particularly in policy making and practice (see Carabine 1992, 1995) and, second, to the invisibility of sexuality within the 'discipline', particularly when sexuality is very visible elsewhere (see Carabine 1996b). 'Normalisation' acknowledges the role of social policy in defining and reaffirming heterosexuality as it is composed at any specific moment as acceptable and appropriate sexuality. 'Constitutive' recognises that sexuality as discourse and knowledge – 'that is, what we know as the "truth" of sexuality – is constituted through social policy. "Contestation" reflects the way that social policy is a focus for political action, a site where the "truths" of sexuality are contested challenged and changed' (Carabine 1996a: 59). Due to lack of space I will concentrate on the effects of normalisation.[3]

NORMALISATION

In *The History of Sexuality* (1990) Foucault outlines, as an alternative to more traditional, sovereign-based understandings of power, a bipolar mechanism of power – disciplinary and biopower – neither dependent on sovereign power nor reducible to law. Power is effected through social policy explicitly by being reducible to law, but also implicitly through more subtle and complex means.

The evolution of disciplinary power with its 'seeing gaze' and 'normalising' techniques meant it was no longer necessary to evoke sovereign power and with it the power to take life. Disciplinary power shifted the focus of control to individuals and attempted to submit them to constant surveillance rather than physical punishment. Foucault identifies three aspects of disciplinary power: the gaze/panopticon, normalisation and examination.[4] For the purposes of this chapter I shall apply just one aspect – normalisation – whereby all individuals are compared and differentiated between according to a desired norm so producing homogeneity. It establishes the measure by which all are judged and deemed to conform or not. In his notion of 'norm' Foucault did not conceive power as being imposed by one section, class or group of society on another. Rather he saw it as a dynamic of knowledge, practised and learnt, which was dispersed around various centres of practice and expertise. Both social policy and sexuality are such centres of expertise and practice.

Taking sexuality first, in *The History of Sexuality* (1990) Foucault investigates the ways in which sexuality has come to be seen and spoken of: the development of knowledges about sex, as a means of understanding the operations of power. For Foucault, not only is sexuality socially constructed and produced by effects of power, but so too are bodies (Ramazanoglu 1993: 6) explicable only in terms of 'truths' which are themselves socially produced. Foucault's interest was not in finding, for example, the causes of heterosexuality or sexual violence or lesbianism, but rather in describing how heterosexuality or sexual violence or lesbianism come to be defined and constructed as the operation and effects of power. Foucault (1972, 1990) argues that power is constituted through discourses. Discourses are historically variable ways of specifying knowledges and truths, whereby knowledges are produced as 'truths', in this case, about sexuality. Discourses function as sets of socially and historically constructed rules designating 'what is' and 'what is not'.

Thus, sexuality not only becomes the focus or object of discourses: the focus of 'experts', of scientific concern and sexologists, sexuality also becomes knowledge itself. Within these 'knowledges', categories or typologies of sexuality, such as homosexual, bisexual, invert and paedophile, which tended to focus on 'abnormal' aspects of sexuality were identified. By focusing on what was considered 'abnormal', that which was considered 'normal' was also constituted in 'expert' accounts of sexuality. It is through this 'normalising' effect, which places 'perverse' sexualities under the microscope for examination, categorisation, regulation and punishment, that a knowledge of 'normal' as well as 'abnormal' sexuality is created. Prevalent discourses of sexuality specify what sexuality is at particular moments in time. They are the means by which what we know to be the 'truths' of sexuality are established.

In his work on sexuality, Foucault (1990) investigates the ways in which it has come to be seen and spoken of and in particular how the development of knowledges about sex and sexuality can be understood as an operation of power. These knowledges tell us what is 'normal' and 'natural' sexuality whilst establishing the boundaries of what is acceptable and appropriate. Although what we know to be heterosexuality at any given time is historically, culturally and socially specific, subject to redefinition and transformation, it is hetero-sexuality that persists as the benchmark of 'normal' and 'natural' sexuality.[5]

In this way ideas about heterosexuality become naturalised in common-place thinking, with the effect that heterosexual relationships are taken for granted as the norm. Social policy as practice and discipline develops within the social, and policy makers, writers and analysts are also influenced by these common understandings about the nature of sexuality.

In relation to sexuality and social policy, normalisation can be identified as operating in four main ways. First, it constitutes appropriate and acceptable sexuality. Second, normalisation operates in a regulatory capacity through which not only is heterosexuality established and secured, but also women's bodies and sexuality are disciplined and controlled. This regulatory function can be seen to operate explicitly through legislation and statutes and implic-itly through:

1 normative assumptions about heterosexuality as 'normal' and natural underpinning and informing social policy;
2 the linking of notions of eligibility to welfare to ideas about appropriate and acceptable sexuality.

Third, the normalisation process produces differentiating effects and frag-mented impacts, being variously regulatory, penalising or affirmative in respect to different groups of women. A fourth aspect is the role of normal-isation in achieving the aims of social policy and welfare. There is not sufficient space to deal with all of these aspects here and therefore I will focus first on the ways in which appropriate and acceptable sexuality is con-stituted through social policy, second on the regulatory capacity of social policy, and third on differentiating aspects and outcomes.

APPROPRIATE AND ACCEPTABLE SEXUALITY

Normalising judgement compares and contrasts, differentiating between all individuals according to a desired norm. It establishes the measure by which all are judged and deemed to conform or not. The normalising effect is a means by which appropriate and acceptable sexuality – hetero- and homo-sexuality – is enforced and regulated. The normalising effect is such that sexuality is understood in terms of what is 'natural' and 'normal' and 'unnat-ural' and 'abnormal'.

In relation to sexuality the normalising effect means that we commonly believe sexuality to be an inherently natural biological drive and the natural and normal direction of the drive to be heterosexuality. Therefore, it is only 'normal' and 'natural' to want to engage in heterosexual sex. Applying the normalising judgement means that it is commonly felt that it is 'normal' to be heterosexual and that it is 'abnormal' to be lesbian or homosexual. The implicit acceptance of heterosexuality as 'normal' sexuality in social policy is part of a process through which measures are established by which all sexualities, behaviours and relations are judged and deemed to conform or not. This normalising effect is the means by which appropriate and acceptable sexuality is enforced and regulated. This 'truth' of sexuality is generally left unchallenged and unquestioned in much of social policy writing, resulting in a notion of heterosexuality as normal, fixed and universal sexuality being established and constituted through social policy.

Social policy (in its widest sense) either implicitly or explicitly conveys messages about appropriate and acceptable sexuality. Some sexual arrangements and relations are favoured over others. By and large, these tend to be heterosexual married relations. For example, if we examine the UK welfare state through the lens of sexuality we can see that its foundations are firmly constructed on the basis of normal heterosexual relations, with the heterosexual family form central to the provision of welfare and women's major role as mothers and carers seen as 'natural' and 'normal'. At the core of postwar welfarism was a series of fundamental and essentially traditional assumptions about the family and motherhood (Weeks 1981: 235). Beveridge expressed a concern about the 'importance of a child being brought up in the proper domestic environment, and was anxious not in any way to encourage illegitimacy, or immorality' (Weeks 1981: 235).

More recently, in the then Lord Chancellor's speech for the twenty-first century, Lord Mackay argued the importance of the institution of marriage as crucial not only to society but also to health, wealth and education, particularly where children were involved (*Newsnight*, 10 February 1997). The Lord Chancellor's speech coincided with the launch of National Marriage Week, which commenced on 10 February. Clare Dyer, reporting on Lord Mackay's speech, stated that '[t]he Government would do all it could to support marriage, and to try and reverse the rise of divorces and unmarried couples living together' (*Guardian*, 11 February 1997). Lord Mackay's speech can also be seen as significant in that it signalled the Conservative government's support for a variety of new schemes to support traditional marriage and parenting. He is reported as saying that 'women should not feel apologetic about describing themselves as housewives ... Caring for children is extremely hard work' (*Evening Standard*, 13 February 1997). Interestingly, in the previous week Peter Lilley, then Secretary of State for Social Security, introduced the 'Parents Plus' initiative which was to use private enterprise to encourage 'lone' parents to move off benefits into work. Taken together these two approaches could be seen as highlighting the contradictory nature of

Conservative government policy. Alternatively, they could be interpreted as reinforcing the respectability of full-time mothering within the context of a long-term, heterosexual, married-couple relationship.

Implicit in the founding policies of the welfare state and subsequent social policies are the 'normalising' effects of these discourses, which have as their object 'active' men and 'passive' women. For example, ideas are reflected within social policy about men as physically, economically and sexually active (going out to work, being the breadwinners and taking the lead in sexual relations) and as dominant (as head of household and sexually). Corresponding ideas which assume women's dependency on men, both financially and sexually, are also evident in social policy and form the basis of not only the welfare state but also the mixed economy of welfare.[6] Normative constructions of women's passive and nurturing femininity are not only incorporated in but central to the public and private provision of welfare and caring, as in, for example, community care policies and women's labour-market involvement in welfare as nurses, teachers, cleaners, social workers and auxiliaries.

But there are inconsistencies. Some countries are demonstrably more tolerant than the UK (although this appears likely to change under the New Labour Government) of diverse family forms and sexual relationships, such as lesbian and gay relationships, same-sex parenting and adoption, and this may be reflected in social policies which make acceptable gay coupling or marriages, or which give immigration rights to gay partners. For example, the Netherlands has anti-discrimination and equal opportunities legislation and legal parity; parts of Australia give such immigration rights; Denmark has anti-discrimination and equal rights legislation and recognition of lesbian and gay couples, but no right to adopt; and Sweden has the Homosexual Co-Habitees Act. However, common in all of these countries is a privileging of heterosexuality.

An analysis of social policy also reveals that the normalising process does not apply to all heterosexuals or even all married couples evenly and equally, but to a narrowly defined 'ideal' of heterosexuality. In this way, all women, including heterosexuals, are compared and differentiated between. The 'ideal' against which all women are measured is white, heterosexual, preferably married or at least in a long-term, stable, heterosexual relationship, non-disabled and, if a mother, aged between 18 and 40 years. Women who do not conform to this ideal, such as older, teenage or single mothers, and those who may also be black and/or lesbian, disabled or working-class, are situated as 'not normal', in need of normalisation.

One example of this is the availability in the UK of fertility 'treatments', particularly where these are provided through the National Health Service. 'Treatment' is usually restricted to heterosexual women within certain age limits who are in stable, long-term, monogamous relations. It is also reported that 'treatments' are usually restricted to women who are married, white, non-disabled and 'firmly attached to an affluent male partner' (Foster 1996:

109). This example illustrates the processes by which discourses about acceptable and appropriate sexuality and motherhood are evoked as a means of
determining eligibility or access to limited welfare resources, illustrating the
complex and contradictory relationship between sexuality and social policy
for women. (The question of eligibility will be considered later.) On the one
hand, women's role as mothers is accepted as 'normal' and is central to much
of social policy; on the other hand, women are simultaneously differentiated
between and against a narrow 'ideal' which at different moments they may or
may not conform to. It is not enough that women are heterosexual, and this
is not to argue that heterosexuality is not privileged, but rather to argue that
it is a disciplinary form of power which affects all women.

Another example can be seen in the way that single mothers are viewed. In
1993 the Welsh Secretary, John Redwood (*The Independent*, 8 March 1993;
Guardian, 3 July 1993), suggested that welfare might best be withheld from
single mothers until the father was found and a financial contribution
secured. The introduction of the Child Support Agency has meant that this
is now a reality facing many single mothers.

Complementary to its defining of acceptable and unacceptable sexuality,
social policy has a related regulatory function. It is through social policy
that acceptable sexuality is regulated, being rewarded or privileged, as in the
case of ideal heterosexuality, or penalised when women fail to conform and
fall outside the 'norm'.

REGULATORY FUNCTION

This regulatory function is an important aspect of the normalisation process,
as is evident in social policy explicitly and implicitly. First, regulation is operationalised at an explicit level through legislation and statutes. In relation to
sexuality the law is a primary mechanism of regulation and social control
which specifies what you can and cannot do, with whom and where. The
normalising effect is such that it informs not only what is natural and normal
sexuality but also the acceptable contexts, behaviours, relationships, ages,
places, etc. In the UK, as in other countries, there are a number of pieces of
legislation which stipulate what is acceptable, legal and illegal sexuality; for
example, the Sexual Offences Act 1967, Section 28 of the Local Government
Act 1988, rape in marriage legislation, control of prostitution, divorce acts,
marriage acts, and age of consent legislation.

Assumptions about heterosexuality

Implicit in much of this legislation are sets of normalising effects and messages which variously support and set the boundaries for heterosexual
relations, whilst confirming the illegality or unacceptability of lesbian and gay
sexuality. Section 28 of the Local Government Act 1988 exemplifies this in

prohibiting local authorities from promoting homosexuality or teaching of its acceptability as a pretended family relationship.

Age of sexual consent legislation is another example which demonstrates how different forms of control and ideas about acceptability concerning heterosexual and non-heterosexual relations exist. For example, in the UK this legislation is applied in different ways, reflecting different forms of control and ideas about the acceptability of when heterosexual and gay male sexual relations may legally commence.[7]

Regulation is operationalised not only through the implicit assumptions about heterosexuality contained in social policy but also by evoking disciplinary power both explicitly, through legislation and statutes, and implicitly, through the taken-for-granted assumptions inherent in social policies about the universal 'normality' and 'naturalness' of heterosexuality. For example, Family Credit claim forms use the neutral term 'partner', defined as 'a person you are married to or a person you live with as if you were married to them'. This could possibly include same-sex relationships, but in Britain normative values are such that to live in a same-sex relationship would not really be the same as living with someone as though you were married. This is confirmed in the sentence – 'The woman should claim – even if the man is working' (Benefits Agency 1993).

Through these implicit assumptions about heterosexuality it is not always necessary for social policy to operate by 'wielding a big stick' (this is considered in more detail later); sometimes it operates by offering 'carrots' or rewards. Women today are not generally 'forced' through legislation and social policies to form heterosexual relations or to get married. But they do, through the combined disciplinary regimes of femininity and heterosexuality. (However, this is not to say that women are not penalised for refusing to conform to heterosexual norms.) Quite recently in the UK, the Archbishop of York, John Habgood, called for tax cuts to support married people and to encourage cohabiting couples to marry. He argued that 'the selfless commitment of marriage needs to be buttressed by social support' and 'the Government could encourage marriage by making it fiscally more attractive' (*Guardian*, 14 February 1995). Almost a year later Peter Mandelson (New Labour) was advocating the payment of £5,000 to first-time married couples.

In this way, social policy can be said to 'watch over sexual practices' (Bell 1993: 21). Through legislation, as in the examples cited above, and social policies concerned with, for example, child care and sex education; through professional responsibilities and codes of practice and conduct for teachers, health and social workers; social policy 'watches over' sexual practices in differentiated ways. All variously delineate and define, implicitly and explicitly, what are acceptable and appropriate sexual relations and behaviours; when and where we can have sex, and with whom.

Eligibility for welfare

Normalising ideas about appropriate sexuality explicitly inform and influence social policy and welfare in other ways; for instance, through an explicit relationship between 'appropriate' sexuality and access to and eligibility for welfare. The normalising effect is also a mechanism by which rights and entitlement and, therefore, eligibility to welfare are determined. For example, in 1988, Margaret Thatcher, the then British prime minister, spoke of the problem of young single girls who were deliberately getting pregnant in order to jump the housing queue and obtain benefits (*Guardian*, 23 November 1988). These ideas were more forcibly endorsed in the run-up to the 1993 Conservative Party Conference and with it a swingeing attack on single mothers. The message came through loud and clear that welfare benefits and housing should only be available to, by implication, 'respectable', married women. It was also believed that welfare worked as a perverse incentive to young girls to become pregnant. Although the British government backed down, rhetorically at least, as a result of public and media pressure, policies were still introduced which resulted in removing a local authority's responsibility to prioritise single mothers' access to public housing. More recently, as a result of changes introduced in the November 1996 budget, the lone parent payment was to be abolished in April 1997. Other examples of the way in which normalising ideas about sexuality influence eligibility for welfare include income maintenance, where a (hetero)sexual relationship, whether married or cohabiting, is a factor in determining eligibility for benefit. Social policy may also be linked to eligibility as a means of enforcing appropriate and acceptable sexual behaviour, as in the USA with the use by some states of Norplant, a contraceptive implant (*World in Action*, October 1993, 'Children having children'; *The Independent*, 7 October 1993).

Another dynamic of the relationship between sexuality and eligibility to benefits and welfare is that even though women may pay full taxes and national insurance contributions, this does not guarantee they will be considered eligible for welfare services and benefits. In some cases, they may be discriminated against or denied access to services or benefits on the basis of their sexuality, as in the withholding of funding to lesbian and gay groups, or the refusal of some councils to give same-sex partnerships joint tenancy agreements, or the recognition of lesbian and gay relations for pension purposes (Wilton 1995: 190). Furthermore, 'older lesbians' ... needs with respect to bereavement or institutional care may ... be neglected' by social work agencies (Cosis Brown 1992: 200).

Additionally, whilst women may gain social rights through, for example, labour-market involvement, those rights will also be mediated by 'race', class, sexuality, age and disability. The nature of women's interactions and experiences of welfare are not simply determined or even guaranteed by their labour-market involvement. Tamsin Wilton (1995: 201–2) illustrates how, in relation to health, lesbian women may experience homophobia, be discounted as potential users, and even have their specific health-care needs ignored. Indeed, in order to avoid discrimination many women may have little choice other than to allow people to assume that they are heterosexual in order to gain access to certain services and welfare benefits.

Social policy can also have powerful normalising effects without 'wielding a big stick'. For example, social policies and the law do not explicitly identify lesbianism as something requiring to be controlled, as gay male sexuality is identified. But nevertheless, lesbians experience social policies as discriminating and excluding. It is not illegal to be a lesbian, but many lesbians have lost their jobs specifically for being lesbian, especially where they work with children or young girls (*Pink Paper*, 26 May 1995). Additionally, lesbian mothers tend to lose child custody cases, where the 'norm' is for mothers to be given custody (Van Every 1991/92: 64) – because they are deemed to be 'unfit' mothers because of their sexuality.

DIFFERENTIATING EFFECTS

Discourses of sexuality also interact with and are mediated by, for example, discourses of 'race', disability, age and class to produce differentiating effects (Bartky 1988: 72; Ramazanoglu and Holland 1993: 240). Ideas about black women being sexually voracious and lacking sexual self-control, or about Asian women as erotic and passive, are reflected in the practice of social policy. Black women have argued that they have always had 'easier access' to abortion, contraception and sterilisation (see Bryan *et al.* 1985: 105). It has been reported (*The Independent*, 7 October 1993) that Norplant is being targeted at teenage mothers and poor women from ethnic minorities in the US. In discourses concerned with women's sexuality, as well as gender, 'race' and disability, there is often a fusion of women's social characteristics with their biological functions, as with reproduction (McNay 1992: 18). Social policy at one and the same time both compounds the defining of the social category of women in terms of biological functions – through focusing on discourses of motherhood, family and caring – whilst also being a means through which to challenge these assumptions. These various discourses – of sexuality, gender, race, disability and femininity – come together to be mediated and constituted in social policy, and become a means of effecting normalisation, of differentiating between different women, and of establishing eligibility to welfare. For example, women who are disabled are seen either as incapable of sex, and as having no sexuality at all, or as sexually vulnerable. In social policy this is reflected in women with learning disabilities being placed on the contraceptive pill and/or being given no sex education at all, and/or being 'protected' from personal/sexual relations, or being invisible in the recognition of sexual abuse or in the need for education about safer sex (Hayes and Wright 1989).

Within social policy, as well as in society more generally, women's subject position is relative not only to men but also to other women. Thus the relative power of women depends on particular practices which differently favour (or not) 'mothers', 'single women', 'married women'(see McNay 1992: 69), 'black women', 'lesbian women', 'disabled women' and 'non-disabled women'. The extent to which women are 'favoured' in social policies is influenced by the extent to which they conform to that which is considered 'normal'. 'Normal' is generally and consistently associated with heterosexuality. The greater the convergence with the 'norm' the narrower the gap between women and entitlement to welfare services and resources. The greater the divergence away from the 'norm' the less, usually, the entitlement as of a 'right'. For example, I would suggest that lesbians and gay men are often denied citizenship rights, if not in reality then often in discursive formation, so that we get the notion that lesbians and gay men are not 'taxpayers' but are somehow 'outside' and not part of the electorate (Carabine 1992b).[8]

CONCLUSION

In conclusion, first, theorising sexuality in relation to social policy requires recognition that prevalent sexuality discourses privilege heterosexuality and affect *all* women in specific and material ways. Sexuality discourses intersect with and are mediated by discourses of 'race', disability, age and class. At the welfare and social policy interface these dimensions of difference produce materially different experiences for women, thereby demonstrating that women's subject position is determined not in sole relation to men but also in relation to other women. Women's power in relation to welfare is dependent on particular and specific practices which differently favour, or not, 'mothers', 'married women', 'black women', 'disabled women' and 'non-disabled women', 'lesbians', and 'single mothers'.

Second, developing such a framework requires recognition of the disciplinary and regulatory role of social policy, particularly the operationalising of this through normalising effects.

Third, theorising sexuality is not simply a matter of 'adding' lesbians and gay men to a growing list of 'isms' and differences, and it is not about reducing sexuality to issues of lesbianism and homosexuality. It is necessary that a framework incorporates sexuality in its widest sense if we are to untangle what all sexuality issues, from abortion and contraception to HIV/AIDS, from lesbian and gay struggles to sex education, etc., tell us about welfare. We need also to ask what welfare and social policy tell us about sexuality.

Social policy has to take account of lesbians' and gay men's needs and their experiences of welfare, but as these are defined and articulated by them. Williams (1987: 24) argues in her critique of racism and the welfare state that 'such struggles are about the politics of need – challenging the state's and administrators' and agency's definition of need' as well as those of the discipline. This means more than adopting an anti-discriminatory approach. It also requires 'intervening in a deep well of socially respectable and institutional prejudice' and recognising that 'this form of oppression is as important to people as economic hardship' (Penna and O'Brien 1996: 58). This means not making assumptions that women, if they are lesbian, will not want children or will have no need for fertility 'treatments', as well as recognising that they may be denied access to such 'treatment' because of dominant discourses of heterosexuality and negative discourses of lesbianism. Including sexuality also means that we need to take care not to accept stereotypical representations of black, disabled and lesbian women's sexualities. This necessitates our working with more fluid notions of identity in order to avoid fixing women on the basis of their sexualised and/or other identities. Correspondingly, this requires that we recognise needs as fluid, not as solely determined by a person's identity or sexuality.

If, as Erskine and Ungerson (1995: 256) argue, 'new giants have emerged in the Social Policy debate: Exclusion, Discrimination, Social Control', an analysis of sexuality/theorising sexuality, which incorporates 'race', class, gender, age and disability, may tell us a lot more about these new giants of welfare than more traditional approaches do. It may tell us not only about these 'giants' but also about the relationship between identity, difference and welfare and about forms of resistance; it may identify multiple sites of power and the changing social relations of power. The interdisciplinarity of social policy is a point in its favour. Whether sexuality is developed and accepted as an important and new theoretical perspective, however, remains to be seen.

NOTES

1 I suggest reasons for including sexuality in analyses of social policy in Carabine (1996b).
2 This point was made by Avtar Brah at a 'Women and Difference' study day held at Loughborough University, 1 February 1997.
3 See Carabine (1996a) for a discussion of constitutive and contestation aspects of this analysis.
4 Vikki Bell (1993: 33–5) provides a clear summary of Foucault's three methods of disciplinary power.
5 See Carabine (1992a, 1996) for more detailed discussion of this.
6 The mixed economy of welfare includes all welfare provision, such as those by the state, voluntary, family and private ones.
7 In the UK the age of consent for heterosexual sexual relations is 16 years and for homosexual relations 18 years. Until February 1994 this latter had been 21 years.
8 In particular circumstances (for example, as with the disability movement) the relationship between 'normalisation' and 'rights' has been reversed.

BIBLIOGRAPHY

Bartky, S. (1988) 'Foucault, femininity, and the modernization of patriarchial power', in I. Diamond and L. Quinby (eds) *Feminism and Foucault: Reflections on Resistance*, Boston: Northeastern University Press.

Bell, V. (1993) *Interrogating Incest: Feminism, Foucault and the Law*, London: Routledge.

Benefits Agency (1993) Claim form FC1: Family Credit.

Bryan, B., Dadzie, S. and Scafe, S. (1985) *The Heart of the Race: Black Women's Lives in Britain*, London: Virago.

Carabine, J. (1992a) 'Constructing women: women's sexuality and social policy', *Critical Social Policy* 34: 23–37.

Carabine, J. (1992b) 'Constructing women: women's sexuality and social policy', unpublished PhD thesis, University of Sheffield.

Carabine, J. (1995) 'Invisible sexualities: sexuality, politics and influencing policy-making', in A.R. Wilson (ed.) *A Simple Matter of Justice?*, London: Cassell.

Carabine, J. (1996a) 'Heterosexuality and social policy', in D. Richardson (ed.) *Theorising Heterosexuality: Telling it Straight*, Milton Keynes: Open University Press.

Carabine, J. (1996b) 'A straight playing field or queering the pitch? Centring sexuality in social policy', *Feminist Review* 54: 31–64.

Cosis Brown, H. (1992) 'Lesbians, the state and social work practice', in M. Langan and L. Day (eds) *Women, Oppression and Social Work: Issues in Anti-discriminatory Practice*, London: Routledge.

Erskine, A. and Ungerson, C. (1995) 'Cultivating social policy in a hostile climate: pressures for change in teaching and research', in J. Baldrock and M. May (eds) *Social Policy Review 7*, Canterbury, Kent: Social Policy Association.

Foster, P. (1996) 'Women and health care', in C. Hallett (ed.) *Women and Social Policy: An Introduction*, London: Prentice Hall/Harvester Wheatsheaf in association with Social Policy Association Women and Social Policy Group.

Foucault, M. (1972) *The Archaeology of Knowledge*, trans. A.M. Sheridan-Smith, London: Tavistock. (First published in French 1969).

Foucault, M. (1979) *Discipline and Punish: The Birth of the Prison*, trans. A.M. Sheridan-Smith, London: Allen Lane. (First published in French 1975; this translation first published 1977, London: Allen Lane).

Foucault, M. (1990) *The History of Sexuality. Vol. 1: An Introduction*, trans. Robert Hurley, New York: Vintage Books. (First published in French 1976; this translation first published 1978, New York: Random House).

Hayes, C. and Wright, A. (1989) 'Preparations for change in North West Hertfordshire', in M. Pike, M. Kapila, G. Buckley and D. Cunningham (eds) *Responding to the AIDS Challenge: A Comparative Study of Local AIDS Programmes in the UK*, Harlow: Longman.

McNay, L. (1992) *Foucault and Feminism: Power, Gender and Self*, Cambridge: Polity Press.

Penna, S. and O'Brien, M. (1996) 'Postmodernism and social policy: a small step forwards?', *Journal of Social Policy* 25, 1: 39–61.

Ramazanoglu, C. (ed.) (1993) *Up Against Foucault: Explorations of Some Tensions between Foucault and Feminism*, London: Routledge.

Ramazanoglu, C. and Holland, J. (1993) 'Women's sexuality and men's appropriation of desire', in C. Ramazanoglu (ed.) *Up Against Foucault: Explorations of Some Tensions between Foucault and Feminism*, London: Routledge.

Van Every, J. (1991/2) 'Who is "the family"? The assumptions of British social policy', *Critical Social Policy* 33: 62–75.

Weeks, J. (1981) *Sex, Politics and Society: The Regulation of Sexuality since 1800*, London: Longman.

Williams, F. (1987) 'Racism and the discipline of social policy: a critique of welfare theory', *Critical Social Policy* 20: 4–29.

Wilton, T. (1995) *Lesbian Studies: Setting an Agenda*, London: Routledge.

Chapter 9

Reopening the gift
Race and the critique of normative social policy

Chris Smaje

INTRODUCTION

In this chapter I examine critically the claim that postmodern theory under-
mines the normative universalism of orthodox social policy, using debates
concerning race as my principal examples.[1] The orthodox approach suggests
that it is possible to make interventions in the sphere of human well-being
which, if not commanding universal agreement, can at least claim plausibly
to be grounded in conventions of human interest which transcend the particular standpoints of given groups. This idea has been vigorously challenged
of late both by the postmodern turn in academic social theory and by popular political activism. Postmodern social theory and identity politics diverge
sharply in many respects, but together articulate a profound critique of the
way that social policy has hitherto been analysed and formulated. Yet while
this critique persuasively identifies a certain theoretical and political rigidity
in the orthodox approach, I suggest that antique dualisms in political theory
such as subject/object and particular/universal remain a compelling basis for
its contemporary formulation, and argue that social policy should be understood both as a potentially liberating or enabling and a potentially repressive
or constraining force. Against a postmodernism which would refuse to recognise such a distinction, I advocate a 'modernist' approach to the politics of
contemporary social policy which reads such dualities as transformations of
one another and, like Simmel's view of culture as 'the way that leads from the
closed unity, through the unfolded multiplicity to the unfolded unity' (1968:
29), continues to insist on an essentially singular – but not necessarily har-
monious – political order.

REASON AND ITS DISCONTENTS

To understand the postmodern critique of normative social policy, we first
need to devote some attention to the idea of *reason*, which developed along
with the consciousness of modernity in Europe and reached its apogee in the
thought of the Enlightenment (Habermas 1979). Its emergence established

abstract and universal principles of description and evaluation by which the supposedly disinterested observer could account for human conduct, and it thus laid the basis for the contemporary social sciences. It also contained emancipatory possibilities, for it broke the connection between the existing social order and a normative commitment to it established in the 'ultimate grounds' of an earlier religious world view. The precarious distinction thus inaugurated between fact and value established an 'objective' relationship between philosophical reflection and practical political action. This relationship – now the preserve of social policy – orchestrates progress towards the ideal society by the application of rational principles to political decision making. Yet, despite the secular grounding of the concept of reason, its sense of a unitary order of things and of progress towards some goal preserves the monism of Judaeo-Christian religious thought. Adam Smith's famous 'invisible hand' of the market nicely captures this religious sensibility underlying the secular rationality bequeathed by the Enlightenment.

Nevertheless, the secularisation of thought in the Enlightenment had profound philosophical and social consequences. Models for the proper organisation of society were no longer authorised by blank tradition, but had to be found within the existing social order. Modernity 'has to create its normativity out of itself' (Habermas 1987: 7). According to Habermas, Hegel (1807) was the first philosopher to grapple with this problem, attempting to rescue the project of a pre-modern metaphysics in describing the dialectical process whereby an increasingly self-aware consciousness progressed, through externalising itself as object and reappropriating itself as subject, towards an 'absolute knowledge' of the world. Karl Marx famously inverted Hegel's idealist dialectic to argue that reason was conditioned by the material activity of human beings (Marx and Engels 1846). In doing so, he showed that the apparently diverse and autonomous fiscal, political and social institutions associated with the complexities of European modernity – and condensed into mysterious forms such as tradable commodities – entertained a higher-order unity, a particular arrangement of social relations constituted by the order of capitalism which, under the cloak of reason, surreptitiously favoured the interests of capital against those of the working class. He thus criticised the unreflective reason of classical political economists such as Smith who, mistaking the logic of capitalism for a theory of society as a whole, sought to establish the subjectivity of the individual as the basis of human interests.

For Marx, the agent of dialectical change was not, as with Hegel, abstract philosophical reflection. Rather, it was objectified in the actual practice of the proletariat. Nevertheless, he saw the proletariat in still fairly Hegelian terms as the embodiment in consciousness of an objective socio-historical understanding, a point perhaps developed most clearly within a Marxist framework by Lukács (1971). Thus, in accordance with Habermas's point about the problematic location of the normative in modernity, Marx attempted to articulate a theoretical standpoint which could grasp not only the enormous social transformations he was witnessing, but also the conditions of its own possibility.

In Hegel and Marx, then, we find a critique of reason which is developed not through a return to the 'ultimate grounds' of pre-modern thought, but through the category of reason itself. Nevertheless, Marx and other classical social theorists preserved the idea of an active historical subject. In this sense, both reason and the critique of reason share a monism which establishes common intellectual categories such as 'structure', 'order' and 'progress'. These devices have more recently been the object of sustained criticism from a variety of positions which can be loosely termed 'postmodern'. For example, Baudrillard (1975) argues that although Marx was able to show how the fetishised commodity form masked the particularity of the social relations which guaranteed its production, he accorded an untenable privilege to productive labour as the site of human self-creation, failing to appreciate the sense in which his model of alienated labour itself rested upon an asocial, universalised concept of utility. In Marx, says Baudrillard, 'work is ... universalised ... not only as market value but as human value' (Baudrillard 1975: 27) and his analysis 'made a radical critique of political economy, but still in the form of political economy' (Baudrillard 1975: 50).[2] In this sense, postmodernism provides a 'metacritique' which attacks the residual dependence of modernist theory on the concept of reason via its transcendent claims to universality. Derrida, for example, posits an excess within every designation of structure, an endless possibility for 'play' which destabilises attempts to found objective understanding without remainder (Derrida 1976, 1978). Lyotard defines the postmodern as 'an incredulity toward meta-narratives' (Lyotard 1984: xxiv) in which the system-building, objectivist orthodoxies by which social science has proceeded are seen as constructing the very objects of their discourse. And Foucault (e.g. 1967, 1976) has probed the contradictory 'double movement of liberation and enslavement' characterising modernity, which at once unlocks ossified cosmologies and, in its centralising and rationalising tactics, seeks to regulate and entrench social relations in accordance with abstract principles of instrumentality, overruling contradiction, imposing consistent social order, and thus driving a disciplining power deep into the social body.

This spectrum from reason to its metacritique finds its corollary in distinctive approaches to social policy analysis. In the mid-1990s, one scarcely needs reminding of the recent political ascendancy of a particular, libertarian version of 'reason' based on an almost religious faith in the singular power of Smith's 'invisible hand' to administer deliverance. More familiar within both academic social policy and postwar British politics are the multiple traditions of what I have termed the critique of reason, with the Fabianism of Richard Titmuss and others the dominant influence. In his book *The Gift Relationship* (1970), Titmuss contested proposals to introduce a system of paid blood donation into Britain, and in doing so provided one of the most eloquent

defences of a social democratic 'commitment to welfare'. Basing his arguments on Mauss's *Gift* (1922), the classic text of anthropological economics,
Titmuss defined social policy as a field of altruism between strangers which –
against the self-interest of market transactions – established the very possibility of the social. He thereby extended to contemporary social policy one of
Mauss's central insights: that the foundational social force of gift exchange
establishes it not as within the purview of some distinctive realm of the 'economic', but as a 'total social phenomenon' in which the categories of the
economic, jural, religious and so on were inseparably combined. However,
Titmuss's rendering of gift exchange as necessary for the good of society
trapped itself via the concept of the 'biological need to give' in a philosophy
of the subject which, though it appealed to altruism rather than self-interest,
was no less individualistic than the economism it opposed. It also contained
an implicit paternalism in appealing essentially to individual altruism in order
to sustain a non-market status quo.

This paternalism was not lost upon either critics in the tradition of liberal
reason or those of a more radical persuasion. Indeed, the intellectual dominance of a social democratic 'commitment to welfare' waned not long after
the publication of *The Gift Relationship*, partly through broadly Marxist
diagnoses of a gathering crisis in the welfare state (Gough 1979; Habermas
1976; O'Connor 1973; Offe 1984). To oversimplify somewhat, these writers
argued that the bourgeois state attempted to mediate the interests of capital
and labour via welfare provision, but it was ultimately unable to resolve the
contradiction between them established by the logic of capital accumulation.
With state welfare provision increasingly unable to ameliorate capitalist
exploitation, the resulting crisis of state legitimacy provided the motor for
progressive historical change.

Postmodernism represents a turn away from any confidence in such historical teleologies, and it rejects attempts to resolve the conflict between
particular and general interests which has been a central preoccupation of
political philosophy up to and including Marx, positioning the 'general interest' as merely a particular interest with the power to universalise itself. The
appropriate response within the framework of social policy is not obvious,
but programmes founded in normative orders such as ameliorative social
democracy or revolutionary Marxism clearly become problematic, and the
possibility of any singular 'narrative' of progress in welfare is questioned.
Later in the chapter, I consider such arguments more closely in order to
examine the possibility of reconstructing a normative project for social policy.
However, before doing so I turn to a consideration of race.

RACE IN SOCIAL POLICY

A belated interest among social policy analysts in inequalities between
racial(ised) groups has revealed substantial disparities in welfare access and

outcome (Law 1996). Yet none but the most extremist of political philosophies finds any place for race as an ethical basis for the ideal social organisation. For some, these disparities suggest that race may be a more fundamental category in contemporary society than is revealed in the latter's political discourse (Goldberg 1993). Others have read a normative commitment to the ideal of a 'race-free' social order as a rebuke to those who continue to invoke race analytically. Thus, Carter and Green suggest:

> studies of ... 'race' and education, 'race' and housing, 'race' and health provision assume the very object which must be explained and treat 'race' as an active *a priori* subject in social relations. Instead, we need to enquire how it is that social relations appear as 'race relations'.
>
> (Carter and Green 1996: 64)

This latter view is, I would argue, flawed in a number of ways which raise issues of great relevance to the broader theme of the discussion. First, on a theoretical point, Carter and Green criticise those who accord race explanatory power as an 'active *a priori* subject', but merely reverse the problem by according the same status to 'social relations'. Yet there is little basis other than longstanding sociological tradition for assuming that social relations in general are prior to any particular category, such as race. In describing racial categories as a 'naturalisation of social relations' (Carter and Green 1996: 59), the authors doubtless offer a useful critique of the essentialism in folk models of race or ethnicity which impute them to an unchanging 'nature', but it is an insufficient theoretical move merely to make an implicit theory explicit. Symbolic classifications do not come 'after' social relations and culture does not come 'after' nature. This view, not dissimilar to Baudrillard's critique of Marxism, can be developed into a symbolic account of social forms – including race – that does not accord ontological privilege to any particular term (Smaje 1997; Strathern 1992; Williams 1995). By contrast, criticising 'race' as an analytical term but then grounding it in an objectivist concept of 'social relations' is still implicitly to construct race as a theoretical object.

A second problem is the slippage between understanding race theoretically as a process of objectification, and adducing the implications of this process for social policy. The point is illustrated in the familiar debate between advocates of 'colour-blind' and 'colour-conscious' policy. Drawing upon arguments similar to those articulated by Carter and Green, the former suggest, properly enough, that the obvious socio-economic disadvantages faced by people in certain 'races' stems not from some inevitable feature of their character, but from particular practices which constitute them as racial beings and allocate their social and economic position accordingly. The appropriate policy response is therefore to concentrate on eliminating those practices and not upon lending spurious credibility to indefensible racial categories by identifying the needs of distinctive 'racial' groups. Advocates of 'colour-conscious' policy may find some common ground here, but might suggest that many years of colour-blind, class-based ameliorative social policy in countries like Britain and the USA have signally failed to equalise the status of groups which remain defiantly racialised. Against the tendency of 'colour-blind' policy to lose itself in abstract principles of universal justice, 'colour-conscious' policy therefore seeks to draw attention to the particularities of the 'real world' where racialised disadvantage, albeit often reproduced implicitly, is all too painfully felt. As Gutman puts it:

> When we are taught to take principles of justice seriously ... we learn those principles that have been developed for an ideal society ... It would be a blatant contradiction for a political philosophy to posit an ideal society that is beset by a legacy of racial injustice. The principles that most of us learn ... are therefore color blind not because color blindness is the right response to racial injustice but rather because color blindness is the ideal morality (for an ideal society).

> (Gutman 1996: 109)

This debate represents a difference of opinion on how to achieve a commonly agreed goal – an ideal state of universal justice. Yet such a goal would be rejected not only by postmodern theory, but also by arguments which emerge from a certain racial identity politics. Here, black people and white people confront each other over a racial chasm which no amount of theory or empathy can bridge. In the extreme, this leads to a separatist politics which historically has been of relatively limited appeal, but there is nevertheless a profound cynicism in much radical black writing on the nature of welfare and little sense of its enabling aspect. For example, Bryan *et al.* neatly capture the way in which racial, gender and class inequalities simultaneously create welfare needs while frustrating their satisfaction, 'because we are [black] women, the Health Service is central to our lives. We cannot avoid using it ... But ... we invariably find ourselves dealing with a profession which is fundamentally patriarchal and racist' (Bryan *et al.* 1985: 90). Here, black people must necessarily use welfare services but have little sense that they are 'for' them. To redress the situation the authors advocate a collective struggle around black identity, but caution, '"Knowing our culture" ... has never been an automatic process, particularly where the dominant influences on our lives are both controlled and determined by white cultural values' (Bryan *et al.* 1985: 231).

This reprises some central Marxist themes, and illustrates certain problems contained therein. In the face of ruling-class hegemony, the working class is not always clear about its 'true' interests (Gramsci 1971). Only in certain circumstances does it realise these interests and its true historical role (Lukács 1971). Nevertheless, the working class will ultimately reject those reified forms of cultural and social organisation which oppress it and bring about a social order which is no longer alienated. The problem of individual versus collective, particular versus universal, mediated in liberal political philosophy from

Hobbes onwards via a discourse on sovereignty is merely a bourgeois problematic expressing the alienating political form of capitalist society. Released from alienated kinds of knowledge, human interests enter free dialogue with one another in a social field no longer distorted by an uneven distribution of power.

There is much in common here with Hegel's project, and the teleology is only saved from a Hegelian idealism through the location of necessary historical agency in the material conditions of production. But even though racial identity politics find frequent expression in Marxist categories, they contain an implicit critique of Marxism and other modernist political traditions, since they reject the possibility of a universal 'ideal world' in which racial distinctions are abolished. One theoretically rather dubious response from radical intellectuals who still wish to operate across particularist identities and the possibility of communism is to inflate the subject of history from Hegel's consciousness, through Marx's proletariat to the clash of whole civilisations. Thus, Sivanandan describes European civilisation as 'destructive of human love and cynical of human life' (Sivanandan 1982: 92), while Rigby argues, 'Fully dialectical forms of knowledge, exemplified in non-capitalist societies, simply cannot produce such deformed and alienated kinds of subject-formation [as racism]' (Rigby 1996: 39).

A further twist to this argument is given in Said's (1978) well-known critique of 'Orientalism', by which the forms of knowledge produced by the 'west' of its 'others' are seen as merely reflecting the colonial interests from which they emerge. Said rather mischievously quotes Marx's famous comment on the French peasantry, that 'they cannot represent themselves, they must be represented' (Marx [1869] 1973: 239), to capture the sense in which colonial power arrogates to itself a knowledge of the 'other'. Yet the somewhat ironic effect of his intervention is that 'western' categories too often become universalised rather than contextualised, since in many writings the step between recognising the colonial *mediation* of indigenous categories and the colonial *construction* of indigenous categories is but a short one (e.g. Inden 1990). Thus, the realities of the non-western 'other' ever recede beyond the horizon of a diseased Orientalist representation, and 'non-western' peoples are invoked merely as mute witnesses to the power of the 'west'. There are continuities here with postmodern critiques of social policy which, as I shall argue below, have some quite problematic implications.

POSTMODERNISM AND THE POLITICS OF IDENTITY

For many progressive academics, the theoretical and political failures of Marxism now seem all too evident, but the high theory of French postmodernism offers nothing to replace it. This provokes much ire from critics who see postmodernism as a self-indulgent academicism which diverts attention from persisting inequalities. Such arguments may offer some comfort to those who regard themselves as activists of a practical bent, but they seem a rather weak objection at a philosophical level and, as Wood cautions, 'the rhetoric of directness, of immediacy, of "action" can be as cruelly misleading in political intervention as it is in philosophy' (Wood 1987: 191). Nevertheless, relieved of its teleology, Marx's critique of capital and liberal reason still seems highly pertinent, not least in the context of contemporary social policy, while the politics of racial and other identities seems to contain a fresh radical force, despite some unfortunate tendencies towards essentialism. Today, many people pin their hopes for a radical intellectual practice upon some kind of synthesis of these rather disparate ideas, and several attempts to distinguish a radical or 'resistant postmodernism' from the more idealist, reactionary or 'ludic' implications of poststructuralist thought have been made (Foster 1983; McLaren 1994; Nicholson and Seidman 1995; Peters and Lankshear 1996). There is much of merit in these efforts and, given the hugely varied characterisation of the 'postmodern', much to be gained by distinguishing carefully between different arguments. However, in this section I oppose those versions of postmodernism which suggest that the potential for radicalism lies precisely in transcending modernist themes.

'Resistant postmodern' writings often focus on struggles around gender, race, ethnicity, colonialism and other forms of power. These are seen as contesting the grounds of a modern reason which establishes its unitary force and constructs its 'common-sense' world through its power to universalise or 'normalise' a particular vision of the proper social order. However, an attempt to build a resistant 'post'modernism around such struggles faces several difficulties. For one thing, it tends to assume that the 'voice' of the oppressed, the minority group, the 'subaltern' is located completely *outside* the discourse of reason which it opposes, and it thus postulates incommensurate 'language games' of the sort described by Lyotard (1984). Yet the very idea of 'resisting' something constructs actors as *within* a particular social configuration. Postmodern critiques of modernity often engage highly linguistic models of the social, such as Lyotard's narrative/metanarrative distinction, but these do not capture adequately the specific *relations* of contradiction between subject positions which are implied in the idea of resistance. A more structuralist approach to the terrain of resistance may be appropriate in this respect, and Bourdieu's distinction between the 'universe of discourse' and the 'doxic' realm of shared understanding (Bourdieu 1977: 168), or Foucault's discussion of the 're-colonisation' which afflicts the 'insurrection of subjugated knowledges' (Foucault 1980: 86), seem rather more promising.

Resistant postmodernism also entertains a problematic interface with the essentialism of identity politics. To argue that one has access to a wellspring of experience denied others through inclusion in a particular social category has some plausibility[3] but, when elevated theoretically, makes a strong ontological claim which effaces other differences between people in the same category (and similarities with people in other categories). Such claims are rarely justified, and often descend into a kind of pre-sociological subject-ivism in which everyone's 'voice' must be treated equally as a valid datum. This *ad hominem* privileging of experience employs the same power move as a universalising reason, and the structure of the argument which establishes the autonomy of the 'voice' indeed bears a strange resemblance to the notion of individual sovereignty in the libertarian reason of classical political economy.

Yet, while the literature on postmodernism has made much of the multi-plicity of 'voices' which are silenced in the discourse of reason, too much is conflated in the concept of the neglected 'voice'. There is no doubt that dif-ferent social locations in terms of race, gender and so on can imply different kinds of experience. What has been less well theorised is the extent to which differences in experience effected by social location always imply differences in the *normative* grasp of experience. This distinction is too easily elided by those who would, for example, read off from the predominance of white decision makers the fact of a 'white' social policy. My point is not to suggest that the interests or standpoints of dominated groups are automatically and equitably incorporated into the policy-making process, but merely to question the extent to which a distinctive view of the appropriate social order neces-sarily flows from any particular social location, and that the grounds of social policy are thus contested between social groups across incommensurate com-municative fields. It may be true that social policy tends to enact the interests of dominant groups, but it does not follow that the interests of other groups cannot be framed within the same discourse, and the intersubjective con-struction of social location calls into question the claim to subvert modern reason from without.

It could be objected, following Levinas (1969), that intersubjectivity need not undermine – indeed may even establish – a radical difference between communicating parties. Yet, as Trey argues, for Levinas 'to maintain the inef-fable status of the other, the possibility of a mediated subjectivity ... has to be excluded' (Trey 1992: 422), and in this exclusion we can discern a 'power strategy' which is exogenous, lying beyond the postulation of the commu-nicative encounter. In a similar way, the 'resistance' appropriated to the dominated subject by 'resistant postmodernism' constitutes a kind of power strategy which privileges certain dimensions of experience in a way which is not easily justified on the basis of postmodern theory, and in this sense tends simply to conflate or reduce different kinds of struggle as 'counternarratives of modernity' despite an ostensible commitment to their plurality. Peters and Lankshear's view that the 'distinctively postmodern stance of *incredulity* evi-dent in global responses to meta-narratives' informs a politics 'more "localised" and "contingent" ... than the transcendent, universalist, ahistoric turf of meta-narratives' (Peters and Lankshear 1996: 30) is an example of this unhelpful reductionism, which fails to recognise the complexity of the ways in which people are engaged by and deploy *both* 'global metanarratives' *and* 'local narratives',[4] a point which emerges strongly in contemporary anthropological research (e.g. Miller 1994; James 1994).

It is also noteworthy that the forms of resistance which 'resistant postmodernism' tends to warrant are struggles which can quite easily be seen as progressive within the terms of an earlier radical politics. The struggles of Orange Order marchers, survivalist militias, religious fundamentalists, mono-ethnic nationalists and other groups which the same antique politics would hold to be reactionary are less commonly appropriated as 'resistant' to the abstract logic of modernity. Yet these groups are just as much involved in disinterring 'subjugated knowledges' and articulating distinctive visions of local communal autonomy. It is easy to use postmodern theory to undermine attempts by any of these groups to establish the validity of their particular identity claims, but less easy on the basis of such theory to elevate just *some* of them to the status of postmodern counternarrative. 'Resistant postmodernism' is silent on how local struggles that subvert grandiose modernist claims of progress and emancipation are in any sense to be welcomed, are in any sense liberating, or in any sense provide appropriately generalisable models of countermodernity, without immediately drawing upon the notions of progress and hence objective standpoint from which it seeks escape. This silence is necessary in order to preserve the possibility of a postmodern radicalism, since rejecting universalism as merely a strategy of the powerful leads to a plurality of potentially conflicting subject positions. Consistent principles for arbitration between their claims cannot be found within this plurality, but to seek them elsewhere is to return to the putatively repressive tactics of a 'rational' metaphysics (Habermas 1979; Laclau 1996). This is a genuine problem, but it is scarcely resolved by an empiricist deflation of the normative.

Uncoupled from modernist teleologies, a postmodernism which does not surreptitiously draw upon the modernist themes it purports to reject offers only a series of deconstructions, revelatory moments which fleetingly illuminate the mechanics of power but then pass on, lest they assume the mantle of power themselves. Thus, McLaren, for example, appears to be satisfied with the 'intermittent, epiphanic ruptures and moments of *jouissance* that occur when solidarity is established around struggles for liberation' (McLaren 1994: 67), but the grounding of such struggles in a view of identity as 'constantly being produced through a play of difference' (McLaren 1994: 52) seems particularly unhelpful. It fails to recognise that political struggles – while sometimes overconflated in both modernist and postmodern politics – are never entirely contingent, and it seems curiously at odds with McLaren's own critique of a politics which 'can imagine only an agonistic relation to real-world liberalism' (McLaren 1994: 69).

It is scarcely surprising that such ideas often fail to impress those who confront the chronic effects reproduced by particular structures of power.

The notion of 'play' which Derrida (1978) uses to such radical effect in his critique of modernist social theory seems less radical when it is manifested in a context like postmodern architecture as merely an ironic assemblage of different styles. Here, if the old modernism was *too* focused upon production, the iconoclastic 'playfulness' of the postmodern architectural form leaves untouched the relations of production which determine who can and cannot have a say in shaping the built environment. In this reading, postmodern architecture becomes merely 'an appropriation of a particular version of the populist by one dominant group' (Miller 1987: 166). It is here that we can discern the inadequacy of much postmodern critique as radical practice, and thus the force of Habermas's comment that 'nothing remains from a desublimated meaning or a destructured form; an emancipatory effect does not follow' (Habermas 1983: 11).

In sum, something is lost in moving from Derrida's *différance* to the notion of a radical difference between social groups which enables a political critique of modernity. The 'resistant postmodernism' implied in the latter is really a kind of primitivism, in which the abstract reason of modernity is seen as entirely oppressive, and various candidates for a basically 'authentic' critique of reason are paraded. Like primitivism, the interest lies less with the actual complexities and contradictions of the people who bear the onus of critique and more with a version of their 'difference' which merely reinscribes the universality of reason by a power strategy which constructs them against it. In this sense, there are continuities between 'resistant postmodernism' and the skein of romanticism which, searching for totality, weaves between Enlightenment and counter-Enlightenment thought, between the critique of incremental politics and the dream of a 'last battle against politics' (Pasquino 1993) upon which universalist claims to progress have been founded, a skein which links the religious eschatology of pre-modern thought to the implicit telos of a radical postmodern 'difference'.

CONCLUSION: REOPENING THE GIFT

In this concluding section, I advocate an alternative approach to 'difference' in the context of social policy which can be excavated from modernist theory and from which I infer a particular normative stance. Although it is hard now to believe in a modernist 'dialectic of enlightenment'[5] which leads to some ultimate resolution, it is the idea of a final enlightenment rather than the idea of a dialectic which should be rejected, and I want to suggest that the grounds for contemporary social policy exist in dialectical relations like unity versus difference. Marx's view of power was certainly too monolithic, but for all that power is a diffuse social force it is also hugely manifested within particular institutions. Earlier, I described Said's quotation from Marx on the French peasantry as 'mischievous' because – out of context – it implies only an elitist programme to represent the inchoate interests of a voiceless multitude, which historically has so often been merely an excuse to install an oppressive political power. However, another reading suggests a different point; the peasants, vertically divided and isolated from access to power, were unable to choose the terms by which they could objectify themselves and thereby contest the power which was held over them. This suggests a dualistic programme in which the ability to create value, to develop independent spheres of local affect and to contest the exercise of arbitrary power depends upon access to putatively universal normative principles and the institutional framework they sustain.

This is precisely an opportunity afforded by modernity, but it is quite distinct from the modern philosophy of the subject articulated by writers as disparate as Adam Smith and Richard Titmuss. As we saw earlier, Titmuss extended Mauss's discussion of the gift to contemporary social policy via a notion of altruism between strangers based on an individualist concept of the 'biological need to give', and he thereby neglected the anti-subjectivist strand to Mauss's argument which emphasised the interchangeability of people and things as the substance of social structure (Lévi-Strauss 1949, 1950). This view does not accord special (indeed, any) analytic weight to 'experience', 'neglected voices' and so on, and it is here that postmodern theorists not unreasonably suspect a certain undeclared interest. But the argument remains useful in enabling us to grasp political power as simultaneously central *and* diffuse.

This point can be exemplified with reference to two texts which, in true postmodern fashion, are reflections upon a particular writer's own refractory relationship to another writer. One is Marshall Sahlins's (1974) discussion of Mauss's *Gift*. The other is Pasquale Pasquino's (1993) discussion of Foucault's 1976 lectures at the Collège de France. In referring their respective authors back to Hobbes's *Leviathan* (1651) both offer a similar but unusual perspective, arguing that Hobbes's famous 'state of nature' is not an asocial human condition whose consequence in the prospect of a 'nasty, brutish and short' life is so unappealing that people willingly surrender themselves to the autocratic power of the Leviathan, but that this state of nature is *already* a social order in which people retain as individuals not only the possibility to use violence but the *right* to use it and thus enter into *legitimate* competition to impose their own version of the normative. *Leviathan* represents the mutual surrender of this 'discourse of war' and establishes the possibility for truth and for arbitration, a space to countenance the rights of the individual, and thus a kind of explicit rationalisation for the proper basis of social relations which annihilates the prospect of war and a permanent fracturing force.

If, for some, Hobbes's writing is a little too closely identified with the development of the modern state for it to be dissociated from a certain complicity with the interests of the powerful, then Mauss's Hobbesian understanding of exchange as the basis for the social in stateless, 'primitive' societies, albeit somewhat romantic, perhaps makes the point more palatably. Here, exchange is not the reified system of equivalencies or exchange values that McLaren sees as the predicate of 'white culture' (McLaren 1994: 61), and others might view more simply as the logic of capital. Instead, exchange is subsumed in an understanding of differentiated social relations as emergent from a broader process of objectification (Miller 1987; Taylor 1994). This is pertinent to the contemporary politics of identity because it questions the possibility of entirely autonomous spheres of value without supposing the existence of a unified cultural order, thus holding together the dualities of universal/particular, conflict/consensus, enabling/constraining, subject/object and so on which postmodern theory too easily believes it has unravelled. *Contra* Norman Tebbit and his ilk, there is no 'British character' to be defended from alien incursions. *Contra* Bryan *et al.* there is no singularly authentic and liberating 'black culture' to be disentangled from 'white cultural values', although there may be reified cultural forms worthy of articulation in the context of asymmetries of power. Instead, perceptions of identity, experience, individuality and social location based upon race, gender, class and so on emerge from the way that people oscillate across such dualities in constructing themselves. As Miller puts it:

> the individual projects out in representation, but in doing so comes to understand personal experience in relation to a set of media ... which contrast people as social beings having certain relationships. The internalization of these externalizations thereby creates the individual's 'being' in relation to age, gender, social group and other familiar social categories.
>
> (Miller 1987: 56)

We can thus formulate questions about the 'reality' of race raised earlier in a sense as empirical ones. In the context of social policy, it has often proved possible to objectify racial identities in struggles to improve the terms within which racial(ised) minorities experience welfare. But efforts to reify race around a clear 'black' agenda have nevertheless proved problematic, and debates within anti-racism between those for or against a singular 'political blackness' (Modood 1994) seem, from the present perspective, both inevitable and irreconcilable. It is no surprise, then, that the specific demands which emerge from these politics rarely offer a compelling alternative to the political categories of modernity, tending either to questionable abstractions such as meeting the often ill-defined 'special needs of minority ethnic groups', or to quite instrumental demands for political representation or basically multicultural service provision. I wish neither to deny the particularity of certain 'needs', nor to trivialise the importance of these demands, nor to underestimate the degree to which they have been frustrated, but I am not convinced that they have undermined the normative basis of orthodox social policy.

Of course, the failure of a certain identity politics to contest an oppressive modernity could be seen via the Marxist tradition as an example of dominated groups being unclear about the nature of their own interests precisely because they *are* dominated groups. But I prefer to invoke Simmel's theory of modernity as a more appropriate sociological lens through which to consider this dynamic. Simmel (1907) characterises the culture of modernity as a tension between the extreme abstraction of money as a representation of human relations and the specificity of culture and consumption as a self-realisation achieved by particular groups. For Simmel, the 'tragedy of culture' lies in the tendency for these specific cultural forms themselves to become alienated, reified and oppressive (Simmel 1968: 30). Political identities, including ethnic or racial ones, often take this form, and it is in political and aesthetic practice that we see a constant attempt to reinterpret and refresh identities at this concrete level of cultural specificity. The instruments of social policy, on the other hand, tend to lean towards the more abstract pole of the money form, or at least towards the provision of services such as health care, which provides the means to objectify culture through keeping people healthy, rather than creating specific forms of value itself. In some sense, many of the really controversial debates around race in social policy – the educational discarding of black children, regulatory mental health services or, more ambiguously, cross-ethnic adoption – have involved struggles by black people to keep the welfare services they receive at a level of abstraction that does not objectify *them* in particular negative ways. Yet such struggles have generally recognised that although welfare institutions reproduce racism and inequality, claims over them by dominated groups remain central because they act as intermediate goods which, when available at an appropriate level of abstraction, enable the creation of value. My argument is not therefore against any kind of identity politics. Rather, I suggest that the specific claims which emerge from these politics should be understood in relation to a wider political process, and not in terms of essentialist notions of 'difference' or the romantic dramatisation of conflict which characterises many putatively postmodern critiques of welfare.[6] Here, I think Titmuss was correct to suggest that the possibility for 'altruistic opportunities' created by social policy institutions renders them as 'generators of moral conflict' (Titmuss 1970: 17). The resolution of these conflicts may be highly problematic, more so than Titmuss himself granted. Nevertheless, I would argue that instead of elevating such conflicts to ontological status and thus reopening the discourse of war, it is more compelling both theoretically and politically to reopen a discourse of the gift.

ACKNOWLEDGEMENT

I thank Geoff Cooper, Martin O'Brien, Bob Carter, Alison Drewett and Colin Tipton for commenting on earlier drafts of this chapter.

NOTES

1   The concept of 'race' is notoriously problematic and I offer no programmatic definition here, an omission which is partially justified in my subsequent argument. A fuller account of my position is provided in Smaje (1997).
2   See Terrail (1985) for a spirited defence of Marx against these charges, and Spivak (1996) for a more sympathetic 'postmodern' critique.
3   Though, as Taylor argues, the idea is a specifically *modern* one, deriving from 'the massive subjective turn in modern culture, a new form of inwardness, in which we come to think of ourselves as beings with inner depths' (Taylor 1994: 77).
4   The global/local duality is also invoked problematically, since opposing only one unit of the dyad draws attention to the impossibility of defining exactly where the 'global' gives way to the 'localised'.
5   Used here in a different sense to Horkheimer and Adorno's (1973) work of the same name, although arguably these authors retained some commitment to a notion of progressive transformation.
6   However, I make no suggestion that the political categories of modernity are a *necessary* prerequisite for founding adequate normative claims. Even so, although Mauss's analysis of 'gift societies' establishes the possibility of understanding 'difference' through homologous political categories, my argument – like the postmodernism I have criticised – does not entirely escape Spivak's critique of a 'continuist, romantic, anti-capitalist version ... [of] use-value' (Spivak 1996: 118), albeit here *within* capitalism itself. Yet despite the extraordinary philosophical sophistication of Spivak's approach to value, the politics she infers from it is based upon a fairly crude understanding of the 'global division of labour'. Perhaps this speaks to a general problem in founding a universal theory of value. A comment from Ricoeur retains its force: 'we are in a kind of lull or interregnum in which we can no longer practice the dogmatism of a single truth and in which we are not yet capable of conquering the scepticism into which we have stepped' (Ricoeur 1965: 283).

BIBLIOGRAPHY

Baudrillard, J. (1975) *The Mirror of Production*, St Louis: Telos Press.
Bourdieu, P. (1977) *Outline of a Theory of Practice*, Cambridge: Cambridge University Press.
Bryan, B., Dadzie, S. and Scafe, S. (1985) *The Heart of the Race: Black Women's Lives in Britain*, London: Virago.
Carter, B. and Green, M. (1996) 'Naming difference: race-thinking, common sense and sociology', in C. Samson and N. South (eds) *The Social Construction of Social Policy: Methodologies, Racism, Citizenship and the Environment*, Basingstoke: Macmillan.
Derrida, J. (1976) *Of Grammatology*, Baltimore: Johns Hopkins University Press.
Derrida, J. (1978) 'Structure, sign and play in the discourse of the human sciences', in *Writing and Difference*, London: Routledge and Kegan Paul.
Foster, H. (1983) 'Postmodernism: a preface', in H. Foster (ed.) *The Anti-Aesthetic: Essays on Postmodern Culture*, Seattle: Bay Press.
Foucault, M. (1967) *Madness and Civilisation: A History of Insanity in the Age of Reason*, London: Tavistock.
Foucault, M. (1976) *The History of Sexuality. Vol. 1: An Introduction*, Harmondsworth: Penguin.
Foucault, M. (1980) 'Two lectures', in *Power/Knowledge: Selected Interviews*, Brighton: Harvester Press.

Frampton, K. (1983) 'Towards a critical regionalism: six points for an architecture of resistance', in H. Foster (ed.) *The Anti-Aesthetic: Essays on Postmodern Culture*, Seattle: Bay Press.

Goldberg, D. (1993) *Racist Culture: Philosophy and the Politics of Meaning*, Oxford: Blackwell.

Gough, I. (1979) *The Political Economy of the Welfare State*, London: Macmillan.

Gramsci, A. (1971) *Selections from Prison Notebooks*, London: Lawrence & Wishart.

Gutman, A. (1996) 'Responding to racial injustice', in A. Appiah and A. Gutman *Color Conscious: The Political Morality of Race*, Princeton NJ: Princeton University Press.

Habermas, J. (1976) *Legitimation Crisis*, London: Heinemann.

Habermas, J. (1979) *Communication and the Evolution of Society*, Cambridge: Polity Press.

Habermas, J. (1983) 'Modernity – an incomplete project', in H. Foster (ed.) *The Anti-Aesthetic: Essays on Postmodern Culture*, Seattle: Bay Press.

Habermas, J. (1987) *The Philosophical Discourse of Modernity*, Cambridge: Polity Press.

Hegel, G. [1807] (1977) *The Phenomenology of Spirit*, Oxford: Oxford University Press.

Hobbes, T. [1651] (1968) *Leviathan*, Harmondsworth: Penguin.

Horkheimer, M. and Adorno, T. (1973) *Dialectic of Enlightenment*, London: Allen Lane.

Inden, R. (1990) *Imagining India*, Oxford: Blackwell.

James, W. (1994) 'War and "ethnic visibility": the Uduk on the Sudan–Ethiopia border', in K. Fukui and J. Markakis (eds) *Ethnicity and Conflict in the Horn of Africa*, London: James Currey.

Laclau, E. (1996) *Emancipation(s)*, London: Verso.

Law, I. (1996) *Racism, Ethnicity and Social Policy*, Hemel Hempstead: Prentice Hall.

Levinas, E. (1969) *Totality and Infinity*, Pittsburgh: Duquesne University Press.

Lévi-Strauss, C. [1949] (1969) *The Elementary Structures of Kinship*, London: Eyre and Spottiswoode.

Lévi-Strauss, C. [1950] (1987) *An Introduction to the Work of Marcel Mauss*, London: Routledge and Kegan Paul.

Lukács, G. (1971) 'Reification and the consciousness of the proletariat', in *History and Class Consciousness*, London: Merlin Press.

Lyotard, J.-F. (1984) *The Postmodern Condition: A Report on Knowledge*, Manchester: Manchester University Press.

McLaren, P. (1994) 'White terror and oppositional agency: towards a critical multi-culturalism', in D. Goldberg (ed.) *Multiculturalism: A Critical Reader*, Oxford: Blackwell.

Marx, K. [1869] (1973) 'The Eighteenth Brumaire of Louis Bonaparte', in *Surveys From Exile: Political Writings, Vol. 2*, Harmondsworth: Penguin.

Marx, K. and Engels, F. [1846] (1970) *The German Ideology*, New York: International Publishers.

Mauss, M. [1922] (1990) *The Gift: The Form and Reason for Exchange in Archaic Societies*, London: Routledge.

Miller, D. (1987) *Material Culture and Mass Consumption*, Oxford: Blackwell.

Miller, D. (1994) *Modernity: An Ethnographic Approach*, Oxford: Berg.

Modood, T. (1994) 'Political blackness and British Asians', *Sociology* 28, 4: 859–76.

Nicholson, L. and Seidman, S. (1995) *Social Postmodernism: Beyond Identity Politics*, Cambridge: Cambridge University Press.

O'Connor, J. (1973) *The Fiscal Crisis of the State*, New York: St Martin's Press.

Offe, C. (1984) *Contradictions of the Welfare State*, London: Hutchinson.

Pasquino, P. (1993) 'Political theory of war and peace: Foucault and the history of modern political theory', *Economy and Society* 22, 1: 77–88.

Peters, M. and Lankshear, C. (1996) 'Postmodern counternarratives', in H. Giroux, C. Lankshear, P. McLaren and M. Peters (eds) *Counternarratives: Cultural Studies and Critical Pedagogies in Postmodern Spaces*, London: Routledge.

Ricoeur, P. (1965) *History and Truth*, Evanston IL: Northwestern University Press.

Rigby, P. (1996) *African Images: Racism and the End of Anthropology*, Oxford: Berg.

Sahlins, M. (1974) *'The Spirit of the Gift' in Stone Age Economics*, London: Tavistock.

Said, E. (1978) *Orientalism*, New York: Vintage Books.

Simmel, G. (1968) 'On the concept and tragedy of culture', in *The Conflict in Modern Culture and Other Essays*, New York: New York Teachers College Press.

Simmel, G. [1907] (1978) *The Philosophy of Money*, London: Routledge and Kegan Paul.

Sivanandan, A. (1982) *A Different Hunger: Writings on Black Resistance*, London: Pluto Press.

Smaje, C. (1997) 'Not just a social construct: theorising race and ethnicity', *Sociology* 31, 2: 307–27.

Spivak, G. (1996) 'Scattered speculations on the question of value', in D. Landry and G. Maclean (eds) *The Spivak Reader*, London: Routledge.

Strathern, M. (1992) *After Nature: English Kinship in the Late Twentieth Century*, Cambridge: Cambridge University Press.

Taylor, C. (1994) 'The politics of recognition', in D. Goldberg (ed.) *Multiculturalism: A Critical Reader*, Oxford: Blackwell.

Terrail, J.-P. (1985) 'Commodity fetishism and the ideal of needs', in E. Preteceille and J.-P. Terrail *Capitalism, Consumption and Needs*, Oxford: Blackwell.

Titmuss, R. (1970) *The Gift Relationship: From Human Blood to Social Policy*, Harmondsworth: Penguin.

Trey, G. (1992) 'Communicative ethics in the face of alterity: Habermas, Levinas and the problems of post-conventional universalism', *Praxis International* 11, 4: 412–27.

Williams, B. (1995) 'Classification systems revisited: kinship, caste, race and nationality as the flow of blood and the spread of rights', in S. Yanagisako and C. Delaney (eds) *Naturalizing Power: Essays in Feminist Cultural Analysis*, London: Routledge.

Wood, D. (1987) 'Beyond deconstruction?', in A. Griffiths (ed.) *Contemporary French Philosophy*, Cambridge: Cambridge University Press.

Chapter 10

Individualisation processes and social policy

Insecurity, reflexivity and risk in the restructuring of contemporary British health and housing policies

Sarah Nettleton and Roger Burrows

INTRODUCTION

This chapter attempts to bring together two strands of social scientific literature which have hitherto not fully engaged with each other – one deriving from the work of Ulrich Beck, Anthony Giddens and others (Beck 1992; Beck *et al*. 1994; Giddens 1991) concerned with the emergence of reflexive modernisation, and another deriving from the political economy of health inequalities concerned with the social impact of the growth of economic insecurity (Wilkinson 1996). It does this within the context of a substantive discussion of developments in aspects of contemporary British social policy. Our main focus will be on housing, although we also draw upon contemporary developments within the health literature where many of the arguments discussed have been more fully theorised.

'MAKING UP PEOPLE' IN A RISK SOCIETY

A key feature of life under 'late', 'high', 'post' or 'reflexive' modernity – call it what you will – about which there seems to be at least some consensus amongst commentators (Beck 1992; Beck *et al*. 1994; Giddens 1991, 1992, 1994; Hutton 1995; Lash and Urry 1994; Pahl 1995) is that contemporary society is increasingly characterised by risk. It is argued that these contemporary discourses of risk impact upon how we think about our*selves*, which, in turn, alters the nature of social relationships and of our capacity to provide social support or 'care' for others.

Following Hacking (1986), we might think about these processes as 'making up people'; as creating new ways for people to be. In the conceptualisation offered by Hacking (1986: 231), when 'new modes of description come into being, new possibilities of action come into being as a consequence'. In this chapter we are concerned with the manner in which descriptions of social life which are inherent in what Beck (1992) refers to as 'individualisation processes' create new social identities, which, as a consequence, lead to reconfigurations of social relationships and patterns of social welfare.[1] A concrete example of this is provided by Pat Carlen in her powerful and eloquent study of the political criminology of youth homelessness, when she writes:

> So often have we been told that the market gives and the market takes away, that a hitherto unacceptable level of unemployment is necessary to bring inflation down, that the homeless on the streets can indicate to us in a very tangible way that the requisite sacrificial lambs are indeed upon the altar, that the market gods are being appeased. Even if people wanted to intervene, how could they when their own jobs have become so uncertain, when a generalised fear of risk and uncertainty, together with the prevailing ethic of individualism, make *it almost immoral to care*?
>
> (Carlen 1996: 80, our emphasis)

The nature and content of contemporary risk are qualitatively different to those of pre-modern or early modern societies. A distinctive feature of contemporary risk is the way in which it permeates our psyche, in terms of both how we think about ourselves and how we relate to other people. Three inter-related conceptualisations, developed by Giddens (1991), neatly capture the key elements of contemporary risk: reflexivity of the self, lifestyles and life planning, and ontological security. For Giddens:

> The concept of risk becomes fundamental to the way both lay actors and technical specialists organise the social world. Under conditions of modernity, the future is continually drawn into the present by means of the *reflexive* organisation of knowledge environments.
>
> (Giddens 1991: 3, our emphasis)

Within this conceptualisation, then, a core feature of contemporary risk culture is the constant habit of assessing and making calculations about potential risks which might affect our lives. We seek out, and are continually presented with information produced by, an increasingly diverse array of 'experts' on virtually every aspect of our lives: what we eat; how we sleep; our finances; our intimate relationships; our health; our leisure; and so on (Nettleton 1997). This is typified by the growth of self-help guides, manuals and other guides for living. The North American academic Barbara Duden was struck by this phenomenon in relation to health in the USA some years ago:

> In a bookstore in Dallas I found about 130 manuals that would teach me 'how to be an active partner in my own health'. For many years now the self-care budget in the United States has been growing at three times the rate of all medical expenses combined.
>
> (Duden 1991: 20)

This is emblematic of the reflexivity of the self: 'a project carried on amid a profusion of reflexive resources: therapy and self help manuals of all kinds, television programmes and magazine articles' (Giddens 1992: 30), and now, we might add, the myriad virtual resources of cyberspace.[2]

Kellner (1992) argues that increasingly it is this reflexivity of the self which determines 'who we are' rather than socio-structural determinants. Whatever the exact calculus of self-determination is, there can be little doubt that social identities *have* become more fluid over time and that we are able to work constantly at and negotiate our notions of the self within the context of an increasing array of options. Giddens goes on to suggest that:

> Because of the 'openness' of social life today, the pluralisation of contexts of action and diversity of 'authorities', *lifestyle* choice is increasingly important in the constitution of self identity and daily activity. Reflexively organised *life-planning*, which normally presumes consideration of risks as filtered through contact with expert knowledge, becomes a central feature of structuring self-identity.
>
> (Giddens 1991: 5, *our emphasis*)

Thus, Giddens argues, we are increasingly required to make lifestyle choices. Such choices may involve decisions about our longer-term life plans, such as choosing to buy a particular house, taking out a personal pension, or sending our children to a particular school. This notion of lifestyle choice is of course fundamentally related to the availability of resources. Furthermore, the lifestyle choices and life planning of some individuals and groups can influence not only their life chances but also those of others. This can have a cumulative effect where the social arrangements are such that we are encouraged to make lifestyle choices and life-planning decisions which limit the life chances of others.[3] Notions of the contemporary self, then, are constituted by way of an ongoing project in which people are bound to make lifestyle and life-planning decisions. Such projects are contingent upon the availability of material resources and can often alter and exacerbate social divisions. But lifestyle choices and life planning are not just activities of the better off; they are made by all members of society.

Giddens links these notions of risk, reflexivity and lifestyle planning to a final, and perhaps more familiar concept: that of ontological security. Giddens derives this term from the work of R.D. Laing. Crudely, this refers to emotional security and is based on the notion that one's self-identity is linked to one's biography – the narrative that can be told about one's life. Hence an ontologically insecure individual is, according to this thesis, a person who displays one or more of the following characteristics (see Giddens 1991: 53–4). First, s/he 'lack[s] a consistent feeling of biographical continuity'. Second, 'in an environment full of changes the person is obsessively preoccupied with apprehension of possible risks to his or her existence, and paralysed in terms of practical action'. Third, 'the person fails to develop or sustain trust in his [*sic*] own self-integrity' and may subject himself/herself to constant self-scrutiny.

SOCIAL POLICY AND THE CONSTRUCTION OF THE REFLEXIVE SELF

What has any of this to do with the traditional concerns of social policy? The answer to this is that transformations in welfare in Britain since the late 1970s have formed an important part of the social processes which have contributed to the constitution of the reflexive self. This has occurred in three related ways. First, educational, environmental, health and social care, housing and transport policies in particular have all encouraged the recipients (or 'consumers') to use the contemporary argot) of such services to make choices. Of course for many people who have limited resources the notion of choice appears, and is, to a great extent facile. Nevertheless choices of some sort are being made, however constrained. This process of consumerisation in welfare has been coupled with a second major development, that of extensive technologies of 'informatization' such as needs assessments (for health, housing and social care), league tables (for schools, hospitals, local authority housing repair waiting times, and the Research Assessment Exercise [RAE] in universities) and myriad other audit reports. This mountain of data is then used by individuals and groups to inform their risk calculations prior to making decisions about provision. Third, welfare has increasingly become underpinned by the notion of prevention rather than the provision of goods and services to all those who are in 'need' (Giddens 1994: 151–73). All three of these developments are most overtly evident in the field of health policy but are beginning to manifest themselves in other fields of social policy as well. With this in mind, we introduce some recent debates in the sociology of health policy (see also the chapter by Bunton in this volume) with the intention of drawing some analytic parallels with the main substantive focus of this chapter, contemporary housing policy.

HEALTH POLICY

In *The New Politics of the NHS*, Klein (1995) has argued that whilst the 1980s saw the advent of 'a new economic policy paradigm', in the 1990s this was replaced by 'a new health policy paradigm'. In short, the government finally acknowledged that it had responsibilities for the health of the population that went beyond the provision of a health-care system (Klein 1995: 210). It argued that the main health problems of the twentieth century were due to personal health behaviours. The *Health of the Nation* White Paper and subsequent documentations set out the government's strategy to improve the nation's health (DoH 1992). The risks to health were conceptualised as predominantly those associated with individual behaviours and lifestyles – especially the holy trinity of risks: smoking, exercise and diet.[4]

Within the health literature there appears to be an emerging consensus that health and medicine work within a new framework or paradigm – one which is governed by notions of surveillance and risk (for more detail see Armstrong 1993; Castel 1991; Nettleton 1995; Ogden 1995; Petersen 1996; Skolbekken 1995). Health and medical care are concerned not just with those who are ill, but more with those who are well. There is an increasing orientation in health policy to the prevention of disease and the promotion of health. This involves the identification, scrutiny and monitoring of risk factors. Exhortations about healthy living originate not only in the activities of state-sponsored health professionals – public health consultants, health promoters, GPs, nurses and so on – but also in a myriad of other sources such as school teachers, community group leaders, supermarkets, TV, radio, magazines and so on (Bunton et al. 1995). There has also been an explosion of health 'resources' (be it goods, such as 'healthy foods' or exercise bikes, or services, such as fitness clubs and a myriad types of therapy) of every kind within the commercial sector. Concerns about the environment are also articulated in terms of individual responsibility: we can 'choose' to buy or not to buy 'green products'; we can take our papers, cans and bottles for recycling; we can use disposable or reusable nappies; we can eat free-range or 'farm-fresh' eggs; and so on. Certain moral and ethical considerations emerge from this. Monica Greco (1993) points out that health which can be 'chosen' represents a very different value and moral dimension to a health which one simply enjoys or has. She writes:

> It testifies to more than just a physical capacity; it is the visible sign of initiative, adaptability, balance and strength of will. In this sense, physical health has come to represent, for the neo-liberal individual who has 'chosen' it, an 'objective' witness to his or her suitability to function as a free and rational agent.
>
> (Greco 1993: 369–70)

Thus in relation to health we are constantly engaging in lifestyle and life-planning choices which in turn constitute our notion of self. But such a self is bound to be precarious, as individuals live in a society where the awareness of risks becomes intensified and where the onus is upon the individual to scrutinise and respond to those risks (Nettleton 1997).

HOUSING POLICY

On the face of it there is no comparable national strategy for housing which is designed to ensure that the population has access to good housing. It is difficult to point to any policies which will prevent homelessness and promote secure shelter. However, the discourses drawn upon within policy statements use similar conceptualisations of the functioning of individuals in relation to society to those found within the disease-prevention and health-promotion documentation.

A key thrust of the housing policies of successive British governments since World War II has been the expansion of home-ownership. A minority were home-owners at that time; now, however, they form about 68 per cent of all households. The policy of increasing home-ownership was significantly accelerated by the Tory governments who were in office between 1979 and 1997. In fact, 3.8 million more households in 1997 own their own home than in 1979, an increase of some 38 per cent (DoE 1995: 6). Three policy initiatives in particular, combined with the formation of more households that wanted to buy their own homes, contributed to the accelerated growth of owner occupation (Hogarth *et al.* 1996). First, council houses were sold to tenants at discounted prices under the 'Right to Buy' (RTB) scheme, which formed part of the 1980 Housing Act. Between 1981 and 1995 1.57 million council houses were sold (Wilcox 1996: 106). Second, restrictions were placed on local authorities, which were unable to use their capital receipts to build new houses. This, combined with the RTB, has resulted in a substantial reduction and residualisation of local authority housing available for rent, and the 'pushing' of some households towards home-ownership as the only viable 'option' open to them. Third, the Financial Service Act in 1985 and the Building Societies Act in 1986 deregulated the credit market. New players came on to the lending scene, expanded the market, and offered mortgages to those groups who had hitherto been regarded as 'riskier' customers.

In sum, housing policy since the late 1970s rests on the notion that individuals, or households, are able and should be encouraged to take responsibility for their own homes. Three themes are made explicit in the official policy documentation: 'opportunity, choice and responsibility' (DoE 1995). But this refers to individual choices within deregulated market contexts wherein individuals remain responsible for the consequences of their actions despite the vagaries of the wider economy. Choice, responsibility, uncertainty, risks, investing in one's self – be it a home or one's health – are themes which transcend both housing and health policy.

A number of parallels between health and housing policies can be deciphered. As illustrated in Figure 1, both aim to foster self-reliance, individual responsibility and investment in the domestic space. Individuals are encouraged to be enterprising, and to take advice so that they may calculate and negotiate their own risks, be they related to health or to finance. As in all spheres of welfare we see here examples of what O'Malley (1992) usefully calls 'the privatisation of risk'. This individualisation, as we discussed above, is one of the key features of the late/postmodern condition. As Beck and Beck-Gernsheim note:

One of the decisive features of individualisation processes ... is that they not only permit, but demand an active contribution by individuals ... if they are not to fail individuals must be able to plan for the long term and adapt to change; they must organise and improvise, set goals, recognise obstacles, accept defeats and attempt new starts. They need initiative, tenacity, flexibility.

(Beck and Beck-Gernsheim 1996: 27)

- Self-reliance
- Individual responsibility
- Investment
- Entrepreneurship and calculation
- Privatisation of risks
- Individualisation

Figure 1 Individualisation processes transcending health- and housing-policy domains

HOME-OWNERSHIP AND ONTOLOGICAL INSECURITY

People have been encouraged to buy, and be financially responsible for, their own homes. At the same time people are being encouraged to be responsible for their own health and the health of their relatives and to care for their kin when they are ill. The extent to which individuals can fulfil these 'household responsibilities' will be contingent on both their own economic resources (for example, their paid work, their savings and their financial obligations) and the forms of capital they possess (for example, their level of education, their health status, their physical prowess, their marketable skills and so on). The fact that individuals have to be flexible and responsive may in turn contribute to the creation of new forms of inequalities. Emily Martin (1994), in her extensive anthropological study of North American culture, found the notion of flexibility to be a dominant motif and organising principle of contemporary society. Indeed, flexibility itself may come to constitute a form of capital. She speculates:

One of our new taken-for-granted virtues for persons and their bodies has come to be 'flexibility'. Arising as a trait to be cherished and cultivated, from corporations and city governments to credit cards and shoes, flexibility is an object of desire for nearly everyone's personality, body, and organisation. Flexibility has also become a powerful commodity, something scarce and highly valued, that can be used to discriminate against some people ...

A conception of a new elite may be forged that finds the desirable qualities of flexibility and adaptability to change in certain superior individuals of *any* ethnic, racial, gender, sexual identity, or age group in the nation.

(Martin 1994: xvii)

Flexibility of course demands the cultivation of a reflexive monitoring of risks and the ability to alter life plans rapidly. The necessity for such flexibility tends to undermine the stability required to generate ontological security. The clear downside of the development of a flexible, reflexive self is the potential for increased ontological insecurity. This is nowhere better illustrated than in the recent history of UK home-ownership.

In the 1990s the chances of home-owners experiencing the 'real difficulties' associated with buying a home were increased due to four factors acting in combination, each of which was outside of the control of any individual home-owner – however reflexive s/he might have been. First, in a low-inflation economy, the long-term (usually twenty-five years) nature of the credit contract means that the entry ratio of mortgage costs to earnings is large. Second, the costs of credit are variable and, in an increasingly globalized market, unpredictable, with interest rates varying between 7.5 per cent and 15 per cent over the late 1980s and early-to-mid-1990s. Third, continuous and secure employment contracts are being displaced by more insecure and short-term employment contracts. Fourth, rising house prices and relatively high interest rates have often meant that entry into sustainable home-ownership now necessitates dual-earner households. These two final features demonstrate the critical nature of the changing labour market for sustainable home-ownership, and it is likely that this constitutes the main reason why the 'problem' of unsustainable home-ownership is going to remain significant during the coming decades.

Social security policies have compounded the situation by invoking even greater levels of insecurity by reducing eligibility and entitlements to benefits. For example, borrowers taking out mortgages after September 1995 who are in receipt of income support (IS) will have to wait nine months before receiving help with mortgage interest (MI). 'Existing' borrowers eligible for IS will also wait longer (two months with nothing, then 50 per cent for four months), but not as long as new borrowers. Borrowers are encouraged instead to make their own arrangements by taking out private mortgage-protection plans. These have been found inadequate because not only are they relatively expensive but they have tight eligibility and claiming criteria. Ford *et al.* (1995) found that of those in arrears only about one quarter could have been helped by private insurance. One of the main reasons for this is that mortgage arrears are not always the consequences of a total lack of income, but a result of reduced income (for example, a new job at lower wages, loss of income earned, etc.), yet there is neither a public nor a private safety net to deal with this situation. The restructuring or 'flexibilisation' of work is resulting in continuous and secure employment contracts being displaced by more insecure and short-term employment contracts and/or increasing rates of self-employment. Mortgages, however, are premised on the assumption of stable employment over a long period of time. There is an increasingly clear disjuncture emerging between the supposed need for flexible labour markets and the ability of people to sustain mortgage costs over long periods (Burrows 1997a). It would seem reasonable to speculate, therefore, that for as long as this disjuncture exists home-ownership will remain problematic and/or unsustainable for a significant proportion of home-owners.

This discussion of the problematic nature of much contemporary home-ownership is, of course, sharply at odds with theorisations of home-ownership as a stable buttress in the private sphere against the risks and uncertainties of the world outside. Paradigmatically, in his book *A Nation of Home Owners*, Saunders (1990) argues that in a world increasingly characterised by change and instability home-ownership provides the major source of 'ontological security, for a home of one's own offers both a physical (hence spatially rooted) and permanent (hence temporally rooted) location in the world' (Saunders 1990: 293). He argues that home-ownership is something to which people universally aspire, and goes so far as to suggest that people have an innate desire to own their own homes. Home-ownership, he argues, enables a greater sense of emotional security and so a stronger sense of self and identity:

> Ownership not only guarantees certain rights which may be denied to tenants, but it also ensures permanency, even across generations. In a world where change is rapid and expectations are forever being turned upside down, the privately owned home seems to represent a secure anchor point where the nerves can be rested and the sense allowed to relax ... When ordinary people own their own homes, they seem to feel more confident and self reliant.
>
> (Saunders 1990: 311)

Saunders's conceptualisation of owner occupation as a source of ontological security now reads as more than a little quaint from the viewpoint of the late 1990s. Whilst the discourse of home-ownership of the 1980s was littered with comfortable, life-planning, biographically undisrupted terms such as 'trading up', 'equity gain' and 'gentrification', the discourse of the 1990s has been dominated by uncomfortable, chaotic, unpredictable and biographically disrupting terms such as 'negative equity', 'arrears', 'repossessions' and 'debt overhang' (Forrest and Murie 1994: 55). Furthermore, as Forrest and Murie point out, these are not just words: 'there are households which are becoming impoverished rather than enriched by their experience of the tenure'.

The decisions and social processes associated with buying a home constitute concrete lifestyle choices and life planning. Buying a 'place of one's own' involves the assessment of a whole series of risks: levels of inflation; trends in the housing market; the condition of the property; government policies; labour-market conditions; the long-term viability of intimate relationships; health; and so on. The house buyer is also confronted with an array of insurances which draw attention to possible risks, such as life insurance, buildings insurance, contents insurance, mortgage protection plans and endowments. There are also plenty of 'reflexive resources' available to help people make their 'choices'. We can turn to the wide range of 'expert' advisors on insurance policies, financial planning, mortgages and endowments, who all claim to offer sound advice.

However, the discourses surrounding home-ownership contain an inherent contradiction. On the one hand buying a home is presumed to be a secure investment and a means of taking control over one's future, on the other hand buying a home is fraught with hazards and risks. A fine balance has to be maintained by lenders who want people to buy homes *and* to insure against all the potential pitfalls. The advertising blurb for one major lender, for example, states that:

> Buying a home is probably the biggest financial commitment you will ever make. So it's reassuring to know that when you talk to General Accident, you'll be talking to one of the largest and most respected providers of insurance and financial services in the UK ... in addition to wise mortgage guidance, we can offer some of the most knowledgeable, trustworthy advice available on related policies, such as endowments and other life insurance.
> (General Accident 1996)

As is well documented (Ford 1997), the risks associated with buying a home are becoming greater as jobs become less secure and the social security 'safety net' shrinks. Mortgage indebtedness in Britain is no longer just a private matter; it is a major public issue. In Britain between 1990 and 1995 over 345,000 households with a mortgage (many with dependent children), containing some one million individuals, were subject to mortgage possession (Wilcox 1996: 139). Currently an additional 900 or so households lose their homes in this way every week. In addition to this, mortgage arrears remain at historically high levels. Although levels peaked in 1991, at the end of 1995 there were still some 85,000 households with mortgage arrears of more than twelve months, almost 127,000 with arrears of between six and twelve months, and almost 178,000 with arrears of between three and six months (Wilcox 1996: 139). These aggregated figures are problematic in a number of ways (Ford *et al.* 1995), not least because they do not reveal the complex patterns of mortgage indebtedness experienced by individual households over time. Recent survey work shows the extent to which mortgagors face financial difficulties with their mortgages but manage to pay, as well as the variety of missed payment patterns that contribute to the arrears figures. They also provide information on the incidence as well as the stock of arrears at any one time. Using the five-year period between 1991 and 1994, Ford *et al.* (1995) have shown that roughly one in five home buyers had been 'at risk' (in terms of either financial difficulties or missed payments) during the period considered: 3 per cent had no current arrears but had previous arrears; 3 per cent were having difficulties paying and had arrears previously; 1 per cent were in arrears again, having cleared previous arrears; 1 per cent had been in arrears for the whole of the period under consideration; 3 per cent had fallen into arrears for the first time in the last three years; and 9 per cent had no arrears over the period but had current payment difficulties.

Like inequalities or 'variations' in health, mortgage indebtedness is strongly socially patterned, and the distribution of risks is the subject of extensive calculation and discussion (Burrows 1997a). Further, it can be shown that patterns of indebtedness are strongly correlated with poor subjective well-being and increased use of primary health-care services, even after controlling for physical health and a range of relevant socio-economic variables (Nettleton and Burrows 1998). This association between problematic home-ownership and mental health problems should come as no surprise. If secure owner occupation invokes ontological security, insecure home-ownership invokes ill health.

In his recent book *Family Connections*, David Morgan (1996) has suggested that home-ownership is as important as it is because it confers identity and may act as a marker of social status:

> The idea of property points both to a location in physical and social space and to an individual or family project which is increasingly bound up with individual identity … To have a 'good' address and to be a home-owner is to make certain kinds of status claims which reflect on one's own sense of personal worth or achievement and often upon the identities of those to whom one is associated.
>
> (Morgan 1996:180)

If entering owner occupation confers such status, it is perhaps not surprising that those people who have difficulties keeping up with their payments often experience feelings of worthlessness and lack of self-esteem (Nettleton and Burrows 1998). For these people home-ownership has not resulted in ontological security. On the contrary, they are more likely to be ontologically insecure, as the fear of losing one's home may disrupt one's feelings of biographical continuity, may sensitise one to possible risks, and may lead one to question one's own self-integrity.

Of course the majority of home-owners do keep up with their mortgage payments and do not have their homes repossessed. However, the spectacle of repossessions, negative equity and growing job insecurity may impact upon everyone's sense of security. It is possible that a rise in mortgage arrears and repossession may invoke a wider sense of unease amongst home-owners, especially at a time of substantial economic and employment restructuring.

Following on from the point quoted from Pat Carlen towards the beginning of this chapter (Carlen 1996: 80), this insecurity is made especially concrete in the social imagery of street homelessness.[5] The problem of homelessness is deeply emblematic of the sort of society we have become. Although not routinely articulated by the lay public in the periodising language of postmodernity, the spectacle of street homelessness certainly invokes a deep feeling of unease about the way we live today. What could better epitomise the end of the modernist project than the pre-modern conditions of existence experienced by so many people who are homeless? Surely it is only under conditions of postmodernity that the obscene juxtaposition of street homelessness and hyperdynamic technological developments could occur within such close proximity? Surely it is only under conditions of post-modernity that societies able to produce the sorts of scientific and technological development we now witness on an almost daily basis are, at the same time, seemingly unable to provide for the most basic needs – shelter, warmth, food – of substantial numbers of 'citizens'? (See Burrows 1997b; Davis 1992; Lash and Urry 1994.) Is not the policy response to homelessness indicative of the postmodern thesis that contemporary discourses are exhausted? It is not only postmodern cultural artefacts (architecture, music, art, novels, cinema and so on) which now so often appear as tired rehashes of older, originally more vibrant, elements. The same also appears to be the case in the fields of politics and social policy (Gibbins 1989). Somehow we now seem powerless at the level of social policy to address even basic human needs. It is as if we have become so embroiled in the complexities of social and cultural life, and so dominated by individualistic discourses, that the recognition of real need has become obscured. Surely it can only be under postmodern conditions that policy interventions based upon providing more affordable and decent housing could have become almost unthinkable (Burrows *et al.* 1997)?

CONCLUSION: INSECURITY, REFLEXIVITY AND RISK – A RECIPE FOR AN UNHEALTHY SOCIETY?

We have argued that, in a society which appears to be increasingly uncertain, individuals are encouraged to make lifestyle choices and life-planning decisions. Such choices and decisions are increasingly made in relation to our health and welfare due to the retrenchment of state provision. They impact upon our sense of self and, in turn, how we can relate to others. For example, as we have seen, whilst we may recognise that our lifestyle choices and life-planning decisions may at once enhance the life chances of ourselves and diminish the life chances of others, the marketisation of welfare makes it increasingly difficult to act in ways which benefit the collective good. There is a correspondent transformation in the nature of social values which makes it increasingly difficult to care. This transformation has been effectively described by researchers working on the political economy of health inequalities, in the work of Richard Wilkinson (1996) in particular. In his book *Unhealthy Societies* Wilkinson argues that:

> Increasingly we live in what might be called a 'cash and keys' society. Whenever we leave the confines of our own homes we face the world with the two perfect symbols of the nature of social relations on the street. Cash equips us to take part in transactions mediated by the market, while keys protect our private gains from each other's envy and greed ... Although we are all wholly dependent on one another for our livelihoods, this interdependence is turned from being a social process into a process by which we fend for ourselves in an attempt to wrest a living from an asocial environment. Instead of being people with whom we have bonds and share common interests, others become rivals, competitors for jobs, for houses, for space, seats on the bus, parking places ... We feel hurt, angry, belittled, annoyed and sometimes superior as the processes of social distinction and social exclusion thread their way between us.
>
> (Wilkinson 1996: 226)

Drawing on social, psychological and physiological research, Wilkinson argues throughout his book that the mechanisms which link social inequalities to health and well-being may not only be those associated with material disadvantage. Rather health, well-being and the overall quality of life may be linked to social cohesion and a social fabric which is in a sound condition. To the extent that reflexivity and risk continue to mark contemporary developments in social policy, we can safely predict that levels of ontological insecurity will increase and that we will shall all be poorer for it.

NOTES

1 Although our concerns here are primarily substantive, the chapter can also be read as a small attempt to contribute something to the debate about the autonomization (Featherstone 1995), or otherwise (Harvey 1989; Jameson 1984), of the 'cultural sphere' in contemporary life, in that it argues that it is impossible to disentangle changes in cultural identity from other changes which are primarily socio-economic.

2 In addition to the resources now available via the World Wide Web, recent years have also seen the development of myriad virtual communities. The notion of a virtual community refers to the use of the new information and communication technologies to link together otherwise disparate individuals by means of various forms of computer-mediated communication, such as e-mail, newsgroups, distribution lists and desktop videoconferencing systems. These virtual communities are based not on spatial proximity but on common interests. Many of these communities are organised with the express intention of providing some form of social support to members. As such, computer-mediated systems of social support provide a major new zone for the working out of reflexive self-identities (see also the chapter by Loader in this volume).

3 This issue has been explored empirically by Jordan and Redley (1994), and has

also manifested itself amongst liberal academic colleagues and Labour politicians who find it increasingly difficult to support their supposedly collectivist inclinations when it comes to making decisions about their own children's schooling.

4 This has now been partially rectified with the announcement of a Department of Health programme of research examining variations in health, which does seem to recognise the more structural determinants of health.

5 For a fictional exploration of this and some of the other themes explored in this chapter see the novel *Therapy* by David Lodge (1994).

BIBLIOGRAPHY

Armstrong, D. (1993) 'Public health spaces and the fabrication of identity', *Sociology* 27, 3: 393–410.

Beck, U. (1992) *The Risk Society*, London: Sage.

Beck, U. and Beck-Gernsheim, E. (1996) 'Individualization and precarious freedoms', in P. Heelas, S. Lash and P. Morris (eds) *Detraditionalization*, London: Blackwell.

Beck, U., Giddens, A. and Lash, S. (1994) *Reflexive Modernization*, Cambridge: Polity Press.

Bunton, R., Nettleton, S. and Burrows, R. (eds) (1995) *The Sociology of Health Promotion: Critical Analyses of Consumption, Lifestyle and Risk*, London: Routledge.

Burrows, R. (1997a) 'Mortgage indebtedness in England: an "epidemiology"', *Housing Studies* 12, 4.

Burrows, R. (1997b) 'Virtual culture, urban social polarisation and social science fiction', in B.D. Loader (ed.) *The Governance of Cyberspace: Politics, Technology and Global Restructuring*, London: Routledge.

Burrows, R., Pleace, N. and Quilgan, D. (eds) (1997) *Homelessness and Social Theory*, London: Routledge.

Carlen, P. (1996) *Jigsaw: A Political Criminology of Youth Homelessness*, Buckingham: Open University Press.

Castel, R. (1991) 'From dangerousness to risk', in G. Burchell, C. Gordon and P. Miller (eds) *The Foucault Effect: Studies in Governability*, Hemel Hempstead: Harvester Wheatsheaf.

Davis, M. (1992) *Beyond Blade Runner: Urban Control, the Ecology of Fear*, Westfield NJ: Open Magazine Pamphlets.

DoE (Department of the Environment) (1995) *Our Future Homes: Opportunity, Choice, Responsibility*, London: HMSO.

DoH (Department of Health) (1992) *The Health of the Nation*, London: HMSO.

Doling, J. and Ford, J. (1996) 'The new home ownership', *Environment and Planning*, 28: 157–72.

Duden, B. (1991) *The Woman Beneath the Skin: A Doctor's Patients in Eighteenth Century Germany*, Cambridge MA: Harvard University Press.

Featherstone, M. (1995) *Undoing Culture: Globalization, Postmodernism and Identity*, London: Sage.

Ford, J. (1997) 'Mortgage arrears, mortgage possessions and homelessness', in R. Burrows, N. Pleace and D. Quilgars (eds) *Homelessness and Social Policy*, London: Routledge.

Ford, J., Kempson, E. and Wilson, M. (1995) *Mortgage Arrears and Possessions: Perspectives from Borrowers, Lenders and the Courts*, London: HMSO.

Forrest, R. and Murie, A. (1994) 'Home ownership in recession', *Housing Studies* 9, 1: 55–74.

General Accident (1996) Buying your home: your guide to the finance involved.

Gibbins, J. (ed.) (1989) *Contemporary Political Culture: Politics in a Postmodern Age*, London: Sage.

Giddens, A. (1991) *Modernity and Self-Identity: Self and Society in the Late Modern Age*, Cambridge: Polity Press.

Giddens, A. (1992) *The Transformation of Intimacy: Sexuality, Love and Eroticism in Modern Society*, Cambridge: Polity Press.

Giddens, A. (1994) *Beyond Left and Right: The Future of Radical Politics*, Cambridge: Polity Press.

Greco, M. (1993) 'Psychosomatic subjects and the "duty to be well": personal agency within medical rationality', *Economy and Society* 22, 3: 357–72.

Hacking, I. (1986) 'Making up people', in T. Heller, M. Sosna and D. Wellbery (eds) *Reconstructing Individualism: Autonomy, Individuality and the Self in Western Thought*, Stanford CA: Stanford University Press.

Harvey, D. (1989) *The Condition of Postmodernity*, Oxford: Blackwell.

Hogarth, T., Elias, P. and Ford, J. (1996) *Mortgages, Families and Jobs: An Exploration of the Growth in Home Ownership in the 1980s*, Warwick: Institute for Employment Research.

Hutton, W. (1995) *The State We're In*, London: Jonathan Cape.

Jameson, F. (1984) 'Postmodernism, or the cultural logic of late capitalism', *New Left Review* 146: 53–92.

Jordan, B. and Redley, M. (1994) 'Polarisation, underclass and the welfare state', *Work, Employment and Society* 8, 1: 153–76.

Kellner, D. (1992) 'Popular culture and the construction of postmodern identity', in S. Lash and J. Friedman (eds) *Modernity and Identity*, Oxford: Blackwell.

Klein, R. (1995) *The New Politics of the NHS*, 3rd edn, London: Longman.

Lash, S. and Urry, J. (1994) *Economies of Signs and Space*, London: Sage.

Lodge, D. (1994) *Therapy*, London: Secker and Warburg.

Martin, E. (1994) *Flexible Bodies*, Boston MA: Beacon Press.

Morgan, D. (1996) *Family Connections*, Cambridge: Polity Press.

Nettleton, S. (1995) *The Sociology of Health and Illness*, Cambridge: Polity Press.

Nettleton, S. (1997) 'Governing the risky self: how to become healthy, wealthy and wise', in A. Petersen and R. Bunton (eds) *Foucault, Health and Medicine*, London: Routledge.

Nettleton, S. and Burrows, R. (1998) 'Home ownership, insecurity and health in the UK', in A. Petersen and C. Waddell (eds) *Health Matters*, Sydney: Allen and Unwin.

Ogden, J. (1995) 'Psychosocial theory and the creation of the risky self', *Social Science and Medicine* 40, 3: 409–15.

O'Malley, P. (1992) 'Risk, power and crime prevention', *Economy and Society* 21, 3: 252–75.

Pahl, R. (1995) *After Success: Fin-de-Siècle Anxiety and Identity*, Cambridge: Polity Press.

Petersen, A. (1996) 'Risk and the regulated self: the discourse of health promotion as politics of uncertainty', *Australian and New Zealand Journal of Sociology* 32, 1: 44–57.

Saunders, P. (1990) *A Nation of Home Owners*, London: Unwin Hyman.

Skolbekken, J. (1995) 'The risk epidemic in medical journals', *Social Science and Medicine* 40, 3: 291–305.

Wilcox, S. (1996) *Housing Review 1996/97*, York: Joseph Rowntree Foundation.

Wilkinson, R. (1996) *Unhealthy Societies: The Afflictions of Inequality*, London: Routledge.

Part IV

Governance and new technologies of control in the new social policy

Chapter 11

Thriving on chaos?

Managerialisation and social welfare

John Clarke

INTRODUCTION

Like all other texts produced under the sign of postmodernity, this is a necessarily idiosyncratic approach to examining the contemporary state of welfare. It addresses the issues of postmodernity and postmodernism through a concern with the analysis of processes of managerialisation in the remaking of the relationship between the state and social welfare.

DISCERNING POSTMODERNITY

Given the pace and scope of change in welfare states since the late 1970s, is it possible to identify features of those changes that could be described as postmodern? I want to sketch an answer to that question that suggests a number of discernibly postmodern elements in the contemporary state of welfare in Britain. For the purposes of this chapter, I have focused on five main strands.

The first would be the break-up or fragmentation of the welfare state itself. With the retreat from direct public provision, the introduction of marketised relations, the elaboration of agency structures for some services, the creation of client/contractor or purchaser/provider distinctions, the notion of an integrated or monolithic state form cannot be sustained. For some, this shift has marked the emergence of 'post-bureaucratic' organisational forms in both corporate and state structures (see Hoggett 1994). Whether or not this designation is the most appropriate, it is clear that the structural arrangements of the state through which social welfare is organised and directed – if not provided – have shifted away from the bureau-professional integrated hierarchies which characterised the postwar British welfare state.

The second transitional feature to be highlighted might best be described as the movement away from 'universalist' social provision. This shift is itself multidimensional. Sometimes it is associated with demands or challenges from social groups and movements for the creation, development, expansion or reformation of social welfare. At others it appears in the form of more individualist or consumerist innovations in service conception and delivery, which place a higher value on adaptation to diversity of need or circumstance. It might be suggested that such a transition is also reflected in – or refracted through – the emergence of professional or intellectual discourses addressing 'postuniversalist' issues or the problems of the intersection of diversity, difference and particularism in the provision of social welfare (for example, Williams 1992, 1996).

The third dimension of change susceptible to postmodernist reading relates to the decline of traditional forms of authority. While this has generally referred to the growing detachment of social subjects from the political and institutional arrangements of modernity (and their grand narratives), one might take the mixture of distrust of, distancing from, and challenges to forms of professional authority institutionalised within the welfare state as a distinct case of this phenomenon. At stake here are both the specific powers of professional domains, which have come under threat from a variety of directions, and the wider aura of social deference historically associated with professional (or even semi-professional) status. One might point to the processes of dedifferentiation that have diminished the claimed distinctiveness of welfare professionalism in particular as significant features of this decline (see du Gay 1996: ch. 8). The organisational subordination of such professional practices and claims to the logics of markets, contracts, customer service or external audit has simultaneously challenged their base of social and occupational authority.

In some respects, the decline of traditional authority might be seen to overlap with the fourth transitional feature: the abandonment of conceptions of social progress or improvement through the agency of the welfare state. The idea of progress is widely viewed as one of the fatalities of the transition to postmodernity, and its connections with the development of the welfare state are integral and intimate ones. Certainly the postwar welfare state has been viewed – in Britain at least – as both evidence of progress and the institutional form through which further progress could – and would – be accomplished. Consequently, the breaking up of the institutionalised forms of progress and the agencies of social expertise expected to ensure its accomplishment defines a particularly condensed moment in the crisis of modernity.

The fifth and final transitional feature involves the articulation of these other elements in the discourse of social policy as an academic/intellectual formation. One might argue that it now bears the marks of these changes imploding into the structure of the field, dislocating the foundational assumptions about history as progress, about the integral relationship between the state and welfare, and about the social composition of the public embodied in ideas of social improvement. These identify the 'internal' elements of a dislocated and uncertain social policy: those elements which arise in the intersection of social policy as a specific field of academic practice and the socio-political formations of the welfare state itself. There are, of course, other elements that can be discerned in the intellectual instabilities of contemporary social policy; in particular, the 'leakages' from other disciplinary formations.

All of these – and more – might be adduced to an analysis of a postmodern relationship between welfare and the state in which the dominance of processes of dislocation, disintegration and differentiation could be identified. But it is precisely this form of plausibility which makes the appearance of postmodernity and postmodernism so frustratingly elusive. The first strand concerns the instantiation of postmodernity. It is possible – and tempting – to tag a trend, change or phenomenon with the label 'postmodern'. In doing so, one treats it as exemplifying a particular feature or tendency of postmodernity. This involves producing a symptomology: an exercise of tracing the manifestations of postmodernity. Here is a collapse of traditional authority; there a multiplication or fragmentation of social identities. This treats postmodernity as a historical condition which is manifested in its epiphenomenal forms.[1]

In the process, the issues of how to conduct the analysis and explanation of what might be called sub-epochal transitions appear to get lost. To put this another way, if the disintegrative processes that have characterised the remaking of the relationship between welfare and the state are not the effects of the postmodernisation of the welfare state, then what are they? If the changing relationships between 'the public' and the authority of welfare bureau-professionals are not merely an example of the decline of traditional authority, then how are we to understand what has happened to the forms of power and authority associated with social welfare? These questions – and others like them – appear absent from the emerging arguments about postmodernity. However, they are also not exactly the heartland of conventional social policy analysis. What follows is addressed to the sense that there may be more to life than a choice between becoming postmodern or remaining locked within a conventional disciplinary paradigm.

THE PROBLEMS OF MANAGERIALISATION

Here I want to use the work I have been doing with others on processes of managerialisation in social welfare to reflect on some of the issues and problems that need to be addressed in making sense of the contemporary relationship between the state and welfare (Clarke *et al.* 1994; Clarke and Newman 1997). I have used this rather ungainly phrase rather than saying 'the welfare state' for a number of reasons. The first, and most mundane, is the problem of empirically identifying such an object when what is being referred to is a political and ideological institutionalisation – a public reference point. The second reason for doing so is that it allows attention to be focused on the fact that recent changes have involved the remaking of what social welfare means and the form of the state in Britain – and the relationship between these two. In trying to think through this multifaceted set of changes, a number of themes have recurred.

One is the problem of how to hold on to the analysis of specific national formations in what is now widely understood to be a global or globalised political economy. This issue has particular salience given that postmodernity – like post-Fordism before it – is represented as wrapped up with globalising processes, particularly those of new communicative integration and disintegration. But it also bears heavily on the place of managerialism in restructuring. Some observers have suggested that a 'new public management' is an international, if not global, phenomenon to be found in most places where the relationships between the state, the public and public services are being reconstructed. In this, they reflect the globalising, or at least imperialist, logic of managerialism itself, which proclaims itself as the universally applicable solution to the problems of inefficiency, incompetence and chaos that characterise the old ways of providing public services (see Osborne and Gaebler 1992, for example). Nevertheless, some rather significant national differences continue to exist in terms of political conceptions of the scale and scope of the state, the levels of public service, and the organisational forms through which such services may be provided. The persistence of these differences is a reminder that globalising processes need to be seen as contextual – shaping the conditions in which different national (and even sub-national) choices can be made. One striking feature of managerialism's relation to social welfare is that 'globalisation' exists as both a material and a discursive condition for change. The changing – and more globalised – context of the UK has shaped its political economy and its political choices but it has also appeared as a legitimating discourse within those choices – explaining the need for changes ranging from privatisation to new management systems or even accounting practices in public services. Change itself is constituted as desirable or necessary as a result of globalisation (Newman and Clarke 1996).

If restructuring is not simply the nationally experienced effect of global changes, there are other problems about how to make sense of the forms it has taken – in particular the processes of managerialisation that have been central to the British experience. One strong tendency within recent social policy analysis has been to treat these changes as the direct result of a specific political-ideological formation: the new right, neo-liberalism and its incarnation in the Conservative Party and governments of the 1980s and 1990s (see, for example, Deakin 1994; Hill 1993). Depending on the weight given to specific party political arrangements, this attention to politics and ideology ranges from an internationalist to a national level of analysis. For example, the stress on neo-liberalism has drawn attention to transnational processes, politics and institutions, whether in the interchange of personnel and ideas in the neo-liberal intelligentsia and think tanks or in the institutionalisation of neo-liberal economic thought in supranational institutions such as the World

Bank. Although this stress rightly emphasises the spread of neo-liberalism, it risks underestimating the complexity of specific national politics – not least in those settings where neo-liberalism has been combined with neo-conservatism (for example, the USA and Britain). In such contexts, it is more difficult to trace a simple acting out of a pristine neo-liberal agenda, and there is also a temptation to force an intellectual unity on the reforms introduced by particular national governments. One part of the legacy of 'Thatcherism' in Britain (and the Reagan era in the USA) has been the unstable mix of neo-liberal approaches to economic and political reform with strongly neo-conservative views of social and moral issues.

For us, though, this view of politically driven reform has had one particular limitation in trying to make sense of the role and place of managerialism. There has been a danger of submerging the specificity of managerialism as an ideological formation and social project within the attention to the new right. Managerialism then appears as a mere 'tool' or proxy of new right politics for enacting the reform of the welfare state. This seems inappropriate in at least two respects. On the one hand, it loses the active contribution of managerialism to the project of state restructuring – the ideological naturalisation of organisational reconstruction; the articulation of modes of organisational power and calculation that have displaced bureau-professionalism as the operating logics of public service organisations; and the creation of dispersed systems of organisational interrelationship and control.

On the other hand, and at the same time, an understanding of managerialism as a distinct and separate formation also enables attention to the instabilities associated with the process of reconstruction. Of course, there are a number of sources of instability: the contradictions within the new right; the persistent social tensions associated with social welfare; and the problems of accommodating to the Thatcherite legacy (Hay 1996). But managerialism adds its own dynamic to these instabilities. Managerialism is an imperialist formation, seeking the enhancement or enlargement of the 'right to manage'. As such it carries a critique of the failings of other claims to power. Whilst this has been primarily directed at the 'old regime' of welfare bureau-professionalism, it is also extended to the failings of political rule. Political rule too readily involves 'interference' in operational matters, is prone to tactical manoeuvring rather than being 'strategic', and too often fails to understand the 'realities of the business'. In the Prison Service and the NHS in particular, it is already possible to see managerialism turning on its political allies, demanding more freedom to manage and less interference from government. More and better management will solve the problems caused by introducing managerialised processes. The intrinsic dynamics of managerialism as a social formation are lost if one treats it solely as the agent of new right politics, rather than as a (possibly junior) partner in an alliance for the reform of the state.

This leads to a related issue about how to characterise the changing form of the state that has emerged from these reforms. We have ended up describing the reconfiguration of the state form as involving 'dispersal' rather than the more widely used (and post-Fordist-derived) idea of 'fragmentation'. Dispersal is a way of signalling such processes as the effect of strategic calculation rather than inevitable occurrences. These are processes through which agency – the power to act – is being distributed from and by a strategic centre. The state delegates its authority to act in specified ways to subaltern organisations. Dispersal does not carry the intrinsically disintegrative connotations of fragmentation. The relations of power that both underpin and act through the processes of dispersal are foregrounded as a result. This stress on the 'relations of power' means that it is necessary to examine not just what sorts of power are 'held' in different places but also what the flows of power are that allocate positions and places in this field. It also means thinking about the power flows involved in enforcing and monitoring the exercise of such delegated agency.

Dispersal as a strategy of reconstruction has had a number of objectives. It aims to either bypass or discipline the old institutional sediments of state organisational power – the 'bureau-professional' organisations of the welfare state. It has subjected them to forms of power dispersed *beyond* them to the citizen as consumer and to new forms of control from the centre through both fiscal discipline and methods of evaluation. It has also tried to recruit them to the exercise of 'self-discipline' through the internalisation of financial and performance targets. Finally, each organisational 'agency' has been repositioned in a field of forces. The vertical axis aligns agencies as delegated authorities between the centralised power of the nation state and the 'consumer' power of the periphery, while also subjecting them to more rigorous forms of financial and performance evaluation. The horizontal axis characteristically repositions them in a nexus of marketised or quasi-competitive relationships. Within this field of forces agencies are typically given the 'freedom to manage' (Birchall *et al.* 1995).

The 'freedom to manage' is a reminder that the dominant organisational agency, and the practical ideology, of this dispersal is managerialism. Managerialism represents the intra- and interorganisational mode of coordination that 'makes sense' of such dispersed power in a practical way. Managerialism is presented as the 'cement' that can hold together this dispersed organisational form of the state and, in its 'customer' orientation, claims to be able to represent and service an individuated 'public'. Managerialised relations aim to provide the 'discipline' necessary for efficient organisation, particularly in relation to the claims of welfare professionalism for discretionary authority. Managerialism articulates a new basis for 'discretion' as attached to a managerial rather than professional calculus – and expressed in the claim to be given the freedom to 'do the right thing' (Clarke and Newman 1993).

The effect of these changes has been to leave old professional or service discourses marginalised – in the condition of being 'lost for words'. The old languages have lost some of their purchase on organisational realities and their capacity to mobilise power and resources. That sense of loss is intensified by the fluidity of managerial discourse in its attempts to stake out the high moral ground of organisational command. Who can deny that organisational commitments to efficiency or quality are desirable objectives? This is probably best manifested in the Peters-and-Waterman-derived demand that we 'learn to love change' – a clarion call that has been taken up across the public services. Being 'against change' is a rather difficult discursive position to occupy, especially when the urgency of organisational change is legitimated by reference to the pace and scale of change in the turbulent 'external environment' (as evidenced in the opening paragraphs of any strategic plan). To be a 'conservative' (or resister) in such circumstances carries the risk of being identified as outmoded, defending elite or sectional interests, being against progress, or threatening the future of the organisation. The fluidity of the discourse of change is an essential precondition of its deployment as a discursive tactic, since any particular change is subject to a process of elision with the (epochal) need for change. Managerialism is intent on promoting the promiscuity of 'learning to love change' (or at least a condition of serial monogamy, since another corporate initiative will soon replace the last one in employees' affections).

But this inspirational and affective discourse of management is overlaid on a harder base of organisational rationalism. The rationalism of managerialism provides a non-partisan (and depoliticised) framework within which choices can be made. Competing values are reduced to alternative sets of options and costs and assessed against their contribution to the organisation's performance. They are subjected to a rational analysis which claims to stand outside and beyond the partisan claims of different 'interest groups'. While different professional or occupational groups may pursue their parochial interests, management represents the organisation's best interests (for example, see Green and Armstrong's (1995) discussion of 'bed management'). The calculative technologies of managerialism thus provide a foundation for enacting the new logics of rationing, targeting and priority setting. Its quantitative and evaluative technologies form the basis for the new roles of contracting, audit and regulation. The scientific knowledges which they deploy position managers as neutral and impersonal. Managers can be trusted: they are not part of the war between different political and occupational interests.

The rational/technical character of managerial knowledge offers the promise of resolving two different forms of 'chaos'. The first is the chaos of the old regime – the irrationality of unmanaged systems in which the decision making of 'street-level bureaucrats' cannot be controlled, and in which bureaucratic control mechanisms proliferate seemingly stupid and irrational systems of rules which get in the way of effectiveness (Peters 1987).

Managerialism represents a way of imposing a rationalised order on this chaos. The second promise of managerialism is that of coping with the complexities and uncertainties of the modern world – the 'chaos of the new' – through the quasi-scientific techniques of strategic management and the delivery of fast-paced change and innovation. Where bureaucracies adapt slowly and in a rather ramshackle fashion, creating new rules and functions to cope with new situations within a framework of getting by and making do, managerialism promises to organise the irrational within a rational framework.

I think it is arguable whether the ability of managerialism to transform the world of social welfare effectively is reflected in a capacity to produce new subjects. This is a rather tricky issue, since it is difficult to establish how one would know if such subjects were being constituted in practice. But I do want to insist that there are some problems attached to simply reading them off from the discourse itself. It is, of course, possible to find the bearers of the new managerialism, in both its trained products and its enthusiastic converts across welfare organisations. It is equally possible to find those who use the discourse conditionally or calculatingly – performing compliance. Finally, it is possible to see those who 'do not believe a word of it' but whose behaviour is nevertheless constrained and constructed by its institutional embeddedness. Indeed, I am tempted to argue that what is most striking about the impact of managerialism is its ability to produce behavioural compliance at the same time as inducing scepticism, cynicism and disbelief. There is a difference between being subjected to a discourse and becoming a subject through it.

A rather different way of thinking about the success of the managerialist discourse is to consider how it has accomplished the TINA effect: 'There is no alternative.' This means paying attention to the transformations in the fields of relationships, processes and practices in which welfare work is embedded and not merely to the field of representations of them. The reworking of organisational regimes, the conditions of interorganisational relationships, the architecture of power within and between them, the preferred modes of calculation and control, and the allocation of resources create a new terrain in which people behave in an increasingly managerialised fashion. They compete for contracts, engage in decentralised decision making, prepare business plans and interact with customers because those are the logics of the organisational and interorganisational field of relationships (see also Hoggett 1996).

The combination of dispersal and managerialised co-ordination in a new state form has established the basis for a potential new political consensus about social welfare and the place of the state. The elementary forms of mixed economies, markets and managers are installed as a paradigm of 'delivering welfare' within which political manoeuvring can take place. The creation of a 'welfare pluralism' involving multiple sectors, primarily linked by contracting mechanisms, forms the basis for a new consensus (Rao 1996).

The importance of 'well-managed organisations' in making this new order work is taken for granted. The basic forms of this political–economic settlement have led Hay to conclude that we are seeing the revival of what used to be called 'managerial politics' – the competition between parties about who can best manage British capitalism (1996: ch. 8). For reasons that will become obvious, we would want to suggest that what is emerging is better described as a *managerialised politics*. This indicates that the promise by governments to 'manage the economy' means something very different in the 1990s to what it did in the 1950s and 1960s. But more importantly, the phrase 'managerialised politics' designates the changed relationships between government, the state and welfare in the 1990s and the distinctive role being played by managerialism within those new relationships. The emergent consensus includes the widespread commitment that government needs to draw on the new managerial techniques and technologies.

The problems which the managerial state is intended to resolve derive from contradictions and conflicts in the political, economic and social realms. But what we have seen is the managerialisation of these contradictions: they are redefined as 'problems to be managed'. Terms such as 'efficiency' and 'effectiveness', 'performance' and 'quality' depoliticise a series of social issues (whose efficiency? effectiveness for whom?) and thus displace real political and policy choices into a series of managerial imperatives. As a consequence, we can see a trend towards major social contradictions and conflicts being experienced at the front line of service-delivery organisations. This is uncomfortable for those working there, but more importantly it points to the limitations of the capacity of new organisational regimes to cope with these problems. This incapacity is most serious in terms of how far the new regime can provide an institutional form for rearticulating the relationship between state and citizens. The instabilities, gaps and legitimacy problems that both led to and resulted from the demise of the social democratic state cannot be resolved in this way. Where champions of the managerial state have celebrated its dynamism, our analysis leads us to a different view. What we see are the instabilities of a form of state that cannot reconcile the social contradictions and conflicts of contemporary Britain within a managerial calculus.

We have not been convinced that it is possible to capture these sorts of shift in concepts of change that operate in terms of the 'from/to' dualisms that currently dominate much of the literature (such as from Fordist to post-Fordist, or from hierarchies to markets). I confess that I feel a similar reluctance to see such changes being submerged by a 'modernity to postmodernity' conceptualisation. I have written elsewhere (Clarke 1996) about the problems of forcing history into binary distinctions articulated around the prefix 'post', not least the travesties that come to represent that which was pre-the-post. In this context, though, I want to approach the arrival of postmodernism in social policy in a rather different way.

AVOIDING THE POMO WARS

One reason for retracing some of these issues about assessing managerialism's place in the remaking of the relationship between the state and welfare is that they stake out a field of problems and set of approaches which refuse to fit the modernist/postmodernist distinction. Indeed, one possible reaction to the previous section is to dismiss it as an incoherent mish-mash of irreconcilable ideas drawn from all over the place – where Gramsci sits uncomfortably alongside Foucault; ideology alongside discourse; structuralist concepts alongside poststructuralist ones and so on. Of course, I prefer to think of it as a developing theoretical repertoire which enables the exploration of different levels of analysis and facets of complex social processes. Nevertheless, I find this set of concerns extremely difficult to reconcile with a theoretical terrain mapped and defined in terms of postmodernism. This difficulty causes me a more general concern about the prospect of social policy as an intellectual area entering a period of 'pomo warfare'. It is difficult to see whether the rather delayed entry of social policy into these struggles is an advantage or a disadvantage. One might hope that it is possible to learn lessons from elsewhere, but if the experience of other domains provides any guide, we can now expect the symbolic or discursive equivalent of trench warfare.

It is already possible to see the beginnings of the earthworks (for example, Hillyard and Watson 1996; Penna and O'Brien 1996; Taylor-Gooby 1994, 1995) where the protagonists begin to dig into defined sites: postmodernists over here; modernists over there. This forms the basis for the classical war of position, with the opponents moving slowly backwards and forwards over the contested terrain: at one point, a yard gained by a ferocious assault on historicism; at another, a futile sortie into enemy-held concepts. From these entrenched locations we can start to lob theoretical shells into one another's positions (25-lb lumps of highly explosive epistemology), and to string out the barbed-wire traps and lay the philosophical minefields into which the opposition will witlessly wander. It will, I hope, be clear that I do not regard this as a very attractive prospect. Once the trenches have been dug and the positions defined, the categories have an alarming tendency to take on a life of their own, so that people are required to announce themselves and their allegiances. Are you now or have you ever been a modernist? The accusatory echoes of previous engagements can be heard: are you an essentialist, a humanist, a structuralist?

While it may be true that (in a postmodernist sense, at least) there are no innocent victims, the tendency to bifurcate positions and enforce these divisions usually implies getting people to sign up for one or the other side. It is, I think, something to be resisted for practical, theoretical and epistemological reasons. Epistemologically, it no longer makes sense to construct a world which is constituted by and through essentialist binary distinctions.

Theoretically, social policy is already unstable – its one-time Fabian core has been eroded, undermined, invaded in multiple ways from different directions.[2] It has become more difficult to discern what the core of social policy now is, in that many of the old foundational assumptions were already displaced or decentred before the emergence of postmodernism. Some of those dislocations are the result of the internal challenges – about subject matter, methodology, theory and politics – but they are also the effect of the new right assault on the welfare state itself, since above all the fortunes of social policy as an academic field appeared to be inextricably bound up with the rise and development of the state's welfare role. The effectiveness of the new right in remaking the relationship between the state and welfare has been at the heart of the intellectual crisis of confidence of Fabian-influenced social policy. The range of political and intellectual shocks and assaults to which Fabianism has been subjected in the last two decades sometimes make me feel that adding to it is like bear-baiting.

But if social policy is already more – and less – than its old conventional heartland, over what is the postmodernist battle to be fought? In part, it will surely be a battle of travesties, reflecting Kate Soper's caricatures of the 'dogged metaphysicians' and 'feline ironists' (1993: 19), transcribed into social policy settings. One of the frustrations of the pomo wars elsewhere has been precisely the combination of splitting and caricaturing of positions, forcing them to fit the binary distinction. In some respects, being an 'applied' social science seems to make social policy more vulnerable to this process. If the experience of a previous 'post' – post-Fordism – is anything to go by, we tend to get simplified appropriations of highly contested arguments from elsewhere. I have a suspicion that this reflects a view that social policy academics should not be asked to cope with difficult or challenging thoughts on the grounds that they are not real social scientists! It will be clear that I would really rather be somewhere else instead of trying to find my way out of this potential wasteland. My escape route, at least for the purposes of this chapter, is to suggest that the sign 'postmodernism' misrepresents or misrecognises a cluster of changes that have already taken place within social policy, and in doing so externalises them as something we should discover.

THE CULTURAL TURN IN SOCIAL POLICY?

Perhaps the most significant cluster of changes in social policy has already taken place around what might be described as a 'cultural turn'. By this I mean to refer to the rather diverse sources of interest in the cultural, ideological, discursive or symbolic formations of social welfare. While there has always been a strand within social policy that has addressed the topic of ideology, this has tended to be in the form of ideology conceived of as a relatively systematic body of politically oriented ideas which have, to a greater or lesser extent, influenced the development of social welfare (Clarke *et al.*

1987; George and Wilding 1976). By contrast, the cultural turn in social policy has addressed the realm of ideology as involving the implicit social assumptions as well as explicit ideological conceptions that have informed the social character of welfare provision. At different times – and using different theoretical means – the class, gendered, familial, racialised, disabling and heterosexualised tendencies of welfare policies and practices have been explored. What most of these have had in common is the intellectual practice of deconstructing the naturalising effects of particular ideological formations and the consequent revelation of the social – rather than natural – relations that are produced or reproduced through ideologies.

Of course, at this point it is important to register the diversity of intellectual resources that have shaped this development. The cultural turn marks the combined effects of a number of different theoretical and methodological strands: structuralist Marxism, particularly in the Althusserian conception of ideology; a pre-structuralist Marxism expressed in the Gramscian concerns with both hegemony and the contradictoriness of 'common sense'; post-structuralist approaches to the arbitrary and conventionalised productive power of language; the Foucauldian excavation of epistemes and discourses together with the knowledge–power relations embedded in them; and the legacy of phenomenological and symbolic interactionist approaches to social construction, particularly in the sociology of deviance. All of these contributed to the anti-empiricist shift in social policy (and the social sciences more widely), symbolised in the epidemic rash of quotation marks that indicate the recognition that the term 'word' is itself a social construct with a provisional and fragile claim to social truth. Social policy has been hugely enriched by this shift and the systematic denormalisation of welfare policy and practice that it has enabled. But the cultural turn does not belong to a specific theoretical, epistemological or even political tendency, and claims about its postmodernist or poststructuralist unity need to be resisted.

One central strand in the cultural turn has been the insistence on the fluidity or plasticity of social arrangements, particularly in explicit contrast to the fixity attributed to 'natural' differences. The socially constructed character of particular sets of norms, relations, differences has become a recurrent thread in the analysis of welfare policies and their institutional expressions. Although there are good reasons – both intellectually and politically – for emphasising the fluid/plastic quality of social constructions, there are points at which I would prefer to see the attention to fluidity tempered with a concern with what might be called solidification. The capacity of words, meanings, constructions and identities to be fluid or polyvalent has emerged as a central understanding within the 'cultural turn' – and is a central tenet of postmodernist epistemologies. Nevertheless, there is a question about how some meanings or constructions take on socially solidified forms, why some differences rather than others become socially valorised, and why some norms become empowered as truth. Fluidity, plasticity and polyvalency identify capacities or potentialities rather than a permanent state of social flux. Rather than polyvalency, many social constructions are characterised by their everyday solidity – their passage into common sense as truth. As usual, managerialism provides a rich field of examples: the solidification of conceptions of efficiency; the institutionalisation of separated, individuated and competitive 'businesses' within fields of public service; and the eternal desirability of change. As examples, what they do is to raise the questions of how to grasp solidification, institutionalisation or sedimentation in examining social constructions, and how to assess the different densities attained by different formations. That is, between the extremes of absolute polyvalency and absolute solidification is a range of different densities or plasticities that social constructions may achieve (and which may have something to do with the extent to which they are contested).

Since Foucauldian analysis has done so well with the metaphor of doing 'archaeology', I would like to propose an additional, and equally metaphorical, endeavour that is needed in developing the cultural turn in social policy. I think that we need cultural geology as well as archaeology.[3] In part, this involves the work of tracing what Gramsci (1971) called the 'sediments' and 'traces' of earlier philosophies that have settled into common sense (for example, all the religious, moral and social deposits that are embedded in the idea of 'desert' in relation to poverty). But it also identifies the task of differentiating the more fluid, changeable and unstable cultural formations from the more densely compressed, socially resilient and resistant ones.

CONCLUSION

I have wanted to pursue this metaphor because of a sense that the cultural turn and the accompanying language of social construction risk giving an unreal lightness – a weightlessness – to the constructions that we find in social policy. By contrast, the geological metaphor aims to recover a sense of solidity, density or massiveness about some of these constructions because they do weigh heavily on us. Put at its crudest, social constructions become solidified into 'social facts' and social facts kill people. Poverty is certainly an ideological formation, it is a truth produced by particular discursive strategies, it is a social construction – and people die from it. One could go on and make similar points about racialised identities and their social consequences or about other forms of constructed social differences. It is those 'solidifications', those weighty social constructions, that may form the common ground between those of us produced by the 'cultural turn' and the founding social concerns of social policy as a field of study. The risk of the cultural turn (and one exacerbated by the prospect of pomo wars) is that of losing the distinctive focus of social policy, of blurring it into a generalised social science concern in which all social constructions are equally interesting objects of study.

In doing so, it might be possible to achieve a richer, more multifaceted approach to studying social policy in which we do not get locked into the security or certainty of one particular level or focus of analysis. Returning to the heartland of conventional social policy, we could perhaps reasonably expect an approach to poverty which was able to:

- count the numbers of people living in poverty (while knowing that the poverty line is itself a social and methodological artefact);
- trace the consequences of living in poverty;
- track the changing social composition of those living in poverty;
- monitor the changing economic gradients of income and wealth distribution;
- understand the ideological and discursive sources of changing policies towards poverty and their practical effects;
- grasp the socially constructed nature of poverty as an ideological formation (or discourse);
- examine the shifting alignments and articulations of ideological/discursive strategies around poverty.

Is it possible to have a social policy which can think difficult thoughts in a multifaceted way without either having a nervous breakdown or dissolving into internecine warfare?

ACKNOWLEDGEMENT

I am grateful to those with whom I have been working on managerialism over the last few years: in particular, Allan Cochrane, Eugene McLaughlin and Janet Newman. Although they have helped to shape my views about all of these issues, they are, of course, not responsible for the end product. Janet Newman suffered a particularly intense exposure to my post-phobia but is expected to make a full recovery.

NOTES

1   It also assumes a degree of stabilised agreement on how to distinguish the features or characteristics of modernity and postmodernity, but that is another – and longer – story.
2   There is also a specific point here about the national formation of intellectual fields and traditions. As a field of study, social policy has a peculiarly British quality rather than just being a product of generic or transnational modernism.
3   It will be immediately clear that I do not know anything about geology. This is not a problem given the metaphorical status of the term here, just as an absence of knowledge of archaeology has not inhibited the circulation of Foucault's metaphor.

BIBLIOGRAPHY

Birchall, I., Pollitt, C. and Putnam K. (1995) 'Freedom to manage? The experience of NHS trusts, grant-maintained schools and voluntary transfers of public housing', paper presented to UK Political Studies Association Annual Conference, York, April.

Clarke, J. (1996) 'After social work?', in N. Parton (ed.) *Social Theory, Social Change and Social Work*, London: Routledge.

Clarke, J. and Newman, J. (1993) 'The right to manage: a second managerial revolution', *Cultural Studies* 7, 3: 427–41.

Clarke, J. and Newman, J. (1997) *The Managerial State*, London: Sage.

Clarke, J., Cochrane, A. and McLaughlin, E. (eds) (1994) *Managing Social Policy*, London: Sage.

Clarke, J., Cochrane, A. and Smart, C. (1987) *Ideologies of Welfare*, London: Routledge.

Deakin, N. (1994) *The Politics of Welfare: Continuities and Change*, Hemel Hempstead: Harvester Wheatsheaf.

du Gay, P. (1996) *Consumption and Identity at Work*, London: Sage.

George, V. and Wilding, P. (1976) *Ideology and Social Welfare*, London: Routledge and Kegan Paul.

Gramsci, A. (1971) *Selections from Prison Notebooks*, London: Lawrence & Wishart.

Green, J. and Armstrong, D. (1995) 'Achieving rational management: bed management and the crisis in emergency admissions', *Sociological Review* 43, 4: 743–64.

Hay, A.C. (1996) *Re-stating Social and Political Change*, Buckingham: Open University Press.

Hill, M. (1993) *The Welfare State in Britain: A Political History since 1945*, London: Edward Elgar.

Hillyard, P. and Watson, S. (1996) 'Postmodern social policy: a contradiction in terms?', *Journal of Social Policy* 25, 3: 321–46.

Hoggett, P. (1994) 'The politics of the modernisation of the UK welfare state', in R. Burrows and B. Loader (eds) *Towards a Post-Fordist Welfare State?*, London: Routledge.

Hoggett, P. (1996) 'New modes of control in the public service', *Public Administration* 74, 1: 9–32.

Newman, J. and Clarke, J. (1996) 'The tyranny of transformation: the discourse of change in public services restructuring', paper presented to International Research Symposium on Public Services Management, University of Aston, March.

Osborne, D. and Gaebler, T. (1992) *Reinventing Government: How the Entrepreneurial Spirit is Transforming the Public Sector*, Reading MA: Addison-Wesley.

Penna, S. and O'Brien, M. (1996) 'Postmodernism and social policy: a small step forwards?', *Journal of Social Policy* 25, 1: 39–61.

Peters, T. (1987) *Thriving on Chaos: Handbook for a Management Revolution*, London: Pan.

Rao, N. (1996) *Towards Welfare Pluralism: Public Services in a Time of Change*, Aldershot: Dartmouth.

Soper, K. (1993) 'Postmodernism, subjectivity and the question of value', in J. Squires (ed.) *Principled Positions: Postmodernism and the Rediscovery of Value*, London: Lawrence & Wishart.

Taylor-Gooby, P. (1994) 'Postmodernism and social policy: a great leap backwards?', *Journal of Social Policy* 23, 3: 385–404.

Taylor-Gooby, P. (1995) 'In defence of second-best theory', paper presented to Social Policy Association Annual Conference, Sheffield, July.

Williams, F. (1992) 'Somewhere over the rainbow: universality and diversity in social policy', in N. Manning and R. Page (eds) *Social Policy Review* 4, Nottingham: Social Policy Association.

Williams, F. (1996) 'Postmodernism, feminism and the question of difference', in N. Parton (ed.) *Social Theory, Social Change and Social Work*, London: Routledge.

Chapter 12

Performativity and fragmentation in 'postmodern schooling'

Stephen J. Ball

INTRODUCTION

This chapter deploys a profane, epistemological eclecticism. It is also rather wide ranging and further it draws promiscuously from the work of three research projects in the area of education policy in an attempt at a 'grounded' analysis of some aspects of current education policy in the UK.[1]

My main concerns are:

1 to unpack and explore some of the incoherence and bricolage which characterises contemporary education policy;
2 to demonstrate how this incoherence and bricolage 'work' in schools and upon teachers;
3 to address in particular the articulation of difference and hierarchy through performativity, which provides a 'kind of diversity' and increasing fragmentation in educational provision.[2]

To forward these concerns I shall deploy concepts and ideas from both Foucault and Lyotard[3] and exemplars and illustrations from the aforementioned research studies. Contextually my discussion is located by an assertion that western societies and their education systems are not yet thoroughly postmodern[4] but are no longer simply modernist – a situation described by some writers as high modernity. The chapter assumes some knowledge of the current state of 'policy chaos' in education (see Ball 1994 for an exposition of these policies).

Barry Smart makes the point that:

> education and learning have become much more subject to the demands of system performance, more oriented towards the provision of 'training' and the inculcation of 'skills' and rather less concerned with what are increasingly denigrated as 'liberal' values and ideas.
>
> (Smart 1992: 174)

He is half right. There are shifts in the direction he indicates, and these shifts are animated by powerful discourses about what education is and is for. And some of these discourses may be seen to be symptomatic of 'the postmodern condition'; but as Lyotard puts it: 'I have said and will say again that "post-modern" signifies not the end of modernism, but another relation to modernism' (Lyotard 1984: 277). Education policy in the UK and other western societies, at all levels, displays a complex, fluctuating disarray of policy strategies, political projects and desires, which are popular and incoherent, totalising and individualising, homogenising and fragmenting.[5] What we refer to as education policy is an ensemble of metapolicies which cannibalise and collate bits of other policies in response to the ebb and flow of public panics, inconsistent research, fashion, expedience and blind hopefulness. This contributes to 'a ... turmoil of understandable nostalgia, crippling indecision, and bewildering prospect' (Nisbet 1980: 329) around educational issues. Education policy has a particular relation to panic and nostalgia. Some policy discourses become possible in response to panic others sustain themselves by constituting panic, around the concerns which they bring into play. As Kroker *et al.* note, panic is 'the key psychological mood of postmodern culture' (Kroker *et al.* 1989: 13). One particularly interesting example of this, and of the incoherence and perversity of policy discourses, is the political press for and responses to 'raising standards' in education. In recent years the UK government has both celebrated the raising of standards in schools, as indicated by increasing percentage pass rates at GCSE, and at the same time condemned these improved pass rates as indicating 'declining standards' in the marking of the examinations. Education policy texts are littered with contradictory tactics and meanings, with notions like control and operativity commonly deployed on the one hand, as against autonomy, 'natural' economic processes and choice on the other.

None the less, it is possible to provide a certain 'logic' to this incoherence, and to 'map' the disarray and tensions which are evident in the education policy ensemble, by considering the political, symbolic and economic purposes which are attributed to and enmesh education (and teachers) at the point of transition from modern to postmodern conditions in western societies, and which relate back to the contemporary problems of the state. This mapping also points up the complexity of the overdetermining paraphernalia of governmentality in play in the field of education. This overdetermination is indicative, I suggest, of the key role of the teacher (and education) in the nexus of change from modern to postmodern conditions, occupying, as they do, an unstable position at the intersection between family, politics and the economy.

In relation to the family, education in late modernity is both an agency of normalisation and a commodity of choice; the education market offers parents an opportunity to choose, although for some there is a significant gap between making and getting a choice. Within this market parents are interpolated and inscribed as competitive consumers (acting in the self-interest of their family and child, seeking social advantage), and the processes and skills of choice play an important part in constituting a model of 'good parenting' (Gewirtz *et al.* 1995). In relation to the economy, education is expected to provide particular and general skills required by capital and to graduate students who are 'fit for work' in a whole variety of ways. More generally, the effectivity of the education system is taken to be one basis of the competitiveness of the national economy in the global marketplace (this is another source for recurring panic around the UK's test performance in various comparative studies).[6] Performativity plays a particular role in reorientating education, educational institutions and students to the competitive needs of the economy. 'Performativity is a principle of governance which establishes strictly functional relations between a state and its inside and outside environments' (Yeatman 1994: 111). This is where Smart is correct.

It is possible to begin to see some of the instabilities and contradictions which work on and through education in the ebb and flow of the politics of the National Curriculum. In its first phase (1987–90) the National Curriculum, particularly in the key subjects of mathematics, science and technology, was driven by the affinity of interest between what I have called elsewhere vocational progressivism and new progressivism, and their 'discourse of competence and inclusion and response to change' (Ball 1990: 113). A relationship of contents, pedagogies and assessment in these subjects to post-Fordist modes of production was discernible (Rustin 1989; Ball 1990: 100–32). New progressivism, while not totally unified and coherent, 'gives emphasis to skills, processes and methods rather than content, and to applications and problem solving rather than abstract knowledge; the teacher is facilitator rather than pedagogue' (Ball 1990: 136). The learner and learning are conceptualised in constructivist terms, with the former as a unique and active meaning maker. It is not unreasonable to argue that, during this phase of curriculum reform, a new form of correspondence was being forged between the requirements of capital accumulation and the reconceptualised forms and processes of schooling. In Bernstein's terms, we were seeing a shift in the principles of social control underpinning the curriculum – a shift from collection to integration, from submission to conformity (Bernstein 1971).

In its second phase (1991–4), the National Curriculum, with a particular emphasis upon struggles around English, history and geography, and accompanied by a sustained campaign against educational progressivism, was dominated by cultural restorationism. The restorationist agenda consists of a regressive traditionalism applied to all facets of educational practice (see Ball 1993); it is a hard-line, old humanism based upon a discourse which links education strongly with traditional social and political values and with social order (Ball 1990: 24). It relies upon a cultural and moral naturalism, a lexicon of essential values, identities and meanings. It thus obscures and defies difference, heterogeneity and struggle. Struggles over class and race, over inequality and oppression are displaced by a discourse of common heritage and the classless society, and subsumed by cultural and legal tactics (as is also the case in immigration and refugee status laws) which carefully define who is a legitimate contributor to the performativity of the state.

Within all this, modernisation, restorationism and entrepreneurial schooling sit in odd and uneasy relation to one another; although there are also various indirect affinities. Taken together they inscribe into education a set of practical dilemmas and irresolvable cultural tensions in terms of what it means to be educated. They represent very different responses to 'the incredulity towards meta-narratives', as Lyotard (1984: xxiv) defines 'postmodern'. On the one hand, education is to play its part in the ideological narrative and organisational strategy of the 'enterprise culture', producing enterprising subjects and subjectivities. On the other hand, as against this, education is required to respond to a political agenda of concerns which are embedded in panic about cultural pluralism, moral uncertainty and the decline of community, by inculcating common values and encouraging a sense of national identity – pedagogic nostalgia and a simulacrumic 'Englishness' play a key role in this project of political legitimacy.

Taking this adumbrated landscape of cannibalised and incoherent policies as my backdrop, I want to consider now how these policies 'work' and 'work upon' education and teachers through what Lyotard calls 'a certain level of terror, whether soft or hard' (Lyotard 1984: xxiv). In particular, I am concerned with the terrors of performance and efficiency – performativity; 'be operational (that is, commensurable) or disappear' (Lyotard 1984: xxiv).[7]

PERFORMATIVITY AND INTENSIFICATION

Performativity 'works' in at least three ways. First, it works as a disciplinary system of judgements, classifications and targets towards which schools and teachers must strive and against and through which they are evaluated. The discourses (or 'language games', in Lyotard's terms) of 'standards' and 'quality' do important work here. The education system is subsumed within the 'quality revolution' (Kirkpatrick and Martinez-Lucio 1995; Oakland 1991). Second, as part of the transformation of education and schooling and the expansion of the power of capital, performativity provides sign systems which 'represent' education in a self-referential and reified form for consumption. And indeed many of the specific technologies of performativity in education (total quality management, human resources management, etc.) are borrowed from commercial settings. Both of these aspects of educational performativity are linked to and 'valorised' within the market form in education. Teachers are inscribed in these exercises in performativity, through the diligence with which they attempt to fulfil competing imperatives and inhabit irreconcilable subjectivities. Third, performativity also resides in the pragmatics of language. An utterance is performative in so far as 'its effect upon the referent coincides with its enunciation' (Lyotard 1984: 9). The addressee is placed within the context created by the utterance. For example, many of

the utterances of educational management and the effective schools movement have these characteristics and they exemplify the instrumental rational
orientation to institutional life. The use of assessment 'statements', the language of inspection and the discourse of 'unsatisfactory teachers' all have
enunciative effects. I want now to make some of this more specific.

Performativity, or what Lyotard also calls 'context control', is intimately
intertwined with the seductive possibilities of 'autonomy'. The 'autonomous'
subjectivity of the productive individual has become a central economic
resource, but, as Lyotard suggests, it has other attractions:

> It cannot be denied that there is a persuasive force in the idea that context
> control and domination are inherently better than their absence. The per-
> formativity criterion has its 'advantages'. It excludes in principle adherence
> to a metaphysical discourse; it requires the renunciation of fables; it
> demands clear minds and cold wills; it replaces the definition of essences
> with the calculation of interactions; it makes the 'players' assume respon-
> sibility not only for the statements they propose, but also for the rules to
> which they submit those statements in order to render them acceptable. It
> brings the pragmatic functions of knowledge clearly to light to the extent
> that they seem to relate to the criterion of efficiency: the pragmatics of
> argumentation, of the production of proof, of the transmission of learn-
> ing, and of the apprenticeship of the imagination.
>
> (Lyotard 1984: 62)

Many of the themes of the remainder of this chapter are sketched out in this
extract. Lyotard's formulation here has a particular relevance to recent UK
education policy (and public sector policy in general). Set within and a key
part of the framework of the market form in education, performativity
requires a number of significant shifts and transformations in identity and
purpose for many schools and individual teachers. Thus, for example, the
public possibilities for metaphysical discourses around social justice and
equality are dramatically closed down (Reynolds 1992) and the fables of
promise and opportunity which attend comprehensive education are marginalised. Pragmatism and cold calculation, as against fable and metaphysics,
inscribe a new kind of public professionalism and a new kind of public professional. Old-style bureau-professional judgement and debate over values are
displaced; performativity replaces micropolitics (Clarke and Newman 1992).
The humanistic commitments of the substantive professional are replaced by
the teleological promiscuity of the technical professional. This shift is underpinned and ramified by the introduction of new forms of deintellectualised,
competence-based training. This is situated within the more general shift
which Cerny (1990) describes as that from a welfare to a 'competition state'.

Furthermore, the school and the teacher are now captured within a complex framework of calculation and judgement valorised by the incentives and
self-interest (a kind of calculation) of the market form. The main aspects of

this framework are: managerialism and its technologies of the self, like total quality management (TQM) (see Ball 1997a); the publication of national tests and examination results and the construction of local league tables; inspection, articulated and enacted on the principles of management, quality and procedure; teacher appraisal, incentive payments and performance-related pay; and parental choice (linked to per capita, formula funding). The act of teaching and the subjectivity of the teacher are both profoundly changed by this overdetermining panopticism. Thus, the observation and classification of individuals are provided for in a number of ways: the rating of teachers by inspectors, performance-related pay, annual appraisals and increasingly complex, often computerised, procedures for systematising, recording, and monitoring teacher activity.[8]

But, again, within all this two apparently conflicting effects are sought: an increasing individualisation, including the destruction of solidarities based upon a common professional identity and trade union affiliation, and the construction of new forms of institutional affiliation and 'community'. The latter take the form, for example, of the articulation of a corporate culture, which, as a new kind of organisational fable (another fabrication – see below), is a new focus of institutional allegiance. In Butler's terms this might be regarded as an 'enacted fantasy' (Butler 1990: 136). The institution rather than the profession or 'service' is the main point of reference for identity. As against this, former colleagues in other institutions are now competitors. Survival is the basis of common purpose – pragmatism and self-interest rather than professional judgement and ethics are the basis for new organisational language games. 'Administrative procedures should make individuals "want" what the system needs in order to perform well' (Lyotard 1984: 62).[9]

> I think TQM has a value in that, in making us think in terms of customers ... which is how I regard my parents, and ... to a certain degree the students now. I don't think it changes the fundamental relationship but I think one is very definitely aware that numbers need to be kept up, that we need to have high targets not only for the students but to make sure that the school goes on functioning as well as it does, and I think the introduction of selection has made this very clear.
>
> (Year Tutor)

> I was kind of lukewarm about TQM, I thought it was great, it was fine, but I wasn't madly keen ... or madly anti ... and I think ... the interesting thing ... I like to be a little sceptical about some of these things, because ... you know, these things come and go ... the pattern of equality doesn't come and go actually, so in that sense I would espouse it fully, but I think some of the techniques are really helpful and ... that whole sort of ... notion of continuous improvement, the continuous search for excellence, the continuous stress on quality, looking at the relationships between people and how they enhance the quality of institution, looking at some of

the problem solving approaches as well ... the sort of barriers and solutions ... stopping us, how we're gonna solve it, and working through those problems. I think it has been very very useful for this school, and I think by and large it may well be seen as a management tool, I don't know whether we've captured the hearts and minds of absolutely everybody.

(1st Deputy)

In all this management, the market, quality, self-surveillance and self-evaluation are tightly tied. As Willmott (1993: 522) suggests, 'employees are simultaneously required, individually and collectively, to recognise and *take responsibility for* the relationship between the security of their employment and their contribution to the competitiveness of the goods and services they produce'. And the restlessness and relentlessness indicated here reflect and incorporate the uncertainties and instabilities (social, political and financial) in which many schools now operate. At the same time, even within the institution, as the competitive market, institutional marketing and corporate culture encourage a centripetal focus on teamwork and a common sense of purpose, the managerial logic of performativity encourages differentiation and internal competition between teams:

I've noticed it this year more than last year ... you come back and you go through the results, and there is a very big thing about ... how has this department done or this cluster against that cluster, you know, it's how are the maths results compared to the science results, and the science results compared to the history results. I mean it may be like that in all schools, but here it seems like, if you've got bad results compared to somebody else ... you are going to be frowned upon by other members of staff at the school ... I don't think it's enough sort of togetherness, if you like, not everyone pulling for the school, for success ... for [the school] as a whole ... it is people pulling for science success or for humanities success.

(Main Grade Teacher 1)

It's very strange, there's kind of a facade of being together, but within it ... as a whole team, yes, we're kind of ... we're against ... you know, we've got to battle and compete against all these others.

(Main Grade Teacher 2)

The cluster team is kind of all empowering and all kind of encompassing and it doesn't really recognise what's going on in other parts of the school much, or other teachers in other areas are treated with a bit of suspicion. They're not really one of us, and the teams are deliberately held up against each other sometimes, like this is good practice, and in the Arts they do this, why aren't you doing it, or in English they've done X, Y, Z, isn't this marvellous.

(Head of Department 1)

> She likes to get people competing against each other in different areas of
> the school, and it works, I don't know how effectively it works all the time
> though, certainly within the school I'd say that applied very strongly, and
> in the first few years it was idiotic really, the sort of things people had to get
> up to.
>
> (Deputy Year Tutor)

> We've got the senior team, got middle managers ... [curriculum] teams,
> cluster teams ... I think that's quite interesting. It seems to me that the lan-
> guage is actually bearing out the reality, and we are more likely to kind of
> be set against one another than functioning as a small team.
>
> (Head of Department 2)

All of this resonates strongly with du Gay's notion of the 'post-entrepreneurial
revolution' which 'provides the possibility for every member of an organisation to express 'individual initiative' and to develop fully their 'potential' in
the service of the corporation' (du Gay 1996: 62).

I want to conclude this section by looking at an account generated by one
young teacher within an interview which illustrates the play of these technologies upon and through a subjectivity and their dislocating and
reorganising effects. Perhaps also these comments display something of the
'existential separation' which Giddens sees as endemic in late modernity
(Giddens 1991: 91).

> So in terms of the systems that have been set up, in terms of the general
> management ... I suppose I am thinking more logistical and financial, yes,
> it puts things in place that make it easier. In terms of the personal and how
> it's making you, the teacher, feel in what you are doing ... that's perhaps
> where I have the problem. But you see, perhaps ultimately you kind of ...
> because you're also focused on the children, cos that's what ... well that's
> what I've come into it for ... you have to put that to one side and it comes
> out at other times, and with the other pluses that come from the system,
> that are beneficial for the children, you then work with, you put your own
> personality if you like, into working with those. So again it's a double-
> edged sword ... yes, it makes things set up in a very practical ... you know,
> it gives good messages to the children, that everything is here and they can
> work and we expect and all of that, but then how you are personally feel-
> ing, I don't know. I'm gabbling, aren't I? I'm really gabbling.
>
> How much personal do you have to sacrifice for having the rest there ...
> is probably what would be my ... You see, I think one of the strategies
> behind it, and I think Peter Waters [the total quality management consul-
> tant] said it, you don't have to like each other, as long as you can work
> within the systems ... well ... I'm sorry, I'm not a product, and I don't ...
> you know, and that really gets me.
>
> (Main Grade Teacher 2)

In these extracts the teacher's commitments, sense of professional identity, sense of self and self-worth are beset by tensions and contradictions. An old and a new subjectivity vie with one another, producing another kind of personal incoherence and dissonance – a fragmentation of the self. The 'nostalgia for the lost narrative' conflicts with new forms of legitimation. Again, my point is that incoherence works through the education system in the form of various but limited discursive potentials, and certain classes of statements are privileged and characterise the discourse of the particular institution (Lyotard 1984: 17) while others are filtered out; although the limits and boundaries of discourse are never fixed once and for all.

PERFORMATIVITY AND FABRICATION[10]

Here also, as Lyotard puts it, there is a tension between 'calculation' and 'essence' which is central to the issue of organisational representation (see below) and concomitantly 'the production of proof':

> The performativity of an utterance, be it denotative or prescriptive, increases proportionally to the amount of information about its referent one has at one's disposal. Thus the growth of power, and its self-legitimation, are now taking the route of data storage and accessibility, and the operativity of information.

> (Lyotard 1984: 47)

Right across the public sector the 'operativity of information' is a key resource and one of the main disciplinary tactics of accountability. In the name of public interest more and more information about public sector organisations is required, recorded and published. In part this provides 'information' for market decision making, but it also increases the performativity of 'official' judgements, like Ofsted (Office for Standards in Education) inspection reports, and enfolds practitioners within the minute arts of self-scrutiny and self-improvement, with the effect of self-intensification. The effects are achieved as a response partly to self-interest, partly to self-esteem, and partly to the 'new professionalism' which is articulated in terms of the mastery of the new performance indicators. Practice becomes subtly refocused upon those tasks which serve and are represented within the 'information' of performance, a process of revalorisation. Tasks and activities which cannot be measured and recorded or which do not contribute directly to performativity are in danger of becoming 'valueless'. Lyotard notes 'the "democratic" university (no entrance requirements, little cost to the student and even to society if the price per student is calculated, high enrolment) which was modelled on the principles of emancipatory humanism, today seems to offer little in the way of performance' (Lyotard 1984: 49).

Enormous energy and effort are devoted to providing a patina of legitimacy for such information – an industry of validity (truth games) has emerged around and in relation to the production and maintenance of performative 'information'. None the less, we should not think of performative 'information' as authentic in any simple sense. Systems of calculability almost always leave latitude for presentational variation. This is particularly pertinent when performative 'information' is implicated in the dynamics of a market form, as is the case in education. Schools are required to publish a variety of types of 'information' about themselves, including brochures and annual reports, examination passes, rates of attendance and students' destinations. In addition Ofsted inspections require documentation about a whole range of 'policies' and systems in use in a school. Both forms of representation invite schools to fabricate themselves. That is to say, performance indicators and other representations are used to 'stand for' or 'in place of' the organisation as a set of day-to-day work practices. They 'fabricate' an organisation that is for external consumption; they provide a focus for the gaze of quality and accountability; they are there to be viewed and evaluated and compared. This is a 'satisficing' process which has an indirect relationship, but a relationship none the less, with the 'core' technologies of the organisation. As in the mainstream economy, the emphasis is increasingly upon the 'sign value' of schooling and 'choice making', and consumption decisions are founded upon these arbitrary but coherent significations. I am not suggesting that the 'core' technologies are insulated from the performative requirements of fabrication, but there is a slippage or mismatch between fabric and core. There are resonances here of the depthlessness and crisis of representation which are key aspects of the condition of postmodernity (Harvey 1989).

As part of this fabrication, within the context of the education market, schools are also increasingly aware of the significance of the way they represent themselves to the relatively naive gazes of 'lay' audiences. There is a general tension in the education market between information giving and impression management. Schools have become much more aware of and attentive to the 'need' to organise carefully the ways in which they 'present' themselves to their current and potential parents. Two of the sixteen schools with which we have worked have employed public relations consultants to help them in this respect. Most schools have marketing committees and devote considerable time, energy and expense to the design of brochures, prospectuses and school events. We explored this is some detail in previous work (Gewirtz et al. 1995) and noted in the case of school prospectuses:

- the use of more sophisticated production techniques and the resulting 'glossification' of school imagery;
- the commercialisation of texts and an associated focus on 'visual images' and explicit indicators of 'quality'; and
- a growing emphasis on middle class symbolism.

(Gewirtz et al. 1995: 127)

The last point refers to the use of drama and music as social class surrogates, both as forms of appeal and indirectly as forms of selection aimed at max-imising middle-class recruitment. It is interesting to note that thirty-five of the forty-one grant maintained (GM) schools which responded to the change of regulations in 1996 concerning selection of students indicated that they would select on the basis of aptitude or talent in music or drama (parlia-mentary answer, 11 June 1996). Also, as indicated, there has been a shift of emphasis in the content and form of marketing material produced by schools, away from text to pictorial representations and thus closer to the immediacy and ease of interpretation which are basic to the aesthetics of advertising. Concomitantly the amount of information presented in such material has reduced considerably:

> Of all the media forms, ads constitute the most formulaic, condensed and overstructured communications in the search for interpretative closure. Unlike reading a book or other printed matter, ads rely on the encoding of visual images; are tighter, briefer, and receive less concentrated attention from readers.
>
> (Goldman 1987: 694)

There is now a high level of reflexivity and planning 'for effect' in the ways in which schools communicate themselves to their audiences. In more general terms, the emphasis on 'selling' schools affects and inflects a whole range of interactions between schools and their social environment. Thus, for example, Carol Fitzgibbon recently drew attention to the increasing use of consul-tants by schools preparing themselves for Ofsted inspections (*Guardian*, 21 June 1996). The management of organisational 'impressions' and appear-ances is subject to enormous care:

> She [the Head] would prefer a much harder sell on the school than actually happens ... at the moment I think what's really happening is that ... she tends to say that sort of thing a lot ... within the school and hopes that it will become reality, whether it actually is reality at present, I'm not at all sure.
>
> (Deputy Year Tutor, GM school)

The concern for favourable 'representation' also confronts subject teachers in the ways in which they are expected to organise and present examination results or 'represent' their subject.

> I'm rushing around like a loony today trying to put together this exam results display she wants ... I didn't have any data to do it with and I've had to collect that and then I've had to find a way of presenting the results in a way that looks good ... GCSEs and A-level results against the national average ... that's presented us with some problems, because obviously with four subjects the results are uneven ... I've found a way of doing the A-level that looks all right, I'm struggling a bit with the GCSE.
>
> (Head of Department)

As a further variation on the fabrication of organisations, many schools have used their new budgetary freedoms to redesign and redecorate their entrance and reception areas – typically in open-plan, 'building-society' style. Again, the purpose seems to be to take control of and change the organisational messages conveyed. There is a detachment and confusion of signs; a shift from bureaucratic to businesslike imagery; from something that is clearly 'represented' as a public service to something that *might be* a consumption good. There is an interarticulation of social signs (Lee 1993), as new forms of signification are coming into play (alongside the reinvention of older forms, such as uniform). We may also want to see all this, and the generation of systems of 'objective' quality indicators, as a response to a general 'crisis of representation' that is part of the postmodern 'structure of feeling' (Pfeil 1988). Together they create a new sense of certainty and 'worth', new forms of recognition of value, within the fuzzy hierarchies of the education marketplace. The reinvention of grammar schooling and the identification and labelling of 'failing schools', as opposite extremes of a hierarchy, work in a similar way to re-establish points of certainty for parents – new classifications and divisions – within the risky business of school choice. Within all this the 'sciences' of inspection (and of school improvement and effectiveness) are at work to objectify, stigmatise and normalise (see Ball 1997b).

EDUCATION AND THE POSTMODERN WELFARE STATE

In a whole variety of senses, only some of which I have touched upon above, education in the UK as a system of welfare provision has become fragmented (while in other ways it has become more monolithic). It is fragmented by the market form. Relations between schools have become increasingly marked by competition, suspicion and even hostility. Co-operation and collaboration between schools have been interrupted by the antagonistic, competitive relations of the market; although there are some exceptions to this. The market, budgetary autonomy and new systems of pay and conditions for teachers combine to break down traditional solidarities among teachers and marginalise and weaken the role of trade unions. Teachers and head teachers are now more clearly inwardly focused upon the survival of their institution within the education market. Budgetary devolution, 'opting out' and the removal of the powers of local authorities (together with effects of market forces) have fragmented many local systems of education (Radnor *et al.* 1995). Alongside this, the introduction of parental choice and school selection work in some circumstances to break down the relationship between schools and their localities and communities. Schools are again inwardly focused and are encouraged to have primary concern for the interests of their clients (those students they recruit/select) rather than the needs of their social community (those students in their social locality).

Furthermore, open enrolment and per capita funding have produced and provided new legitimation for systematic inequalities in funding and other support between schools. The differential valuing of students in relation to the systems of performativity in the education market, and the relation of this to selection and enrolment, have exaggerated societal patterns of social fragmentation and inequality. (In general terms, girls, high-achieving students, and those with 'motivated' and 'supportive' parents are valued and sought after; students with special educational needs, emotional or behavioural difficulties, social disadvantage, and English as a second language are not.) There are various indications from research, although partial and inconclusive, of increased social segregation between schools (Echols and Wilms 1993; Gewirtz *et al*. 1995; Lauder *et al.* 1994). The dedifferentiating effects of comprehensivism, such as they were, have been reversed. Against this fragmentation, the imposition and cultivation of performativity in education, together with the importation and dissemination of managerialism, also require and encourage a greater commonality of organisational forms and institutional cultures in schools and bring education closer to the forms of regulation and control which predominate in the private sector. This is part of what is termed 'mainstreaming' in the new institutional economics (Dale 1994: 27).

However, the market form produces and reproduces fragmentation in a further sense. It calls up and reinforces a particular kind of relationship between citizens – that of competitive individualism. Indeed, it interpolates a new kind of consumer citizen. The market 'not only designates a kind of organisational form ... but more generally provides an image of a mode of activity to be encouraged in a multitude of arenas of life' (Rose 1992: 145). Rose's formulation of the 'enterprising self' is equally appropriate, I suggest, for thinking about the competitive parent. Relationships within and between schools, between schools and their 'clients', and among 'clients' themselves are all changing in response to the new political economy of signs and values at work in education. 'These new practices of thinking, judging and acting are not simply "private matters". They are linked to the ways in which persons figure in the political vocabulary of advanced liberal democracies' (Rose 1992: 142).

To return to my initial interlocutor Barry Smart: in a discussion of 'after progress' he argues that:

> Like it or not, we are increasingly having to learn to live with contingency, to face up to the mixed blessing of modernity, both the new opportunities and the new risks. The implication of this is neither nostalgia, nor panic, but rather the necessity of coming to terms with the consequences of modernity, in particular, of understanding why it is that the generalising of 'sweet reason' [has] not produced a world subject to our prediction and control.
>
> (Smart 1992: 25)

But in many respects (not all, but many), as I have tried to suggest, education policy is organised and driven by a potent combination of nostalgia (a grammar school in every town, Englishness and the National Curriculum: see also Fitz *et al.* 1997), panic (UK test performance, standards of reading) and the reassertion of 'sweet reason' (National Curriculum, Ofsted, managerialism).

CONCLUSION

Are these new policies for new times? In the muddle and dissonances of educational reform it is possible to discern distinct patterns: difference is replaced by individualism and by value (the differences between students now reside in their potential contribution to performativity); relevance (in relation to culture and heritage) by specialisation (in relation to talent and future labour-market opportunities) and a 'classless' curriculum; inclusivity and intrainstitutional diversity by selection (and concomitantly exclusion) and interinstitutional diversity (and concomitantly exclusivity). Pluralism is more apparent than real in all this. As Yeatman puts it: 'The performative state is a response of vertically integrated control agendas to the conditions of postmodernity' (Yeatman 1994: 112).

The provision of schooling in the UK has begun to resemble a post-Fordist economy of education in so far as educational institutions are moving away from mass production and mass markets (comprehensivism) to niche marketing and 'flexible specialisation' (selection, specialisation and privatisation). It has begun to resemble a postmodern economy of education in so far as the devolutionary and deregulatory imperatives represented in the education market are clearly part of a 'wider retreat from modern bureaucratised state education systems', which are seen to be 'inappropriate to societies of the late twentieth century'; these imperatives offer 'new ways of resolving the core problems facing the state' (Whitty 1991: 41), while perhaps at the same time creating new ones. This is the shift, noted earlier, from a welfare to a competition state. Furthermore, education, as I have tried to indicate, is increasingly subject to and a subject of the power and emptiness of the image; from the panics orchestrated by the media, through the proliferation of handbooks of choice, to the complex fabrication of institutional identities and representations and the importation of pop-management corporate fantasies. Education is also increasingly imbricated in the flow of commodities within these secondary economies of 'self-production' and cultural production. Schools are on trajectories of convergence with other service industries, particularly perhaps those, like the theme park, that blend nostalgia with high technology.

However, within all this there are powerful continuities in evidence, not least the continuity and indeed the ramification of basic modernist structural inequalities founded upon social class. In the 'reform' of education, new class opportunities are made available, new cultural arbitraries are in play, which reprivilege the 'practical knowledge' of the new and old middle classes (Ball *et al.* 1996). 'The market' in education may be read as a new metadiscourse, with its own particular foundations for knowledge, morality and aesthetics.

ACKNOWLEDGEMENT

I am grateful to Trinidad Ball, Doreen Chen, Diane Reay and Carol Vincent for their comments on an earlier draft of this chapter.

NOTES

1 ESRC Project reference nos. 232858, 23251006 and 235544.
2 This is not indicative of a postmodernist celebration of 'difference'; rather it is driven by the reinvention of traditional hierarchies and status differences.
3 I am 'raiding' Lyotard and my use of *The Postmodern Condition* does not indicate a commitment to other aspects of his work.
4 Postmodernity is here taken to denote new forms of discipline, representation, identity and relationships.
5 However, it is still possible and tempting to put this complex of policies together and see them as constituting a coherent and oppressive edifice, a modernist conceit of control, surveillance and discipline. I take up this possibility and temptation later in the chapter, but remain sceptical about the integrity of such an analysis and do not want to 'close down' the contradictions by settling upon a single, clear motive and logic in all this, despite a certain force and coherence in the concatenation of policies.
6 As one example, a *Daily Mail* headline (12 June 1996), commenting on government responses to an international comparison of literacy and numeracy performance, reported 'College crackdown as study highlights Britain's slide'.
7 While I am focused here on secondary education, virtually all aspects of the analysis could be equally well applied and explored in further and higher education (Cowen 1996), or in other sectors of social welfare where performativity is in play.
8 The appraisal interview and its documentation require teachers to fabricate a version of themselves which accommodates and articulates with the performative objectives of the organisation and positions them within its corporate culture. As a confessional event the appraisal is a means of disciplining and an adjustment of the self.
9 The research project extracts used in the text are presented solely as illustration, to provide a grounding for some of the arguments put forward.
10 I find that Judith Butler uses the same term in relation to the performativity of gender: 'acts, gestures, enactments, generally construed, are performative in the sense that the essence or identity that they otherwise purport to express are fabrications manufactured and sustained through corporeal signs and other discursive means' (Butler 1990: 136). I am grateful to Diane Reay for drawing this to my attention.

BIBLIOGRAPHY

Ball, S. J. (1990) *Politics and Policymaking in Education*, London: Routledge.
Ball, S. J. (1993) 'Education, Majorism and the curriculum of the dead', *Curriculum Studies* 1, 2: 195–214.

Ball, S.J. (1994) *Education Reform: A Critical and Post-structural Approach*, Buckingham: Open University Press.

Ball, S.J. (1997a) 'Good school/bad school', *British Journal of Sociology of Education* 18, 3: 317–36.

Ball, S.J. (1997b) 'Policy sociology and critical social research: a personal review of recent education policy and policy research', *British Educational Research Journal* 23, 3: 257–74.

Ball, S.J., Bowe, R. and Gewirtz, S. (1996) 'School choice, social class and distinction: the realisation of social advantage in education', *Journal of Education Policy* 11, 1: 89–112.

Bernstein, B. (1971) 'On the classification and framing of educational knowledge', in M.F.D. Young (ed.) *Knowledge and Control*, London: Collier-Macmillan.

Butler, J. (1990) *Gender Trouble*, London: Routledge.

Cerny, P. (1990) *The Changing Architecture of Politics: Structure, Agency and the Future of the State*, London: Sage.

Clarke, J. and Newman, J. (1992) *The Right to Manage: A Second Managerial Revolution*, Milton Keynes: Open University.

Cowen, R. (1996) 'Performativity, postmodernity and the university', *Comparative Education* 32, 2: 245–58.

Dale, R. (1994) 'National reform, economic crisis and "new right" theory: a New Zealand perspective', *Discourse* 14, 2: 17–29.

du Gay, P. (1996) *Consumption and Identity at Work*, London: Sage.

Echols, F.H. and Wilms, J.D. (1993) 'Scottish parents and reasons for school choice', Vancouver: Department of Social and Educational Studies, University of British Columbia.

Fitz, J., Halpin, D. and Power, S. (1997) 'Opting into the past? Grant maintained schools and the reinvention of tradition', in R. Glatter, P.A. Woods and C. Bagley (eds) *Choice and Diversity in Schooling: Perspectives and Prospects,* London: Routledge.

Gewirtz, S., Ball, S.J. and Bowe, R. (1995) *Markets, Choice and Equity in Education*, Buckingham: Open University Press.

Giddens, A. (1991) *Modernity and Self-Identity: Self and Society in the Late Modern Age*, Cambridge: Polity Press.

Goldman, R. (1987) 'Marketing fragrances: advertising and the production of commodity signs', *Theory, Culture and Society* 4.

Harvey, D. (1989) *The Condition of Postmodernity*, Oxford: Blackwell.

Kirkpatrick, I. and Martinez-Lucio, M. (1995) 'Introduction', in I. Kirkpatrick and M. Martinez Lucio (eds) *The Politics of Quality in the Public Sector*, London: Routledge.

Kroker, A., Kroker, M. and Cook, D. (1989) *Panic Encyclopaedia: The Definitive Guide to the Postmodern Scene*, London: Macmillan.

Lauder, H., Hughes, D., Waslander, S., Thrupp, M., McGlinn, J., Newton, S. and Dupluis, A. (1994) 'The creation of market competition for education in New Zealand: The Smithfield Project phase one', First Report to the Ministry of Education, Wellington: Victoria University.

Lee, M.J. (1993) *Consumer Culture Reborn*, London: Routledge.

Lyotard, J.-F. (1984) *The Postmodern Condition: A Report on Knowledge*, Manchester: Manchester University Press.

Nisbet, R. (1980) *A History of the Idea of Progress*, New York: Basic Books.

Oakland, J. (1991) *Total Quality Management*, London: Heinemann.

Pfeil, F. (1988) 'Postmodernism as a "structure of feeling"', in L. Nelson and C. Grossberg (eds) *Marxism and the Interpretation of Culture*, London: Macmillan.

Radnor, H., Ball, S.J. and Henshaw, L. with Vincent, C. (1995) *LEAs: Accountability and Control*, Stoke: Trentham Books.

Reynolds, K. (1992) '"Equal opportunities" and the local management of schools – what happens now?', *Gender and Education* 4, 3: 289–99.

Rose, N. (1992) 'Governing the enterprising self', in P. Heelas and P. Morris (eds) *The Values of the Enterprise Culture*, London: Routledge.

Rustin, M. (1989) 'The politics of post-Fordism: or the trouble with "new times"', *New Left Review* 175: 54–78.

Smart, B. (1992) *Modern Conditions, Postmodern Controversies*, London: Routledge.

Spybey, T. (1984) 'Traditional and professional frames of meaning for managers', *Sociology* 18, 4: 550–62.

Whitty, G. (1991) 'Recent education reform: is it a post-modern phenomenon?', Paper presented at the conference Reproduction, Social Inequality and Resistance: New Directions in the Theory of Education, University of Bielefeld, Germany.

Willmott, H. (1993) 'Strength is ignorance; slavery is freedom: managing culture in modern organisations', *Journal of Management Studies* 30, 4: 215–52.

Yeatman, A. (1993) 'Corporate managerialism and the shift from the welfare to the competition state', *Discourse* 13, 2: 10–17.

Yeatman, A. (1994) *Postmodern Revisionings of the Political*, London: Routledge.

Chapter 13

Post-Betty Fordism and neo-liberal drug policies

Robin Bunton

INTRODUCTION

Lance: This ain't Amsterdam, Vince. This is a seller's market. Coke is fuckin' dead as disco. Heroin's comin' back in a big fucking way. It's this whole seventies retro. Bell bottoms, heroin, they're as hot as hell.
(Tarantino 1994: 41)

The above text from the film *Pulp Fiction* displays a number of features of contemporary western conceptions of drug use which differ from those of previous decades. Firstly, drug use in the film is portrayed as normal, routine and unextraordinary. Though apparent throughout the film, drugs neither dominate the story line nor significantly impinge on characterisation and plot. Secondly, drugs are acknowledged as goods that are subject to fashion and social process. Like bell bottoms and hairstyles, drugs can be a fashion accessory, and people can make choices for fashionable effect. Thirdly, the film acknowledges that drug users may switch between use of one or more drugs. Finally, there is a significant absence of any reference to addiction. In one sub-plot, for example, Vince (played by John Travolta) does encounter difficulties when his dance partner for the evening Mia (played by Uma Thurman) mistakes heroin for cocaine and is severely ill. This use of drugs is not habitual in any clinical sense and it has no connotations of addiction. It is merely a fact of life and one element of risk taking that, on occasion, might go accidentally wrong and need management.

The non-judgemental, dispassionate and underplayed significance of drugs in *Pulp Fiction* distinguishes it from previous cinema representations of drug and drug problems. Previous film portrayal of drug use has focused on tragic 'alcoholic heroes', for example, in films such as *Rio Bravo*, *I'll Cry Tomorrow* and *Days of Wine and Roses* (Cook and Lewington 1979). Films such as *The French Connection* have had a persistent interest in the degradation of addiction and Hollywood has repeatedly focused upon drugs as tragedy in such films as, *The Lost Weekend* or *Underneath the Volcano*. Distinct therapeutic discourses can be identified in the history of such films, according to their age and the therapeutic fashion particular to the period (Cook and Lewington

1979). The subsequent abandonment of the tragic figure of the drug user in contemporary film, I argue here, is indicative of shifts in problem drug-use discourses which are in turn characteristic of neo-liberal governance and current social policy. Such shifts also show similarities to broader cultural, social and organisational shifts attributed to 'post' or 'late' modernity.

NEO-LIBERALISM AND DRUG POLICY

Much recent social science has emphasised the increasingly crucial role expertise plays in the socio-political rule of modern societies through mechanisms such as documentation, classification, evaluation and calculation (Johnson 1993). Successful government of liberal capitalist societies has required not simply the increased use of monetary calculations to make planned use of raw materials and human activities to achieve profit but also, as Weber documented (1930), the co-ordination of the 'psycho-physical apparatus' of human individuals (Rose 1989a). Expert discourse has played an important role in shaping the thoughts and actions of subjects in these societies to render them useful and 'governable'. Recent theoretical work influenced by Michel Foucault has drawn attention to the connections between specific techniques of governance, particular forms of knowledge and the formation of subjects. Such work has been critical of 'humanist' assumptions that knowledge necessarily serves to 'liberate' us and help us discover the nature of human subjectivity and has stressed, rather, the potential of such knowledge to define or fabricate a particular, 'governable' subjectivity. Such work provides an important critical perspective on welfare that has pointed to its compatibility with 'neo-liberalism'. This perspective offers a critical slant on recent changes in drug policy. Lying at the intersection of a number of different expert knowledges, including medical, criminological, the social-psychological and moral, the discourse on drugs constructs or fabricates specific types of subjectivity particular to the late twentieth century.

At one level, analysis of neo-liberal governance has devoted critical attention to numerous western governments to reinstate liberal government principles, including the promotion of enterprising, self-regulating individuals and communities; a privileging of market organisational principles for private and public service provision; a deregulation and restructuring of economic organisational units (typified as a shift from Fordist to post-Fordist organisation); the 'rolling back' of state intervention into social and economic life; and a decollectivisation of welfare. A number of such policies have frequently been attributed to the influence of political groupings of the 'New Right'. At another level, reference has been made to underlying shifts in the nature of the rationality or 'formula of rule' of recent thinking, which in some ways differentiates it from nineteenth-century liberalism. In his later years Michel Foucault began to account for western neo-liberal thought in postwar years and examined fundamental challenges to the idea of the welfare state (Gordon 1991). Rose (1993) has developed this analysis, describing what he refers to as 'advanced liberalism', the features of which can usefully be applied to contemporary discourse on drug use. Such distinctions, I will argue, can help us identify salient features of recent drugs discourse and differences in regimes of drug policy. I will refer to these changes as 'abandoning the addict', 'reconfiguring expertise', and 'pluralising technologies'.

ABANDONING THE ADDICT

In an influential article on the re-emergence of the concept of addiction, Levine refers to the emergence of a postaddiction model of alcohol (and drug) misuse which he dates to the late 1960s (Levine 1978). Postaddiction replaces a medically orientated conception of drug problems which had driven North American and European policy for the previous thirty years. The emergence of addiction under 'modernity', it might be argued, (in medical and other somatic discourses in particular), fashioned the desiring body to suit particular socio-cultural circumstances. Addiction discourses have been linked to the quest for the control of the self and of population, through the control of desire and craving (Alasuutari 1992; Giddens 1992). The temperance movement at the turn of the twentieth century, for example, originated as an attempt to engender bourgeois self-discipline amongst the new urban working classes to rid them of 'in-temperance' (Gusfield 1963; Levine 1978). Fears of potentially threatening 'others' were apparent and played a part in the discourses regulating drug use, well illustrated by the cocaine scares of the early twentieth century in the UK and in the USA (Kohn 1992). These early attempts to instil self-discipline demonstrate a more general strategy of liberal governance to form the liberal subject.

Rose's account of the rationale of liberalism describes a dependence upon an active subject of government (Rose 1993). Liberalism invests a great deal in the existence of free individuals and seeks to shape and regulate that freedom in a social form, specifying what is acceptable 'civilised' behaviour, to be rewarded with the rights of citizenship, and what is not, sanctioned by exclusion. The drug addict was an ideal form of liberal subjectivity, whose existence called for moral and bodily restraint whilst it, simultaneously, legitimated prophylactic interventions that reached families, communities and individuals via new 'microtechniques' of power. A number of individualising discourses came to bear upon populations during the nineteenth and twentieth centuries, constructing them as individuals within a broader territory of 'the social'. The social emerged as a strategy to resolve a number of fragmentation and individualising processes characteristically produced by industrialisation and urbanisation. Social insurance for health and welfare care introduced technologies of government by which it could guarantee the freedoms of the individual and of capital whilst, simultaneously, harnessing the role of professionals and their authority (Rose 1993: 293). It is these features of liberalism which can be recognised in the emergence of the 'welfare state' in the nineteenth and twentieth centuries, characterised by Donzelot as the 'socialisation of society' (Donzelot 1979).

Public health initiatives of the nineteenth and early twentieth centuries illustrate the concern for the regulation of population and the active and healthy citizen (Petersen and Lupton 1996; Lupton 1995; Kendal and Wickham 1992). Health became a concern in the seventeenth and eighteenth centuries of modern European states that had interests in maintaining national economic and military targets. Within this concern, new sets of relationships were established between the state individuals and expert discourse – new relations of welfare. A 'biopolitics of the population' was instituted, attempting to order bodies across space, particularly the new urban spaces. Modernisation and the need for self-restraint could be found in a number of movements at the turn of the century, such as Tolstoy's notions of youth training and sexual restraint. These endeavours are congruent with Elias's account (1978) of the 'civilising processes' of the Middle Ages, and with the nobles' attempts to internalise outer constraints and to control animality and the emotions associated with the grotesque, uncivilised body (Stallybrass and White 1986). Elias points to the ways in which culture was increasingly privileged over nature, giving the oppositions civilised/primitive, healthy/pathological, and civilised/sinful. The temperance movement is typical of these general public health strategies of governance, and produced a new type of secular citizenship and the regulation of 'intemperance'.

If the above developments in drug-addiction policy matched more general governmental strategies associated with the construction of the classical liberal subject, then, there are also parallels to be made with the new specification of the subject under neo- or advanced liberalism. Under advanced liberalism, a new specification of the subject of government has emerged whereby the client has become a customer and risk management is privatised. This shift is apparent in a number of fields. O'Mally (1992) has described the ways in which citizens are increasingly obliged to adopt a calculative and 'prudent' personal relationship to risk and danger. Social work or physician-based care gives way to the self-help group and the help line, and citizens take on a new authority of their own. The power effects of this style of governance are different to those experienced under liberalism. People do not posses or seize power and power cannot be calculated as a 'zero sum', as modern citizens are very definitely agents of their own government (Hacking 1986; Rose 1989b). There is a significant change here in the nature of the populations to be governed. Rather than creating highly differentiated populations, and excluding and 'treating' particular categories of individuals such as addicts, the mad, bad or sad, the whole population is surveyed and interventions are organised as part of a population-wide strategy. This strategy of governance relies on the analysis on risk on the one hand and upon a more flexible identity on the other.

Drug risks

Some of the new strategies of liberal governance can be seen in relation to notions of risk and drug use. Castel, echoing Foucault's concerns with the 'dangerous individual' (Foucault 1988), has suggested that we can identify a transformation in health- and social-care regimes from those based upon 'dangerousness' to one based upon 'risk' (Castel 1991). The new strategies involve replacing the unit of subject or a concrete individual with a combination of factors of risk. Interventions essentially are no longer a matter of face-to-face contact between the professional and client. Rather, the concern of the professional is for the flow of populations and a range of abstract factors deemed liable to produce risk in general. A system of welfare for those individuals in need is transformed into a system for monitoring the health and welfare of populations. Under the regime of risk, epidemiological survey data become the main tool of the health professional, and the dispensary becomes the focus of a new, extended medical gaze (Armstrong 1983). New modes of surveillance, aided by technological advances, make the calculation of probabilities of 'systematic pre-detection' more and more sophisticated. Populations are increasingly being managed on the basis of their risk profiles in relation to factors such as their age, social class, occupation, gender, relationships, locality, lifestyle and consumption, and interventions take more diverse forms.

Health risk discourse has become dominant in the study of social aspects of health, public health, and in particular, health promotion and has received some critical attention in recent years, especially with reference to its regulatory potential (Baum 1993; Bunton 1990b, 1992; Gillick 1984; Greco 1993; Green 1995; Lupton 1995; Nettleton and Bunton 1995; Petersen 1996; Petersen and Lupton 1996; Prior 1995; Stevenson and Burke 1991). The regulation of risk allows the development of population strategies but also individualising foci. Although a collective concept (Ewald 1991), in a great deal of health-promotion discourse risk has been made an 'internal' attribute of the individual. This treatment of risk contrasts to 'external', environmental risk highlighted in the work of Beck and Douglas (Lupton 1995). In such discourse 'risk takers', such as smokers, drinkers or those that practise unsafe sex, become demonized as new, secular 'sinners' (Douglas 1992). Forms of group identification, exclusion, marginalisation and regulation are practised, defining some as 'at risk', some as 'Self' and some as 'Other' (Figlio 1989). Drug 'scares', again, are a good example of the use of risk in this way. 'Chinamen' were made 'other' during the cocaine scare of the early twentieth century (Kohn 1992) in a similar manner to the way that black youths have been marginalised in more recent anti-drug campaigns in the USA and

Australia (Balsham *et al.* 1992; Reaves and Campbell 1994). Plant and Plant (1992) have identified young drug users as 'risk takers', placing them alongside practitioners of other behaviours such as dangerous sports, violence and crime. This serves to broaden the nature of drug misuse as a type of behaviour in need of regulation.

Drug-user identities

Alongside the development of interventions aimed at whole populations has been the construction of a more flexible drug-using identity. This identity is based not upon the relatively enduring persona of the addict but on an essentially 'normal' drug user who will, from time to time, experience problems related to particular practices in particular circumstances. The postaddiction model to which Levine referred (1978) is in fact a number of models that have been around since at least the early 1970s (Robinson 1976). The shift matches broader shifts in discourses on health and illness, and can be typified by what has become known as the drug-related problem approach Berridge (1989b). This approach emerged in the late 1970s and 1980s, pioneered by behaviourally orientated psychologists in particular, offering an alternative to the medical model of drug problems. Berridge has concluded that:

> In the 1980s problem drug and alcohol use are part of the 'new public health' with its emphasis on primary care, individual lifestyle, health planning, indicators and information. Planners, epidemiologists and health economists, ... play their part in defining problem use; psychologist and clinicians still retain the basic core of dependence.
>
> (Berridge 1989b: 39–40)

The shift in WHO categorisation of the nature of the drug problem is indicative of this change. Whereas in 1952 WHO literature had drawn heavily on medical expertise to define alcoholism and drug addiction, by 1969 it had moved towards the definition of drug dependence, and by 1979 to an even looser definition of alcohol and drug dependence syndrome (Heather *et al.* 1985; WHO 1952, 1969). The use of psychological states and social context to define problem drug use is significant. Space prohibits detailed documentation here, but we can summarise this shift as one which moved from a taxonomy based primarily on somatic 'physical dependence' in the 1950s, influenced by the work of medical experts such as Jellinek, to one based upon a more open notion of psychological dependence (Heather *et al.* 1985).

Contemporary discourse dealing with drug use and drug behavioural modification uses a more fluid and flexible drug-taking identity. Such discourse identifies 'drug-taking behaviour' as one part of a repertoire of behaviours engaged in by the population at large and linked to other forms of social behaviour. Orford, for example (1989) has placed drug use within other 'excessive appetites', along with gambling, eating, and excessive sexual activity. Being a risk taker is a not lifelong identity location but a stage particular to age and social circumstance. Equally, 'excessive appetites' come and go and are not necessarily a constant feature of one's biography. Whilst these behaviours have some regularities (they are gender- and class-relative, for example), they are not tied to the individual to the same extent as those of the addict. The more recent popularity of motivational change theory is also indicative of this change (Davidson 1992; Prochaska and Di Clemente 1983). This approach to drug-problem intervention has won considerable popularity in the UK and in Australia and relies upon a taxonomy of motivational potentialities. 'Readiness to change' is a feature that guides intervention. Interventions are guided by the patterning of such potential, not by the long-term, more static personality types, typical of addiction or dependence approaches. Personality is immaterial to this approach, which allows more flexible interventions to be developed and applied to whole populations.

It might be possible to place this relaxation of identity within more general changes related to health and illness under late or postmodern health. Recent emphasis on health rather than illness means that individuals no longer experience health and illness as a highly socially segregated and episodic role set, as defined in Parsons's classic description of the sick role (Parsons 1951, 1958, 1975). Under older 'modernist' institutional forms of health care, being ill often involved fundamental shifts in individual identity. Particular moral careers could be plotted as entry to the sick role and involved a rewriting of the narrative of self (Bunton 1997; Epstein 1995; Frank 1993; Porter and Porter 1988). Under more recent forms of health regimen, health status is not necessarily episodic or a form of deviancy. Equally, under the postaddiction regime the narrative is increasingly transient and resembles more a series of anecdotes than a single plot.

In summary, current problem drug-use discourse constructs a more enterprising, prudent, risk-managing subject that differs from the classical liberal subject of late nineteenth- and early twentieth-century discourse. Drug-user identity is more fluid than that of its predecessor – the addict – and facilitates a range of more flexible intervention strategies aimed at the reduction of risks in populations rather than the treatment of individual needs.

RECONFIGURING EXPERTISE

Under neo- or advanced liberalism as it has developed in the postwar Anglo-Saxon world, there would appear to have been a significant change in the relationship of professional expertise and politics. Liberalism instituted a new mode of authority, which tied government to positive knowledges of human conduct. The growth of expertise in the human sciences directed at solving a series of social problems made individuals governable. Government essentially invested in the truth of scientific endeavour (Osborne 1993, 1997). Rather than totally respecting professional sources of expertise on human conduct, however, advanced liberalism has penetrated these with a series of new techniques that exercise critical scrutiny and budgetary discipline, including accountancy and audit. Calculative regimes and financial management have entered the relationship between professional and state. Audit and marketisation are rendering expertise governable by eradicating the uncertainty of truth claims propagated by the professions. An apparent devolution of power is achieved by handing over decisions to consumers.

A significant change has involved the increased use of the market principle to organise and distribute services and to regulate expertise in the delivery of health care. In the UK the introduction of the market was led by the 'new right' thinking of Conservative administrations. Documents such as the Griffiths Report (DHSS 1983) examining the NHS were typical of this thinking, and they represented a significant move away from a largely consensus-led approach involving teams of doctors, nurses and administrators, towards a system of business management borrowed from the commercial sector which turned administrators into business managers (Harrison *et al.* 1990; Hunter 1991). The introduction of the principles of an 'internal market' into the NHS, with a separation between the purchasers and providers and increased use of private contractors in health-care delivery, has been seen as a major threat to clinical autonomy and the system of professional dominance (Gabe *et al.* 1994).

Principles of economic rationalism were introduced and have had an effect upon drug policy in the UK, through community care provision, policing and crime prevention activities. The retreat from a classic alliance between state and professional has had a different trajectory to that of other areas of health and welfare. The recognition of professional expertise for drug misuse occurred far later than in other areas. One of the reasons for this was the favouring of product eradication policies in relation to alcohol and drugs around the turn of the century. As late as 1951 a WHO expert committee made it clear that 'It is only within comparatively recent years that a medical and scientific outlook on the problem has developed which makes a public health action possible' (WHO 1951).

Medical expertise appeared to offer little therapeutic optimism on which to claim authority. Significant authority had emanated instead from direct policy interventions, such as temperance legislation and that under the Defence of the Realm Act to deal with cocaine and other drugs (Dorn 1983). It was not until later that therapeutic optimism emerged, from the 1930s onwards, once the more centralised, authoritarian measures of the liberal state had changed. The alignment of medical and criminal expertise with governmental strategy became enshrined in the 'British system' of drug policy as late as the 1950s, only to be transformed under the neo-liberal rationale in the 1970s.

A crucial feature of modern societies is that the state is not positioned in dominant, repressive, authoritarian relation to subjects, but rather is a part of a set of institutions and agencies that are directed at enhancing personal freedoms and individual development (Rose 1993). Foucauldian analysis has provided a reversal of traditional, predominantly top-down conceptions of power. Such analysis would seem appropriate to much of social and welfare development at the turn of the century, which has been characterised as an 'anato-politics' that disciplined the individual body and a 'bio-politics' of the population that regulated groups of bodies across predominantly urban space (Hewitt 1991). There would appear to have been a delayed onset of such systems in relation to drugs and governance. Strong moral and religious discourses have been important in defining a strategy of interventions and would appear still to be doing so.

The period of a loose alignment of state and professional expertise typical of liberal governance and drug policy has been a relatively brief one. The influence of moral discourse, foreign policy and racism would seem to have been combined to limit the freedom of professionals to define the truth of drug use and design intervention strategies. Throughout the late nineteenth and early twentieth centuries there has been significant centralised policy making in Europe and North America, and states have not given free licence to professional authority. As Reaves and Campbell note (1994), by defining drug transgression as a disease and a crime, the state and the medical profession have made illegal drug users into 'super deviants', subject to quarantine, imprisonment, involuntary treatment and mandatory sentencing. The language of war characterises drug regulation as a battle over control – the control of the Enlightenment project. The authority of professions has been taken up in high-profile national campaigns, using medical metaphors such as plague, epidemic, contagion, infestation and cancer. Professional authority is taken up by the state in such exercises, but under tight control. The authors quote William Bennet, President Bush's former 'drug Czar', who defined the modern drug problem as one of modern government: "The Drug Crisis is a crisis of Authority – in every sense of the term "authority"" (Reaves and Campbell 1994: 26). Whilst we would expect there to be inconstancy, contradiction and discontinuity in the discourse on welfare in general, and drugs policy in particular, we might also suspect that there are peculiarities relating to governance of drug use that might confound a typification of advanced liberalism.

PLURALISING TECHNOLOGIES

A further feature associated with neo- or advanced liberalism is a pluralisation of technologies for governance. Rose (1993) refers to the ways that social technologies of the welfare state are reconfigured and detached from centralised regulating technologies in favour of various autonomised agencies.

Under classic liberalism, there was a fairly clear contract made between state and professional associations which facilitated the development of institutional solutions to health and social problems with centralised planning and organisation. Under neo- or advanced liberalism, however, norms of service, dedication and alliance between state and professional have substantially disappeared along with the arrival of competition and customer demand. Similarly, there has been a noticeable pluralisation of technologies in western and antipodean drug-care systems. Indications of this can be found in: the shift to incorporate different and more ambitious prevention activities; in the increased range of therapeutic options available; in the adoption of a multi-sectoral approach; in the use of local and community knowledge and expertise; and in the use of notions of the management of 'at-risk' populations. Many of these advances have moved alongside developments in health.

Typically, UK drug policy in the 1970s began to resemble the pluralised statements appearing on preventative health. *Drinking Sensibly* (DHSS 1981) reiterated a number of features of the policy statement *Prevention and Health: Everybody's Business* which came from the Department of Health and Social Security in 1976. The former document not only specified the social and economic costs of alcohol misuse, but to deal with the problems it called on all sectors, including: central government, the health professions, the business sector, trade unions, voluntary bodies and 'the people in the United Kingdom as individuals [to] recognise and play their separate part' (DHSS 1981: 40). The Advisory Council on the Misuse of Drugs reports on treatment and rehabilitation, and on prevention, also reiterated these sentiments (ACMD 1982, 1983). These reports called for regional and district problem teams to ensure the co-ordinated development of services at a local level suited to local needs.

Most important is the recognition in all of these documents that response to the drug problems needed to be broad and diverse. They called for a range of solutions that far outstripped the proposed solution (no plural) of caring for and/or punishing the addict, a solution that dominated drugs policies from the 1930s up until the early 1970s. This shift in drug policy has been documented by a number of commentators, particularly the retreat from the singular medical model and the advent of 'harm minimisation' (Rhodes and Hartnoll 1996). The emerging public health concerns surrounding HIV/AIDS in the mid-1980s gave further impetus to the development of broad-based harm-reduction strategies, involving schemes such as syringe distribution and exchange, community-orientated responses, and other innovatory practices (Rhodes and Hartnoll 1996; Stimson and Donoghue 1996). The policy on illegal drugs from the late 1980s has been typified by Dorn and South (1989) as 'If you must inject'. The arrival of HIV/AIDS, then, further contributed to a reconceptualisation of the drug user which depathologised drug use and constructed the drug user as a potentially rational subject capable of choosing health-related behaviour (Stimson 1995). This reconceptualised drug user was more amenable to varied interventions.

The policy-making community shifted along with such changes throughout the 1980s, in the UK and Australasia at least, and included the expertise of new sets of professionals and the increased involvement of the voluntary sector. Drugs and alcohol policy initiatives in the UK around this time began to favour locally determined, multisectoral, co-ordinated action (Bunton 1990a, 1990b). The UK White Paper *Tackling Drugs Together* (DHSS 1995) reinforced many of the basic approaches of the drug-prevention initiatives of the previous decade. There have been calls for the establishment of local drug-prevention teams in an attempt to recruit the efforts of communities and encourage them to resist and deal with the use of illegal drugs in a variety of ways. The progression of this type of drug policy might be seen as distinctively moving away from the highly centralised, 'socialised' solutions to governance of the liberal period.

CONCLUSION

I have argued here that recent postaddiction technologies have developed that suit more flexible and effective means of governance, focusing on the body and the regulation of habits – a type of 'post-Betty Fordism'. The concept of addiction has largely been abandoned and supplemented by more flexible identities. Drug problems are dealt with instead by more varied means, drawing upon behavioural-change technologies that are at work in broader public health initiatives. These new technologies are reconfiguring the relationships between state and profession in significant ways. The changes in drug-misuse regimes, apparent in popular culture, in the discourse of problem drug use and in policy statements, can be analysed as examples of shifts that have been theorised between liberalism and neo- or advanced liberalism. The broader distinctions Nicholas Rose (1993) has made between these two rationales or formulas of rule or governance usefully highlight the features of new strategies of drug policy, and illustrate new relationships between subjects, expertise and government. These features have been analytically separated here, though in fact they are likely to interact or be seen to act simultaneously in a number of sites. For example, the introduction of the market into health and welfare has affected not simply the nature of knowledge and the regulation of professional practice but also the nature of self-help and self-care, in the form of the commodification of health. In contemporary culture, health, welfare, identity and consumption are inextricably entwined. This analysis, I would argue, provides a much-needed critical perspective of the 'relations of welfare' formed in some recent developments in drug policy.

This analysis has not focused on the main theme of this collection – on postmodernism in social policy. In attempting to account for some underlying changes in contemporary discourse on drugs, I have drawn upon not the oppositions of modernism/postmodernism, but essentially two forms of modernism. With Foucault, rather than anticipate post-, late or high modernity, I have chosen to examine what might be newer forms of modernism. This is not to argue against the use of late-modern, high-modern or other forms in developing a critical social policy. Debates surrounding such terms have usefully informed this analysis.

Recent discussion of postmodernity in the social sciences has drawn attention to a number of developments in the fields of health and social welfare that have a bearing upon current concerns. John Clarke's chapter on managerialisation in this volume identifies five features of postmodernity under discussion in social policy debates: the break-up or fragmentation of the welfare state and the development of 'postbureaucratic' organisational forms; the retreat from 'universalist' social and health-care provision and the recognition of the demands and challenges made by social groups and individuals for more diverse services; a decline in traditional forms of authority, such as those engendered by health-care professions and institutions, and the subordination of professional practices to the logic of the rational calculation of the market; the abandonment of simplistic conceptions of social progress and improvement through the intervention of the welfare state; and finally, shifts in the intellectual field reflecting these changes and introducing uncertainties to areas previously considered established or routinised. Much of the above analysis of the strategies of governmentality relates specifically or tangentially to such issues.

Another alleged feature of postmodernisation, and one not addressed in Clarke's chapter, is the decentring of the subject. The emergence of a new, more fluid, reflexive and potentially precarious subjectivity under post- or late modernity has been postulated in a number of recent theoretical works. Giddens (1991) has referred to the ways that expert knowledge systems allow the assessment of risks and dangers which are negotiated in self-tragectories. Therapeutic, quasi-therapeutic and self-help literature act as resources to the reflexive monitoring of self. Self-medications, body shaping and mood management, as well as the regulation of the pleasures of drug use, are aspects of the contemporary awareness of self. Addiction, according to Giddens (1992), is a modern concept and makes little sense in pre-modern societies. Whilst not necessarily agreeing with this bold statement, we can observe that the numerous therapeutic techniques and preventative interventions currently directed at drug users are acting to specify a particular, modern, liberal and/or neo-liberal subjectivity, and simultaneously a particular notion of civil society. Postaddiction discourses have created technologies to manage intoxicated bodies in ways that produce more flexible forms of social identity than those of the addiction regime.

BIBLIOGRAPHY

ACDM (Advisory Council on the Misuse of Drugs) (1982) *Treatment and Rehabilitation*, London: HMSO.

ACDM (Advisory Council on the Misuse of Drugs) (1983) *Prevention*, London: HMSO.

ACDM (Advisory Council on the Misuse of Drugs) (1988) *Aids and Drug Misuse. Part 1*, London: HMSO.

Alasuutari, P. (1992) Desire and Craving: a Cultural Theory of Alcoholism, New York: State University Press.

Armstrong, D. (1983) *Political Anatomy of the Body: Medical Knowledge in Britain in the Twentieth Century*, Cambridge: Cambridge University Press.

Balsham, M., Oxman, G., van Rooyen, D. and Girod, K. (1992) 'Syphilis, sex and crack cocaine: images of risk and morality', *Social Science and Medicine* 35, 2: 147–60.

Baum, F. (1993) 'Healthy cities and change: social movement or bureaucratic tool?', *Health Promotion International* 8, 1: 31–40.

Berridge, V. (1989a) 'Historical issues', in S. MacGregor (ed.) *Drugs and British Society: Responses to a Social Problem in the 1980s*, London: Routledge.

Berridge, V. (1989b) 'History and addiction control: the case of alcohol', in D. Robinson *et al.* (eds) *Controlling Legal Addictions*, Basingstoke: Macmillan.

Bunton, R. (1990a) 'Changes in the control of alcohol misuse', *British Journal of Addiction* 85: 605–15.

Bunton, R. (1990b) 'Regulating our favourite drug', in P. Abbott and G. Payne (eds) *New Directions in the Sociology of Health*, Basingstoke: Falmer.

Bunton, R. (1992) 'More than a woolly jumper: health promotion as social regulation, *Critical Public Health* (Summer): 1–8.

Bunton, R. (1997) 'Popular health, advanced liberalism and *Good Housekeeping* magazine', in A. Petersen and R. Bunton (eds) *Foucault, Health and Medicine*, London: Routledge.

Bunton, R., Nettleton, S. and Burrows, R. (eds) (1995) *The Sociology of Health Promotion and the New Public Health*, London: Routledge.

Burke, F. (1989) 'Panic drugs in America', in A. Kroker, M. Kroker and D. Cook (eds) *Panic Encyclopedia*, London: Macmillan.

Castel, R. (1991) 'From dangerousness to risk', in G. Burchell, C. Gordon and P. Miller (eds) *The Foucault Effect: Studies in Governability*, Hemel Hempstead: Harvester Wheatsheaf.

Cook, J. and Lewington, M. (1979) *Images of Alcoholism*, London: British Film Institute.

Davidson, R. (1992) 'Prochaska and Diclemente's model of change: a case study', *Addiction* 87: 821–2 .

Denzin, N.K. (1987) *The Recovering Alcoholic*, London: Sage.

DHSS (Department of Health and Social Security) (1976) *Prevention and Health: Everybody's Business*, London: HMSO.

DHSS (Department of Health and Social Security) (1978) *The Pattern and Range of Services for Problem Drinkers: A Report by the Advisory Committee on Alcoholism*, London: HMSO.

DHSS (Department of Health and Social Security) (1981) *Drinking Sensibly*, London: HMSO.

DHSS (Department of Health and Social Security) (1983) *NHS Management Enquiry (Griffiths Report)*, London: HMSO.

DHSS (Department of Health and Social Security) (1995) *Tackling Drugs Together: a Strategy for England 1995–98*, London: HMSO.

DoH (Department of Health) (1991) *The Patient's Charter*, London: HMSO.

DoH (Department of Health) (1992) *The Health of the Nation: Key Area Handbook; Coronary Heart Disease and Stroke*, London: HMSO.

Donzelot, J. (1979) *The Policing of Families*, London: Hutchinson.

Dorn, N. (1983) *Alcohol, Youth and the State: Drinking Practices, Controls and Health Education*, London: Croom Helm.

Dorn, N. and South, N. (1989) 'Drug research and policy in Britain: a contemporary history', *International Journal of Drug Policy* 1, 1: 8–12.

Douglas, M. (1992) *Risk and Blame: An Analysis of Concepts of Pollution and Taboo*, London: Routledge and Kegan Paul.

Douglas, M. and Wildavsky, A. (1982) *Risk and Culture*, Oxford: Blackwell.

Elias, N. (1978) *The Civilizing Process*, New York: Urizon.

Epstein, J. (1995) *Altered Conditions: Disease, Medicine and Storytelling*, London: Routledge.

Ewald, F. (1991) 'Insurance and risk', in G. Burchell, C. Gordon, and P. Miller (eds) *The Foucault Effect: Studies of Governability*, Hemel Hempstead: Harvester Wheatsheaf.

Figlio, C. (1989) 'Unconscious aspects of health and the public sphere', in B. Richards (ed.) *Crisis of the Self: Further Essays on Psychoanalysis and Politics*, London: Free Association Books.

Foucault, M. (1988) 'The dangerous individual', in L.D. Kritzman (ed.) *Michel Foucault: Politics, Philosophy, Culture*, New York: Routledge.

Frank, A.W. (1993) 'The rhetoric of self-change: illness experience as narrative', *Sociological Quarterly* 34, 1: 39–52.

Gabe, J., Kelleher, D. and Williams, G. (eds) (1994) *Challenging Medicine*, London: Routledge.

Gabe, J., Calnan, M. and Bury, M. (eds) (1991) *The Sociology of the Health Service*, London: Routledge.

Giddens, A. (1991) *Modernity and Self-Identity: Self and Society in the Late Modern Age*, Cambridge: Polity Press.

Giddens, A. (1992) *The Transformation of Intimacy: Sexuality, Love and Eroticism in Modern Society*, Cambridge: Polity Press.

Gillick, M.R. (1984) 'Health promotion, jogging, and the pursuit of the moral life', *Journal of Health, Politics, Policy and Law* 9, 3: 369–84.

Glassner, B. (1989) 'Fitness and the postmodern self', *Journal of Health and Social Behaviour* 30: 180–91.

Glassner, B. (1992) *Bodies: The Tyranny of Perfection*, Los Angeles: Lowell House.

Glassner, B. (1995) 'In the name of health', in R. Bunton, S. Nettleton, and R. Burrows (eds) *The Sociology of Health Promotion and the New Public Health*, London: Routledge.

Gordon, C. (1991) 'Governmental rationality: an introduction', in G. Burchell, C. Gordon and P. Miller (eds) *The Foucault Effect: Studies in Governability*, Hemel Hempstead: Harvester Wheatsheaf.

Greco, M. (1993) 'Psychosomatic subjects and the "duty to be well": personal agency within medical rationality', *Economy and Society* 22, 3: 357–72.

Green, J. (1995) 'Accidents and the risk society: some problems with prevention', in R. Bunton, S. Nettleton and R. Burrows (eds) *The Sociology of Health Promotion and the New Public Health*, London: Routledge.

Gusfield, J.R. (1963) *Symbolic Crusade*, Urbana IL: University of Illinois Press.

Hacking, I. (1986) 'Making up people', in T. Heller, M. Sosna and D. Wellbery (eds) *Reconstructing Individualism: Autonomy, Individuality and the Self in Western Thought*, Stanford CA: Stanford University Press.

Harrison, B. (1971) *Drink and the Victorians: The Temperance Question in England, 1815–1872*, London: Faber.

Harrison, S., Hunter, D. and Pollitt, C. (1990) *The Dynamics of British Health Policy*, London: Unwin Hyman.

Heather, N. and Robertson, I. (1981) *Controlled Drinking*, London: Methuen.

Heather, N., Robertson, I. and Davies, P. (eds) (1985) *The Misuse of Alcohol: Crucial Issues in Dependence Treatment and Prevention*, Beckenham: Croom Helm.

Hewitt, M. (1991) 'Bio-politics and social policy: Foucault's account of welfare', in M. Featherstone, M. Hepworth and B. Turner (eds) *The Body: Social Process and Cultural Theory*, London: Sage.

Hunter, D. (1991) 'Managing medicine: a response to "the crisis"' *Social Science and Medicine* 32: 441–9.

Johnson, T. (1993) 'Expertise and the state', in M. Gane and T. Johnson, *Foucault's New Domains*, London: Routledge.

Kendal, G. and Wickham, G. (1992) 'Health and the social body' in S. Scott, G. Williams and H. Thomas (eds) *Private Risks and Public Danger*, Aldershot: Avebury.

Kohn, M. (1992) *Dope Girls: The Birth of the British Drug Underground*, London: Lawrence & Wishart.

Levine, H.G. (1978) 'The discovery of addiction: changing conceptions of habitual drunkenness in America', *Journal of Studies on Alcohol* 39: 143–74.

Lupton, D. (1995) *The Imperative of Health: Public Health and the Regulated Body*, London: Sage.

Nettleton, S. and Bunton, R. (1995) 'Sociological critiques of health promotion' in R. Bunton, S. Nettleton and R. Burrows (eds) *The Sociology of Health Promotion and the New Public Health*, London: Routledge.

O'Brien, M. (1995) 'Health and lifestyle: a critical mess? Notes on the dedifferentiation of health', in R. Bunton, S. Nettleton and R. Burrows (eds) *The Sociology of Health Promotion and the New Public Health*, London: Routledge.

O'Mally, P. (1992) 'Risk, power and crime prevention', *Economy and Society* 21, 3: 252–75.

Orford, J. (1987) 'The need for a community response to alcohol related problems', in T. Stockwell and S. Clement (eds) *Helping the Problem Drinker: New Initiatives in Community Care*, London/New York/Sydney: Croom Helm.

Orford, J. (1989) *Excessive Appetites: A Psychological View of Addictions*, Chichester: Wiley.

Osborne, T. (1993) 'On liberalism, neo-liberalism and the "liberal profession" of medicine', *Economy and Society* 22, 3: 345–56.

Osbourne, T. (1997) 'Of health and statecraft', in A. Petersen and R. Bunton (eds) *Foucault, Health and Medicine*, London: Routledge.

Parsons, T. (1951) *The Social System*, Glencoe IL: Free Press.

Parsons, T. (1958) 'Definitions of health and illness in the light of American values and social structure', in E. Jaco (ed.) *Patients, Physicians, and Illness*, New York: Free Press.

Parsons, T. (1975) 'The sick role and the role of the physician reconsidered', *Health and Society* 53, 3: 89–102.

Patton, C. (1996) *Fatal Advice: How Safer Sex Education Went Wrong*, London: Duke University Press.

Petersen, A. (1993) 'Re-defining the subject? The influence of Foucault on the sociology of health and illness', in B. Turnere, L. Eckermann, D. Colquhoun and P. Crotty (eds) *Annual Review of Health Social Sciences: Methodological Issues in Health Research. Vol. 3: 1993*, Geelong: Centre for the Study of the Body and Society, University of Deakin.

Petersen, A. (1996) 'Risk and the regulated self: the discourse of health promotion as politics of uncertainty', *Australian and New Zealand Journal of Sociology*, 32, 1: 44–57.

Petersen, A. and Lupton, D. (1996) *The New Public Health: Health and Self in the Age of Risk*, St Leonards NSW: Allen and Unwin.

Plant, M. and Plant M. (1992) *The Risk Takers*, London: Routledge.

Porter, R. and Porter, D. (1988) *In Sickness and in Health: The British Experience 1650–1850*, London: Fourth Estate.

Prior, L. (1995) 'Chance and modernity: accidents as a public health problem', in R. Bunton, S. Nettleton and R. Burrows (eds) *The Sociology of Health Promotion and the New Public Health*, London: Routledge.

Prochaska, J.O. and Di Clemente, C.C. (1983) 'Stages and processes of self-change of smoking: towards an integrative model of change', *Journal of Consulting and Clinical Psychology* 51, 3: 390–5.

Reaves, J.L. and Cambell, R. (1994) *Cracked Coverage: Television News, the Anti-Cocaine Crusade, and the Reagan Legacy*, London: Duke University Press.

Rhodes, T. and Hartnoll, R. (eds) (1996) *AIDS, Drugs and Prevention: Perspectives on Individual and Community Action*, London: Routledge.

Robinson, D. (1976) *From Drinking to Alcoholism: a Sociological Commentary*, London: Wiley.

Room, R. (1981) 'The case for a problem prevention approach to alcohol, drug and mental problems', *Public Health Reports*, 96: 26–33.

Room, R. (1985) 'Dependence and society', *British Journal of Addiction* 80: 133–9.

Rose, N. (1989a) 'Individualizing psychology', in J. Shotter and K. Gergen (eds) *Texts of Identity*, London: Sage.

Rose, N. (1989b) *Governing the Soul: The Shaping of the Private Self*, London: Routledge.

Rose, N. (1993) 'Government, authority and expertise in advanced liberalism' *Economy and Society* 22, 3: 283–98.

Stallybrass, P. and White, A. (1986) *The Politics of and Poetics of Transgression*, London: Methuen.

Stevenson, H.M. and Burke, M. (1991) 'Bureaucratic logic in new social movement clothing: the limits of health promotion research', *Health Promotion International* 6: 281–96.

Stimson, G.V. (1987) 'British drug policies in the 1980's: a preliminary analysis and suggestions for research', *British Journal of Addiction* 82: 447–9.

Stimson, G.V. (1995) 'AIDS and drug injecting in the United Kingdom 1987 to 1993: the policy response and the prevention of the epidemic', *Social Science and Medicine* 41, 5: 699–716.

Stimson, G.V. and Donoghue, M.C. (1996) 'Health promotion and the facilitation of individual change: the case of syringe distribution and exchange', in T. Rhodes and R. Hartnoll (eds) *AIDS, Drugs and Prevention: Perspectives on Individual and Community Action*, London: Routledge.

Stimson, G.V. and Oppenheimer, E. (1982) *Heroin Addiction: Treatment and Control in Britain*, London: Tavistock.

Tarantino, Q. (1994) *Pulp Fiction*, London: Faber and Faber.

Weber, M. (1930) *The Protestant Ethic and the Spirit of Capitalism*, London: Allen and Unwin.

WHO (World Health Organisation) (1951) *Expert Committee on Mental Health, Alchoholism Sub-Committee: Second Report*, Tech. Rep. Ser. 42, Geneva: WHO.

WHO (World Health Organisation) (1952) *Expert Committee on Mental Health, Alchoholism Sub-Committee: Second Report*, Tech. Rep. Ser. 84, Geneva: WHO.

WHO (World Health Organisation) (1969) *Report of Expert Committee on Addiction-Producing Drugs*, Tech. Rep. Ser. 407, Geneva: WHO.

WHO (World Health Organisation) (1988) *Towards Healthy Public Policies on Alcohol and Other Drugs: A Consensus Statement*, Report of Expert Working Group Meeting, Canberra, Australia, 28–31 March, Canberra: WHO.

Chapter 14

Welfare direct

Informatics and the emergence of self-service welfare?

Brian D. Loader

INTRODUCTION

Whilst the pervasive role of new information and communications technologies (ICTs) as a means of changing the management of liberal democratic welfare states has been recognised (Pollitt 1990; Hoggett 1990), the prospect of their intrinsic catalytic qualities facilitating entirely new social relations of welfare delivery has been largely ignored. This chapter explores the contention that the advent of technologies like smart cards, CD-ROMS and sophisticated computer networks such as the Internet, with their ability to deconstruct time and space boundaries, represent a profound and significant challenge to postwar models of social policy. In particular, I wish to focus upon the proposition that ICTs may be underpinning a fundamental shift away from the conception of welfare as based upon rationally administered state provision, paternalistically and professionally determined needs, and bureaucratic organisational delivery systems, towards an emphasis upon fragmentation, diversity and self-reliance. More specifically, self-service technologies such as those emerging in the private sector finance and retail industries may be regarded as a prelude to their adoption in creating a self-service welfare system.

Clearly, notions of plurality, diversity and fragmentation have a resonance in the literature of postmodernist writers, and indeed the importance of ICTs for social change has been a consistent theme in much of their work.[1] Perhaps for this reason it might be tempting to assume that technologically driven changes to welfare constitute the impending arrival of a postmodern conception of welfare. Instead, the argument proposed here is that profound technological developments are grounded in late-modernist ideologies, scientific understanding and universal proclamations. This is not, however, to deny that a consideration of postmodern insights may help to illuminate processes of social change and provide us with understanding: a somewhat traditional, Enlightenment approach upon which to make better policy choices one would have thought.

As almost seems customary in discussions of this type, it is necessary to include a 'technological determinism' disclaimer at this early juncture. To suggest that the new ICTs have such force for social change is not to concede that technology determines our future. Rather it is to suggest that ICTs are both developed within a social, economic and political context and in turn create the opportunity for both the intended and unintended transformation of that context. Thus the suggested emergence of self-service welfare systems is not meant to imply a particular outcome but rather a broad conception within which competing formulations may struggle for ascendancy.

Throughout this chapter, my basic premise is that the development of ICTs and their effects upon social welfare relations are mediated by issues of power, class, gender, race, culture, economy and ideology. The largely unpredictable but rapid changes in these social and economic structures ensure that the technological shape of things to come will remain difficult to specify with any degree of certainty.[2] What is important for an understanding of social and public policy developments, however, is analysis of how these mediating factors interact with the process of technological configuration.

The deterministic nature of much of the current debate about social and economic restructuring arises in part from an overemphasis upon technological artefacts which are dislocated from human imagination, and from the cultural and moral contexts which produced them. Thus the impressive capabilities of ICTs are often paraded by management and communications consultants and by some policymakers as producing the transition to a new paradigm of global business opportunities.[3] Failure to join this inevitable force is regarded as courting exclusion, political and cultural isolation, and financial disaster at all levels of human endeavour. For many discussants it is only the encumbrance of the past which prevents us from embracing the technological utopia which will be our 'virtual' future.[4]

Whilst still focusing upon the awe-inspiring qualities of ICTs, an alternative, dystopian vision of tomorrow's world emerges from the disparate work of science fiction writers, postmodernist commentators and technological luddites. This might be described as the 'Blade Runner' syndrome after Ridley Scott's film of that name, which depicted a dark, ghettoised urban existence overlaid by technological instruments of social control in the guise of replicants. Whilst the various utopian and dystopian commentaries which figure prominently in the polemic on social change are regarded as opposites, they arguably share the same deterministic tendency to regard technology as something which is beyond our control but instead controls us. Understandably, such stark juxtapositions may make for enjoyable debate and provide thoughtful tableaux of social change (see Burrows 1997), but such representations are often overdrawn and pay insufficient attention to both continuity with past social and political factors and the role of social action in influencing outcomes.

TECHNOLOGY AND WELFARE

The increasing role of informatics[5] in the provision and delivery of welfare services is becoming more noticeable. Much of the organisational restructuring occurring in the British welfare state can indeed be said to be predicated upon the alleged potential of ICTs to create flexible and decentralised forms (Hoggett 1990; Kelly 1991). The introduction of quasi-market mechanisms (Le Grand 1990) into the NHS and community care programmes, for example, is heavily dependent upon the development of highly sophisticated information networks between a range of statutory, voluntary and private sector agencies. So too in local government, discussion has focused upon the potential of computer networks to facilitate organisational forms responsive to 'customer' demands (Taylor and Williams 1989; Audit Commission 1990). Undoubtedly an increasing motive for utilising ICTs in the public domain has been the growing financial pressures upon the welfare state and the prospect held out of technological solutions increasing productivity and controlling public expenditure.

For the most part, the Petri dish for the growth of the new technologies has been the private sector. The importance of the profit-making sector for developing models which are often later absorbed by the public domain has been observed by several writers (Hoggett 1991; Stoker 1989). Stoker, for example, remarks that 'developments pioneered in the private sector open up the possibility of increased productivity in the service sector' (Stoker 1989: 159). Such prospective transformations are often associated with a broad range of literature which might collectively be called post-Fordist, and which has been responsible for emphasising significant changes in both production processes and the nature of consumption patterns on the basis of technological innovation. 'The availability of information technology in all its forms – data processing, communications and control, computer-aided design, office automation – offers the possibility of recasting traditionally labour-intensive service activities. And one major use of such technology is to reduce the aggregate cost of a particular service and the employment within it' (Stoker 1989: 160). Likewise information technologies, from library stock-control systems to touch-screen kiosks, are able to meet the differentiated and increasingly informed and articulated demands of welfare 'customers'.[6]

Whilst post-Fordist models have been useful for placing welfare reforms within a wider economic mode of restructuring, they have none the less been subject to a range of severe criticisms (Carter and Rayner 1996; Williams 1994). First, they are often regarded as technologically and economically deterministic, due to the lack of attention given to agency and social struggle in influencing social relations of welfare (Bagguley 1994). Second, and relatedly, 'post-Fordist analyses are rooted in a white, male, able-bodied experience of welfare which ignores or marginalises the significance of other social relations'(Williams 1994: 57) such as gender, race or disability. Third, by focusing upon the most startling new organisational forms, such as Benetton's (Clegg 1990), which are developed around highly sophisticated information technology networks and are predicated upon radically different, post-bureaucratic control structures, they have a tendency to stress paradigmatic discontinuity with a Fordist welfare state past.

Welfare services have of course always been heavily information based, and arguably a defining characteristic of the modern welfare organisation, be it a hospital, school or benefits office, has been its tendency to transform people into information before processing them through the system. As a consequence perhaps we should be little surprised that the new ICTs should be eagerly adopted for use, with their promise of faster and more reliable processing capacity. In this context the pervasiveness of ICTs is no more than an example of the continuity (Pierson 1994) of previous practice. Christopher Pollitt, in his review of the development of managerialism in the public sector, highlights the similarities between Frederick Taylor's preoccupation with bureaucratic control procedures, through the 'scientific' measurement of working practices in the early part of this century, and 'the recent epidemic of electronically-mediated public-service systems of performance indicators, individual performance review and merit pay' (Pollitt 1990: 16).

Certainly it may be fair to suggest that the rhetoric of the transforming qualities of the ICTs has yet to be matched by practice in many of the new quasi-markets in the UK. In health care the example of Wessex Regional Health Authority is usually raised fairly early in any discussions of computer systems failure, closely followed by those of the Birmingham health authority and the London Ambulance Service and the more recent debacle of the HISS (Hospital Information System) initiative. In education also the highly complex information systems underpinning modular programmes are seldom matched by the software required to run them. So too, in numerous other examples in the public domain, implementation failure of computerised information systems has been the order of the day (Keen 1994; Margetts 1996; Mays and Dixon 1996).

When one considers the reasons for such technological unfulfilment, however, a significant gulf may be discerned between the culture and structures of the organisations within which the ICTs are implanted and the social and economic context within which the technologies are developed. It is instructive to consider the most common reasons given for the limited success of such initiatives (Audit Commission 1990):

- lack of understanding of the complexity of the public domain by computer companies keen to sell their products in a large market;
- a gap between the 'language' of computer specialists and those responsible for service delivery;
- resistance from professionals to informatics designed to reduce their traditional freedoms;

- fear from employees of job losses;
- too much emphasis upon technology and insufficient attention to information systems.

Any explanation of such failure must take account of the complex social relations which militate against the simple transfer of post-Fordist flexible firm models into the welfare domain. The notion of public service organisations becoming 'Benettonised' (Stoker 1989: 166) implies something more fundamental than merely seeing ICTs as an appendage to an improvement of the efficiency of existing welfare organisations. It suggests a 'new public management' strategy (Hood 1991) devoted to introducing information systems which challenge the heterogeneous and contested organisational cultures of welfare institutions. The NHS Information Network, for example, has faced considerable opposition from interested parties such as professional groups, trade unions and citizens' rights groups over issues such as clinical autonomy, patient confidentiality and privacy.

In this context information is not an independent organisational resource the shape of which all will be agreed upon. Rather it is a negotiated and contested construct which may be designed with a purpose and used in such a way as to impact significantly upon the social relations of welfare. So too the shape and style of the communications network which conveys such information will act to influence the nature of social control mechanisms. Any information system must therefore act to influence power relations between competing agents and be regarded as an important tool in such social and economic struggles. It may be used to decide who is included and excluded; to reinforce existing patterns of inequality; or to define the terms of engagement.

Since computer-mediated information systems cannot be regarded as 'value-neutral', they may be seen as an important site for studying the interrelationship between the state, the economy and civil society, and its consequences for the social relations of welfare. We will return to this later in the chapter, but for now it is important to recognise that post-Fordist accounts have tended to be technologically reductive by paying too little attention to the complex role of informatics in the social relations of welfare. If the limitations of new public management in introducing post-Fordist organisational forms into the welfare state are regarded as merely a 'flawed' version of the real thing (Jessop 1994), this may point not only to the theoretical looseness of the model but also to its inability to incorporate resistance from welfare professionals from within the system, and opposition to welfare regimes from groups who have continually felt marginalised by its class-based, white, male, able-bodied orientation.

THE 'EXTERNALISATION' OF WELFARE

What makes the new ICTs such a catalyst for change is their potential to change radically the power relationships between welfare organisations, subjects and nation states. That is, they may alter the focus from internal organisational information systems based upon bureaucratic control mechanisms to one where new control patterns transform the interstices between the service deliverer and recipient. In particular they may act to transform the way people consume welfare and the way they may perceive their own needs.

Writing from what they describe as a neo-Fordist perspective, Blackburn and his colleagues (1985) have discussed the way that information technologies in the service sector can be used to increase profitability by what they term the 'externalisation of service labour'. That is, 'rather than provide the service "in full", service production takes the form of providing the users with the means to provide the service, to varying degrees, for themselves. The user contributes some of the labour, unpaid, whilst capital provides the means of production' (Blackburn *et al.* 1985: 171). This form of self-help is now fairly widespread in the retail sector, with perhaps the supermarket being the most common manifestation. Consumers effectively enter a warehouse of goods and with the use of a shopping trolley contribute their own unpaid labour to the collection and transportation of goods to their own homes. This process is augmented by a computerised stock-control system which ensures that consumer demand for particular products and their replacement on the shelves are accurately recorded and executed. Until recently the only significant block to increasing labour productivity through self-service was the need to employ people on the check-out. The development of portable bar-code readers, enabling consumers to input their own purchasing data into the system and thereby keep a check on the running total, which is currently being introduced into some supermarkets may increase the scope of self-service still further.

The potential for externalisation of welfare service labour through the adoption of appropriate technologies has only more recently been considered. Thus public information kiosks and electronic village halls act to enable clients to access some public services for themselves. Such initiatives have tended to be driven by the desire to improve the quality of public services, increase democratic participation, provide greater freedom of access to public information and raise productivity. As we stated elsewhere, however (Lauritzen and Loader 1995), the degree to which such projects represent a significant change of control is limited. Typically the extent of externalisation has been restricted by the kinds of social and political resistance which we considered above. These include such factors as:

* the confidentiality of public information;
* the lack of interactivity and a tendency for standardised information to be

provided *to* the public rather than welfare agencies responding to requests *from* the public;
- the definition of public information by public service organisations;
- professional control over expertise and knowledge.

SOCIAL INNOVATION, SELF-SERVICE AND WELFARE DIRECT

We can see from the post-1987 welfare reforms in the UK that ICTs have been limited in their impact upon traditional, modernist welfare institutions, and that even patterns of externalisation to be found in the private sector have not made much impression on public welfare services. There is, however, an alternative form of self-serving technology identified by Gershuny and Miles (1983) which they describe as 'social innovation', a process which requires the transformation of the service so that it is almost completely produced by consumers in their own home, locality or community. One of the most significant impacts of ICTs in service delivery in the private sector has been the rise of direct banking and insurance businesses, which enable a high degree of self-service consumption using telephony. The consequence of this technology has been a rapid closure of many high-street branches and the laying off of thousands of employees: a trend which has no doubt a lot further to go.

The technology required for social innovation is developing at a very fast rate. Whilst not including all citizens, most European countries have a high level of telephone connection, and cable companies are rapidly connecting millions of urban households to a range of digital communications services. Together with smart-card technology and the global communications network of the Internet, these ICTs constitute the infrastructure which may provide the setting for the renegotiation of social relations of welfare.

For such social innovation to lead to a 'welfare direct' model, not only does the technology need to be available but the nature of welfare consumption would need to be significantly transformed from one based upon dependency and standardisation. As with the post-Fordist thesis we must, however, be cautious about assuming a simple transplantation of technology developed in the private sector into the welfare domain, without recourse to the complex social relations which will militate against its development. At the present time there does indeed appear to be a growing consensus emerging across a large section of the political spectrum in the UK that welfare provision should be directed at helping recipients to help themselves. For example, the then Shadow Chancellor of the Exchequer, Gordon Brown, suggested that Labour policy will be less directed towards asking 'what the state can do for you, but rather what the state can do to help you do things for yourself' (*Guardian*, 11 February 1997). Conservative social policy was for some time using the language of consumer choice and 'enabling' welfare agencies. Such exhortations to self-help provide an important context within which the new

ICTs may be used to attempt to hard-wire the perceptions of welfare recipients, but they do not guarantee the outcome.

In part, technological development becomes embedded in the political and social deliberations of 'empowerment', 'citizenship' and 'consumerism' as well as driven by financial restraints. For many citizens the message may be read that if they do not look after themselves then the state is not going to be there, at least not all the way to the grave. Thus an increasing market may emerge for insurance, pensions and other financial forms of direct self-service, which will further provide opportunities for technological development.

A different dimension to the drive towards a self-service welfare system comes from the privatisation of government information systems such as the IT section of the Department of Transport (DVOIT) and the IT Office of the Inland Revenue. Both these tenders were won by the US company Electronic Data Systems (EDS). This process of 'outsourcing' gives a clear indication that public information systems represent a significant market for the small number of private sector international data-processing companies (Margetts and Dunleavy 1995). It is not unreasonable to assume that companies like EDS will be keen to utilise ICTs to maximise their profitability through social innovation.

SOCIAL POLICY FOR THE INFORMATION AGE

The primary characteristics of self-service welfare may be summarised as follows:

• The welfare service commodity is transformed to enable it to be produced in the home or local community.
• The recipient is responsible for taking on almost all the labour costs for the service.
• The system may facilitate the transfer of capital costs to individuals, voluntary organisations or teleworkers.
• The system is built upon highly sophisticated informatics applications.
• The recipient may (at least in appearance) be empowered to contest the authority of professionals.

A number of recent initiatives would suggest that the conditions for social innovation to usher in a further stage in the restructuring of the welfare state may be about to happen. The introduction of voluntary identity cards is but a short step from the more widespread use of smart cards containing personal information which can be used for identification, health care, education or benefits transactions. Large bureaucratic organisations such as the Benefits Agency seem about to embark upon the 'downsizing' experienced in the private sector service industries. Indeed, the privatisation of government information systems may well include those for the Child Support Agency, the DSS, the NHS and the administration of the Home Office's National

Identity Card Scheme, to add to the Inland Revenue and DVOIT mentioned above.

The application of self-service welfare to particular policy areas is not difficult to speculate about. Community care by its nature is based upon the notion of supporting people to live in their own homes. Distance-learning technologies may facilitate educational opportunities for those unable or not wishing to attend traditional time- and space-constrained educational institutions. In health care also there is the potential benefit of enabling people to challenge the 'medical model' and assume responsibility for their own health.

The movement towards a self-service welfare system is not likely to go uncontested. At its very heart is a reconstitution of power relationships between consumers, professionals and the state. Foucault has argued that in the past much information was constructed by governments for the administrative control of increasingly large populations (Foucault 1991). Self-service welfare implies a strategy of 'remote control' whereby individuals take on the responsibility for controlling their own actions (Hoggett 1994). The empowerment achieved through the acquisition and manipulation of knowledge has an implied corresponding responsibility to solve one's own problems. Aspects of health promotion may provide an illustration of how so-called informed and responsible citizens take care of themselves through exercise and watching what they eat and thus avoid becoming a burden upon others in the community.

As I have been at pains to stress, the precise configuration of social relations will be less the product of technological development and more the outcome of social contestation. The sentiment is captured best by Carolyn Marvin, who states that the development of ICTs 'is less the evolution of technical efficiencies in communication than a series of arenas for negotiating issues crucial to the conduct of social life; among them, who is inside and outside, who may speak, who may not, and who has authority and may be believed' (Marvin 1988: 4).

What might be the factors which contribute to the shaping of a self-service welfare model? First, it is important to realise that 'welfare direct' is not a uniform phenomenon. By its very nature it is likely to be fragmentary and take diverse forms which may act to reinforce existing inequalities. Some individuals and localities may be better placed to take advantage of the potential opportunities for empowerment and advancement afforded by some ICTs. Other technological applications, such as the use of closed-circuit television (CCTV), electronic tagging and identity cards, may have more potential for social control and be perceived as excluding more disadvantaged members of society. Moreover, the possible trend towards 'direct welfare' may have significant consequences for women where 'the home' is considered as a female domain. In this context, technology which provides flexible part-time teleworking to enable predominantly women to both earn an income and care for dependents can be regarded as a means of 'keeping women in their place' (Williams 1993) rather than giving them access to 'cyber-space'. A similar 'social imprisonment' may be the consequence of heralding the advantages of ICTs for disabled people as empowerment through home shopping, distance learning or teleworking.

Yet, secondly, it is necessary to recognise that the advent of 'welfare direct' is not simply a neo-liberal desire to return to Samuel Smiles's Victorian values of self-help.[7] The institutions and practices of the welfare state have been much criticised by those championing a recognition of difference and diversity on grounds of gender, race, disability and sexuality. Here the new ICTs may be adopted as a means for groups to break free from state-imposed identification, and seek alternative forms of expression and support through computer-mediated communication (Haraway 1991: 149–81). The feeling of anonymity experienced by using the Internet has led some women and black people to remark on the non-discriminatory nature of discourse and social interaction in remote, networked communications.

Last and relatedly, a growing number of self-help groups are beginning to utilise the Internet as a means to provide computer-mediated social support (CMSS) networks. Here we may be seeing the spontaneous development of social action whereby individuals and groups form themselves into loose associations which we might describe as 'virtual community care'.[8] These CMSS networks are global in nature and enable the voluntary interaction of people clustered around a range of possible areas of support, such as a particular disease (MS, HIV, etc.), a common experience (alcoholism, child abuse, etc.) or a state of mind (depression, shyness, etc.). As sites of exchange for 'lay knowledge', CMSSs may also act as an example of how ICTs may be used by welfare recipients as a means to challenge the dominant professional discourses of health and welfare.

CONCLUSION: THE MODE OF INFORMATION AND WELFARE PROVISION

As mentioned at the outset, the position adopted here is that the trajectory of technologically driven change is not determined by, but rather the consequence of a multitude of competing economic, political and social factors. They are not equal; some exercise more influence than others. I have suggested that current developments can lead one to speculate that we will witness the development of some form of self-service welfare system yet to be worked out in detail. Postmodern analysis, however, suggests that such structural change will lead to a paradigmatic breach with the past. They point to a disillusionment with grand universal theories based upon Enlightenment conceptions of progress, and suggest that nation states based upon territory, hierarchical managerial control of populations and policing are being eroded (Crook et al. 1992: 106) by globalisation. They further maintain that social class and patriarchal and racial modes of political organisation are being replaced by a diverse range of new social movements, championing social difference and emancipation from subjection.

Clearly such assertions have important implications for traditional welfare state models of social policy. Unlike Peter Taylor-Gooby, who asserts that 'postmodernism functions as an ideological smokescreen, preventing us from recognising some of the most important trends in modern social policy' (Tayor-Gooby 1994: 385), I would like to suggest that it may at least be responsible for foregrounding the importance of informatics as a significant force affecting policy outcomes. As such, a consideration of postmodern insights may be useful as a means of ascertaining the extent to which such technologically driven developments represent a disjuncture with past models of welfare provision. Whilst any such consideration must be cursory, I would like none the less to foreground one area which may be fruitful for social policy analysts to consider.

The recent work of Mark Poster (1990, 1995) in attempting to articulate the complex relationship between postmodern discourse and the new technologies of communication is perhaps a useful point of departure. His contention is that a consideration of communications suggests a historical periodisation of what he describes as the 'mode of information'.

> Every age employs forms of symbolic exchange which contain internal and external structures, means and relations of significance. Stages in the mode of information may be tentatively designated as follows: face-to-face, orally mediated exchange; written exchanges mediated by print; and electronically mediated exchange.
>
> (Poster 1990: 6)

The study of the mode of information requires that we examine the manner in which information is processed. 'Each method of preserving and transmitting information profoundly intervenes in the network of relationships that constitute a society' (Poster 1990: 7). The welfare state embodies a particular mode of information derived from the need for large governments to control expanding populations by means of written records and bureaucratic organisation. The hypothesis is that new configurations of communication arising from the ICTs give rise to a 'radical reconfiguration of language, one which constitutes subjects outside the pattern of the rational, autonomous individual' (Poster 1995: 57). 'What is at stake are new language formations that alter significantly the network of social relations, that re-structure those relations and the subjects they constitute' (Poster 1995: 60). I have made clear that it is far too speculative to suggest that the movement towards a self-service welfare system represents the advent of postmodernity. However, Poster's formulation does foreground the need to consider how such social innovation may alter social networks. The widespread use of such technologies may indeed create new language formations. Most significantly, the study of social policy must include the analysis of the restructuring of social relations and subjects which are mediated by the new ICTs.

NOTES

1 I am thinking predominantly here of Jean-François Lyotard (1984) and Jean Baudrillard (1983).
2 Indeed I recognise that some of the main contentions in this chapter are somewhat speculative in nature.
3 A cursory glance at the promotional literature of the telecommunications industry, or Tapscott and Caston's *Paradigm Shift* (1993), will give a flavour of this perspective. Policy makers too are trusting to the determining qualities of ICTs through such programmes as the UK government's Information Society Initiative or as outlined in Bangemann (1994), a report produced for the European Commission.
4 I have tried to deal elsewhere with the limitations of what I describe as the cyber-libertarian perspective (Loader 1997).
5 This is the synthesis of digital communications systems with computer processing power to create new modes of information retrieval, manipulation, dissemination and simulation.
6 For a fuller review of the debate about social policy and post-Fordism see Burrows and Loader (1994).
7 It may be remembered that the doyen of Thatcherite welfare policies, Sir Keith Joseph, wrote the preface to the reprinted Penguin edition of Smiles's *Self Help*.
8 The term 'virtual community care' was coined by Roger Burrows.

BIBLIOGRAPHY

Audit Commission (1990) *Preparing an Information Technology Strategy: Making IT Happen*, London: HMSO.
Bagguley, P. (1994) 'Pioneers of the Beveridge dream? The political mobilisation of the poor against contemporary welfare regimes', in R. Burrows and B. Loader (eds) *Towards a Post-Fordist Welfare State?*, London: Routledge.
Bangemann, M. (1994) 'Europe and the global information society: recommendations to the European Council prepared by members of the High Level Group on the Information Society', Brussels: European Council.
Baudrillard, J. (1983) *Simulations*, New York: Semiotext(e).
Blackburn, P., Coombs, R. and Green, K. (1985) *Technology, Economic Growth and the Labour Process*, Basingstoke: Macmillan.
Burrows, R. (1997) 'Virtual culture, urban social polarisation and social science fiction', in B. Loader (ed.) *The Governance of Cyberspace: Politics, Technology and Global Restructuring*, London: Routledge.
Burrows, R. and Loader, B. (1994) *Towards a Post-Fordist Welfare State?*, London: Routledge.
Carter, J. and Rayner, M. (1996) 'The curious case of post-Fordism and welfare', *Journal of Social Policy*, 25, 3: 347–67.
Clegg, S.R. (1990) *Modern Organisation*, London: Sage.
Crook, S., Pakulsk, J. and Waters, M. (1992) *Postmodernisation: Change in Advanced Society*, London: Sage.
Foucault, M. (1991) 'Governmentality', in G. Burchill, C. Gordon and P. Miller (eds) *The Foucault Effect: Studies in Governability*, Hemel Hempstead: Harvester Wheatsheaf.

Gershuny, J.I. and Miles, I. (1983) *The New Service Economy: The Transformation of Employment in Industrial Societies*, London: Frances Pinter.

Haraway, D. (1991) *Simians, Cyborgs and Women: The Reinvention of Nature*, London: Free Association Books.

Hoggett, P. (1990) *Modernisation, Political Strategy and the Welfare State: an Organisational Perspective*, Studies in Decentralisation and Quasi-markets 2, Bristol: SAUS, University of Bristol.

Hoggett, P. (1991) 'A new management in the public sector', *Policy and Politics* 19, 4: 143–56.

Hoggett, P. (1994) 'The politics of the modernisation of the UK welfare state', in R. Burrows and B. Loader (eds) *Towards a Post-Fordist Welfare State?*, London: Routledge.

Hood, C. (1991) 'A public management for all seasons?', *Public Administration* 69, 1: 3–19.

Jessop, B. (1994) 'The transition to post-Fordism and the Schumpeterian workfare state', in R. Burrows and B. Loader (eds) *Towards a Post-Fordist Welfare State?*, London: Routledge.

Keen, J. (1994) 'Should the NHS have an information strategy?', *Public Administration* 72: 33–53.

Kelly, A. (1991) 'The enterprise culture and the welfare state', in R. Burrows (ed.) *Deciphering the Enterprise Culture*, London: Routledge.

Lauritzen, B. and Loader, B.D. (1995) 'On the way to the electronic forum?', in J. Lovenduski and J. Stanyer (eds) *Contemporary Political Studies. Vol. 2*, London: PSA.

Le Grand, J. (1990) *Quasi-Markets and Social Policy*, Studies in Decentralisation and Quasi-Markets 1, Bristol: SAUS.

Loader, B.D. (ed) (1997) *The Governance of Cyberspace: Politics, Technology and Global Restructuring*, London: Routledge.

Lyotard, J.-F. (1984) *The Postmodern Condition: A Report on Knowledge*, Manchester: Manchester University Press.

Margetts, H. (1996) 'Variation on modernism: 50 years of computerisation in government', paper presented at the Computing Study Group in Public Administration, August.

Margetts, H. and Dunleavy, P. (1995) 'Public services on the world market', *Demos Quarterly* 7: 30–2.

Marvin, C. (1988) *When Old Technologies Were New: Thinking about Electric Communication in the Late Nineteenth Century*, New York: Oxford University Press.

Mays, N. and Dixon, J. (1996) *Purchaser Plurality in UK Health Care*, London: Kings Fund.

Pierson, C. (1994) 'Continuity and discontinuity in the emergence of the post-Fordist welfare state', in R. Burrows and B. Loader (eds) *Towards a Post-Fordist Welfare State?*, London: Routledge.

Pollitt, C. (1990) *Managerialism and the Public Services*, Oxford: Blackwell.

Poster, M. (1990) *The Mode of Information*, Cambridge: Polity Press.

Poster, M. (1995) *The Second Media Age*, Cambridge: Polity Press.

Stoker, G. (1989) 'Creating local government for a post-Fordist society: the Thatcherite project?', in J. Stewart and G. Stoker (eds) *The Future of Local Government*, Basingstoke: Macmillan.

Tapscott, D. and Caston, A. (1993) *Paradigm Shift: The New Promise of Information Technology*, New York: McGraw-Hill.

Taylor, J. and Williams, H. (1989) 'Telematics, organization and the local government mission', *Local Government Studies* May/June: 75–93.

Taylor-Gooby, P. (1994) 'Postmodernism and social policy: a great leap backwards?' *Journal of Social Policy* 23, 3: 385–404.

Williams, F. (1993) 'Women and community', in J. Bornat, C. Pereira, D. Pilgrim and F. Williams (eds) *Community Care: A Reader*, Basingstoke: Macmillan.

Williams, F. (1994) 'Social relations, welfare and the post-Fordist debate', in R. Burrows and B. Loader (eds) *Towards a Post-Fordist Welfare State?*, London: Routledge.

Part V

Citizenship amid the fragmented nation state

Chapter 15

The delivery of welfare

The associationist vision

Paul Hoggett and Simon Thompson

INTRODUCTION

A radical vision of a welfare society must seek to combine the universalism and commitment to equality of the old labour movement with the particularism and commitment to social diversity of the new social movements (Thompson and Hoggett 1996). In other words, what we require are 'universal services which are capable of meeting diverse and differentiated needs' (Williams 1989: 215).

If a system of governance is to respond effectively to the diversity of human requirements, individuals and groups must have real power to articulate and define their needs and determine the manner in which they will be met. In order to see how this might be achieved, many recent discussions of empowerment have returned to the seminal work of Hirschman (1970). Put simply, according to Hirschman, where citizens feel dissatisfied with the performance of an institution, they have two major options: they can either leave it – Hirschman would describe this as the exercise of 'exit'; or they can complain, protest or argue with it – this option he calls 'voice'. (Alternatively, they can do nothing in the conviction that things will sort themselves out over time – so displaying what Hirschman labels 'loyalty'.)

Compared to most other European countries, neo-liberal attacks upon the welfare state came early to Britain. As a consequence, Hirschman's concept of exit has become strongly associated with the arguments of the pro-market right. Parts of the left, by contrast, have sought to develop what might be called the democratised welfare state model which gives primary emphasis to the voice mechanism (Burns *et al.* 1994). Hirschman himself did not counterpose these two empowerment mechanisms but saw them as complementing each other. This is the lead we follow here: on the assumption that the time has come to re-evaluate the potential utility of exit and voice as empowerment mechanisms that work best in tandem, the principal aim of this chapter is to try to find an institutional framework capable of combining exit and voice, and so meeting the complex welfare objectives we have specified.

We will examine the proposition that some form of associative democracy is the most appropriate institutional framework in which such principles could be embodied. The idea of associative democracy, developed recently by writers such as Cohen and Rogers (1995) and Hirst (1994), offers a vision of the future in which there is substantial devolution of power down from the centralised state to a system of voluntary, self-governing associations. The innovativeness of the model lies in its promise to decouple the right of exit from the market; thus the consumer is replaced by the member seeking to join or leave associations located within civil society. In this system, citizens would join a number of welfare associations in order to provide as many as possible of their welfare services for themselves through these associations. Voluntary, self-governing associations would become the chief mechanism through which citizens received housing, health care, education, pensions, and so on.

The associationist vision tends to be rather abstract, so it is useful to pause for a moment to get a more concrete idea of what it might look like in practice. First, and perhaps most important, the idea of a membership association points to something more like a 'welfare' trade union or automobile association than a traditional voluntary organisation. These organisations would get virtually all of their funds from the membership fees of their members, which might be paid for by personal contributions or via state benefits in the form of associational vouchers (Le Grand 1989; Schmitter 1995).

Hirst's model seeks to provide for the independence of the associational sphere. Since associations are not tied to contracts or dependent upon huge grants or subsidies from government, associations stand or fall on the support of their members. On the other hand, while the associational sphere exists alongside a devolved apparatus of representative government (Hirst speaks of regional and municipal forms of government), structures would also be developed through which associational and institutional forms of government could interpenetrate (Hirst's regional assembly is partly composed of representatives elected via the associations).

THE INTERNAL STRUCTURE OF ASSOCIATIONS

The first issue we focus on concerns the internal structure of associations. What form should the relationship of individuals to their associations take? Both Hirst and Cohen and Rogers opt for a combination of exit and voice rights. Let us consider each type of right in turn.

Exit rights

Associational democrats contend that the basis of citizen empowerment lies in the right to join or leave an association – that is, in the right of exit (Hirst 1994: 196; Cohen and Rogers 1995: 65, 69, 71). Exit has a number of beneficial features. First, it operates as an essential last resort: if things go badly in an association, members can always vote with their feet. Second, it is relatively cheap: the association gets a clear signal that something is going wrong without, for example, having to engage in extensive consultation with all its members. Third, considering the objection that a considerable degree of cultural capital is needed to participate effectively in associations, it can be argued that an exit right enables ordinary members – that is, those without such capital – to exercise effective control over their association's elite group.

There are, however, a number of obstacles to the effective exercise of exit rights which caution against overreliance on this mechanism on its own. The first obstacle is financial: if individuals lack the necessary material resources to survive outside of the association they belong to, then exit will be extremely difficult for them. Here the guaranteed minimum income that Hirst proposes, and which is provided directly by the state rather than through associations, forms a vital safety net for individuals wanting to get out of their association (Hirst 1994: 179–88). A second obstacle is that presented by the absence of alternatives. In some – particularly rural – areas, alternatives to the local education or health association may simply not be available. In other circumstances, associational monopolies may arise as a result of the behaviour of the associations themselves; for example, one may be in a position to exploit economies of scale in order to acquire monopolistic power. Here two possible solutions suggest themselves: first, the legal-political framework should make it easy for small numbers of citizens to set up new associations – perhaps special financial aid should be available; second, there need to be procedures for limiting the size of associations (a kind of anti-trust legislation for the associational sector: Hoggett 1994).

Another problem, caused by the vulnerability of some people, presents a serious difficulty for any associational scheme. Many citizens are necessarily placed in situations of great dependency on the welfare state because of their physical or emotional difficulties. It is simply not realistic to speak of vulnerable hospital patients or confused elderly people directly exercising the right of exit or voice. Here it may be that the development of forms of user advocacy are necessary in order to provide them with a way of indirectly exercising such rights. A final obstacle is created by the ties that many people have to their particular social group. Here Hirst's answer seems to lie in his hope that processes of modernisation are undermining what he sees as traditional 'communities of fate' (Hirst 1994: 54). As a contribution to this process, he advocates a system of compulsory liberal education which informs all individuals of the choices open to them. It could be argued that this provides a vital part of a cultural infrastructure in which the right of exit can enhance individuals' autonomy (Hirst 1994: 58).

Voice rights

In the light of these problems with exit, it seems to us that there is a good case for valuing voice. Hirst argues for the introduction of a body of associational law under which all associations would adhere to 'minimal procedures' of self-government (Hirst 1994: 194) in order to make them 'accountable' to their members (p. 168). In the case of welfare associations, this involves providing every member with one vote in elections of representatives onto a management council (p. 192). Cohen and Rogers's account runs along very similar lines. They argue that associations' patterns of internal decision making should combine centralised power over their members with accountability to those members (Cohen and Rogers 1995: 55, 58, 59, 61). Both schemes are, in effect, microcosms of a conventional liberal representative political system: government *of* and *for* – but not *by* – the people.

Voice has at least two important advantages over exit. First of all, it is much more information rich. When people leave an association this does not in itself give the remaining members any clue about what is going wrong; only if members stay and complain – that is, use their voice rights – can the things that are causing the problems be identified and so put right. Moreover, exit cannot provide users of a service with control over that service. This can only be achieved when users are involved as co-producers in the decision-making process that governs a service – again, when they exercise their voice (Pestoff 1994).[1] Although democracy may be time consuming, it is arguable that the quality of decisions which eventually emerge is improved, and that they have a far greater chance of being effectively implemented by citizens who have a sense of ownership of them.

Of course, voice has certain problems of its own. It is questionable whether a significant element of democracy is always valued by members of an association so long as it delivers the goods. Here we are reminded of Warmley Golden Hours – a membership-based group of elderly people in east Bristol. Here the incumbent officers grew so tired of being 'elected' unopposed at an empty annual general meeting that one year they sprang the AGM upon an unsuspecting membership which had turned out en masse for a Christmas social. The point is that not all people at all stages of their lives value the active exercise of voice. In this particular case, members saw their continued loyalty as a more important value than voice.

Second, the common supposition that democratically structured associations function as schools of democracy for the broader political system can also be brought into question. This assumes that associations are microcosms of the system as a whole, creating what could be seen as a case of felicitous institutional isomorphism – that they are places where people learn to be more other-regarding by working co-operatively with others. The potential significance of this argument is pointed up by recent British research (Moyser *et al.* 1992), which reveals that a much larger and more diverse range of people participates in voluntary associations than in political parties. All the better, then, if such participation instils virtues in citizens that strengthen and stabilise the broader democratic political system.

There are, however, at least two counters to this notion that associations have educative value. The first of these simply challenges the evidence. Thus

Rosenblum (1994) argues that there is scant support for the claim that the consciousness-raising benefits of participation cross over from one area of social life to another – for example, from a particular association to the wider political system. Moreover, she unpicks the argument that democratic virtues can be learnt in 'social identity groups', pointing out that such groups are highly diverse in character, and hence – most relevant in this context – they need not be at all democratic (Rosenblum 1994: 87–94). The second reason to be sceptical about the school-for-democracy claim lies in the argument that the decentralisation of political power to associations will in fact stimulate a narrow and negative form of particularism. It will thus make people *less* other-regarding, and so erode the consensual basis on which democracy depends.

To summarise this section, note Hirst's claim that 'the core ethical claim of associationism ... is justified on essentially individualistic terms' (Hirst 1994: 50); associations are therefore 'communities of choice'. But we have seen that there are factors which will tend to make the illusion of choice more powerful than the substance. Thus we would conclude that there are a number of reasons for regarding voice as a vital, indispensable supplement – rather than a wholesale alternative – to exit. The essence of voice is that it draws people to act in concert, and it is therefore an essentially collectivist method of empowerment. The value of a system of associational governance lies in its capacity to combine individual choice with collective action – through a combination of the mechanisms of exit and voice.

ASSOCIATIONS AND OTHER SOCIAL GROUPS

The second general issue that we wish to address concerns the relation of associations to other social groups. To put the problem in the form of a single question: to what extent is it desirable and judicious to permit or encourage the formation of associations on particularistic lines? For example, we would not want to rule out forms of association based upon sexuality, cultural identity, lifestyle or common values, since these are one important means of achieving sensitivity to cultural difference. But in order to defend this position, we must deal with a number of criticisms of particularism. We will approach this general question by using ethnically based particularism as an exemplar in order to consider a number of the specific problems that particularism raises.

Internal governance

One set of problems concerns the possible variation of internal structure in the light of particularism. To what extent should the rules and practices of an association be allowed to diverge from the standard liberal democratic norms which the associational system itself is intended to embody? Should variation of values be permitted on the grounds of cultural particularism? Or should it be ruled out since it violates certain basic values which the system is supposed to enshrine?[2] Consider two examples.

First, the issue of entry: what rules of inclusion and exclusion should an association be permitted to enforce? Could associations exclude members they did not regard as part of 'their' group? For example, could there be a black housing association which excludes those it sees as non-black people?[3] Here Hirst is somewhat ambivalent. On the one hand, he says that under his scheme it would be possible to license a group with 'a strong regional concentration on ethnic, linguistic or cultural lines' (Hirst 1994: 194). But, on the other hand, he maintains that 'individuals cannot be excluded from associations except on the conditions that they can choose to accept or reject' – for example, they can choose Catholicism but not (ascribed) 'blackness' (p. 58). Hence it is possible to set up an exclusively Catholic, but not an exclusively black, housing association. But if, going back to Hirst's first claim, ethnically and culturally based associations are to be permitted, then for Hirst the implication seems to be that culture and ethnicity are purely a matter of choice rather than circumstance. This is clearly an account that many sociologists and others would find hard to swallow.

One point worth making here is that, to some extent, this problem is created by Hirst's focus upon the autonomous individual, which leads him to pose the dilemma of inclusion and exclusion too sharply. We would argue that, by seeing the associational sphere as engaging in practices which are culturally embedded, the question of inclusion/exclusion can be redefined as the extent to which an association encompasses the population of potential members or beneficiaries who share in the cultural meaning of that activity (compare Cohen and Rogers 1995: 55, 58, 59, 61). The fact that there are no Asian members of the Ashley Down Allotment Society in north Bristol is not evidence of their having been excluded. Rather it is evidence that the activity has no cultural meaning or relevance for them at the moment. This is a case of what Hoggett has called 'nonclusion' (Hoggett 1994). Since individuals join associations according to the cultural meanings attached to them, a black housing association may well remain black even where general rights of entry are ensured. What is likely to change, and indeed does constantly change, is the meaning given to 'blackness'.

A second question concerns the possible variation to voice rights. Certain ethnic groups may endorse norms and follow practices that may be considered undemocratic, where, for example, not even the requirements of one-member-one-vote are adhered to. Does respect for cultural forms and lifestyles entail respect for a diversity of forms of participation, representation and accountability? One solution would be to say that such variation should be permitted – but only on the proviso that a very strong exit right is in place. But the problem here is that a strong democratic culture – including strong voice rights – could be one of the necessary conditions for the effective exercise of exit rights as well. Another objection is simply that the proposed undemocratic practices violate fundamental individual rights.

Freezing ethnicity

A further question concerns the relationship between ethnically based associations and the ethnic groups which stand behind them. If associations are allowed to form along ethnic lines, would this contribute to a 'freezing' of ethnic groups into particular forms? Officially recognising such associations could aggravate this process by encouraging previously disparate sets of people to consolidate themselves into ethnic communities in order to win recognition and hence to obtain the resources that may follow such recognition. The danger with such processes of what could be called 'ethnic consolidation' are twofold. First, to freeze ethnic identities is to arrest artificially the process of change which an ethnic group would otherwise go through. Second, facilitating the consolidation of such groups will also aid and abet the processes of assimilation of insiders (and exclusion of outsiders) which such consolidation involves (Anthias and Yuval-Davis 1992: 2-4; Banks 1996: 158). If, as Unger believes, hierarchies are only stable in conditions in which it is difficult to initiate social change, then freezing collective identities will facilitate the stabilisation of hierarchies within such groups (Unger 1987: 516, 532). Clearly this represents a serious threat to the autonomy of individuals, which the rights of voice and exit in associations are intended to protect.

Despite such difficulties, we maintain that associationalism represents a better way of recognising ethnic particularism than do the alternatives currently on offer. The principal rival to associationalism as a way of responding to ethnic particularism is some form of what Dryzek calls 'difference democracy' (Dryzek 1996: 476). Schemes like that proposed by Young (1990) employ a wide range of devices with which to incorporate ethnic (and other) groups directly into the political system. These include 'institutional mechanisms and public resources supporting ... self-organisation of group members' and 'group analysis and group generation of policy proposals in institutionalised contexts' (Young 1990: 184). By dealing directly with ethnic groups in this way, a now familiar set of problems arises. Prominent among these are difficulties identifying the groups which deserve recognition, and the danger – with which we are particularly concerned here – of freezing ethnic groups into particular forms.

In the light of these reflections, it seems to us that associationalism has a distinct advantage over difference democracy. Since it deals only with ethnically based *associations*, rather than ethnic *groups* directly, associationalism can employ a variety of devices for ensuring that the associational system does not fall victim to what Cohen and Rogers call 'sclerosis' (Cohen and Rogers 1995: 66). Thus effective voice and exit rights – already discussed in some detail – are expressly designed to empower individuals in a way that ensures the fluidity of the associational system. Second, some form of what Cohen and Rogers call 'sunset legislation' (Cohen and Rogers 1995: 71) could be used to ensure that associations have to be regularly reratified by the broader political system. Third, Unger's 'destabilisation rights' (Unger 1987: 531–3) could prevent the consolidation of hierarchies within associations. The aim of these various devices is to make it harder to freeze associations – by, for example, allowing a faction from within an existing ethnic group to split off from the main body and set up its own association with relative ease – hence making it less likely that ethnic communities standing behind associations could be frozen either.

Practical consequences

A final question asks whether a system which allows associations to form along ethnic lines increases the dangers of divisive particularism. For example, would it exacerbate the 'mischiefs of faction' that worry Cohen and Rogers? Their fear is that:

> The groups that form typically seek to advance the interests of their members and not any more comprehensive interest (including the interest in maintaining democracy itself). With powers exerted in both public and private arenas, unrepresentative and particularistic groups promote a politics far removed from the democratic ideal of popular control, by equal citizens, of a government promoting the general welfare.
>
> (Cohen and Rogers 1995: 41)

This, then, is the danger of the tenant associations which will not seriously consider the needs of homeless families, of competition between different ethnically based groups for inner-city resources on the basis of an imagined hierarchy of oppression, of the Nimbyism of many neighbourhood communities, and so on.

Cohen and Rogers's solution to this sort of danger is to deploy what they call a 'deliberate politics of association', which involves 'using public powers to encourage less factionalising forms of secondary association – engaging in an artful democratic politics of secondary association' (Cohen and Rogers 1995: 9). They aim to use the state to tinker with the environment in which associations exist, in order to produce associations less prone to divisive conflict with their rivals. While such a solution may work, we have considerable problems with it. Above all, it risks undermining the autonomy and vitality of associations, which are essential to the health of a system of associational democracy.

Hirst's answer to this fear of factions is much more to our liking. He hopes that the decentralisation of power to associations – including those based on ethnicity – will actually reduce the dangers of destructive factionalism. His argument is that associationalism empowers individuals, and that this feeling of empowerment leads to a decrease in the hostility that some citizens might otherwise feel towards others – thus making a peaceful democratic order a greater practical possibility (Hirst 1994: 69). It seems to us that this argument, while not likely to cover all cases, has considerable plausibility. It chimes in, for example, with Habermas's suggestion that, if a 'minority struggling for recognition' come to feel esteemed, then there is less likelihood that their 'tendencies to self-assertion' will 'take on a fundamentalist and separatist character' (Habermas 1994: 118). Thus the ability of ethnic groups to establish ethnically based associations helps to defuse the danger that they will feel disrespected and hence resort to resentful communalist politics.

GOVERNMENT AND THE ASSOCIATIONAL SPHERE

The final issue that we will examine concerns the role of the state in a system of associative democracy.

The claims of representative government

Any devolved system of welfare governance must be able to respond to the centrifugal forces released by associative democracy. This suggests an important role for a residual state. In particular, a reasoned case can be made for the argument that representative government is one of the few agencies available with the potential to transcend particularism. First, it can be argued that political parties are primarily concerned to offer competing definitions of the general good. Whilst such definitions undoubtedly give expression to the particular group interests upon which a party's support is based, within a complex society no party is able to obtain political power without seeking to appeal to a broad range of interests. Whilst a party may prefer the populist strategy of majoritarian politics, there are always advantages to be gained by not being particularist. Second, it can be argued that the apparatus of the state embodies a set of administrative values (Hood 1991) which are generally universalistic in the sense that they give emphasis to procedural impartiality and rectitude (Thompson and Hoggett 1996). These values, sometimes referred to in terms of a 'public service ethos' (Pratchett and Wingfield 1996), now appear to be undergoing a process of rehabilitation in the UK, after mounting public disquiet about partiality and corruption within the enterprise state led to the creation of the Nolan Committee (Committee on Standards in Public Life 1995).

On the other hand, against such arguments for the impartiality of the state, it is necessary to consider the tendency for government itself to be captured by particular interests. Hirst, Cohen and Rogers, drawing on the experience of contemporary American politics, are acutely aware of the way in which government can be captured by external pressure groups such as the gun lobby, but they seem less sensitive to the way in which the modern welfare state has also been prone to capture from within. Thus Hirst seems to overlook the role of the professions as a particular form of 'producer-interest', who can and do occupy spaces not just within 'government' formally and narrowly defined but also within what might be called the 'extended state' of the voluntary, not-for-profit and private sectors. Constitutional independence from the institutions of government is by no means a sufficient condition for autonomy.

Administrative methods of state intervention

In the light of these tensions criss-crossing the state, more thought must be given to the role of the state within a system of associational governance. Statist assumptions, particularly the idea that political issues can be managed by administrative methods, have been a constant feature of British social democracy. It is therefore important to remember that government always has the choice of using administrative or political methods of social intervention. The former involves the use of law, procedure, incentive and sanction whilst the latter relies upon argument, debate and public persuasion. We want to argue that a truly democratic society would seek to use political methods of intervention wherever possible.

At some points, Hirst seems to have in mind a minimalist role for the state which involves steering rather than prescription. It is worrying therefore to find him at other points advocating the use of some quite powerful administrative methods of state intervention. For example, is a steering role compatible with the idea that the 'state would retain major reserve powers, to curb excessive growth in aggregate spending and to challenge standards of provision' (Hirst 1994: 177)? Moreover, federal and regional government would continue to have the ultimate fiscal powers and would therefore control the total level of the welfare budget (p. 186), common minimum standards of welfare would also be decided at federal level and government would remain the chief regulator, ensuring that those standards are met (p. 190). The state would retain powers of inspection too; it would have the capacity 'to act as the guardian of the public in matters touching on financial competence and probity, and on service quality' (p. 192). Having damned the administrative state and its agencies in the early pages of his book, towards the end one begins to feel Hirst is allowing the state to creep back in.

Can administrative methods of social intervention be developed in a way which does not lead to a centralised or technocratic state? One possibility, subject to much contemporary debate, pictures the state as one locus of power among many. Hence its role becomes one of orchestration (Clarke and Stewart 1994) or steering (Kikert 1993, 1995) rather than control and direction. Steering is about establishing frameworks and boundaries, setting norms, shaping behaviour through the use of incentives and setting metalevel rules (Kikert 1995; Rhodes 1996). It requires the use of influence rather than authority and the realisation of policy through the co-ordination of interorganisational networks. Here a state, largely shorn of its service-delivery role, operates in an environment in which power has been dispersed into a myriad agencies and networks. Such ideas are part of the emerging discourse of governance, something Rhodes (1996) has recently described as 'governing without government'.

Regarding frameworks and boundaries, as Hirst notes, the role of government would be to establish a common legal framework within which associationism would develop. Hirst's associative law would establish a set of rules, universal in their application, relating to the conduct of associational life – including probity in financial procedures, openness of associational government, fair employment practices and non-discriminatory professional practices. Running in parallel to this body of associative law, there would have to be a universal charter of membership rights giving all members of associations an unambiguous benchmark outlining the minimum standards of conduct to which all associations would be accountable. Finally, a small number of powerful government agencies with investigatory, appeal and advocacy functions would be required as mechanisms of final resort to ensure compliance with this body of associational law.

Unlike Hirst, we do not believe government should have a continuing role in setting minimum standards or in regulating the quality of service. The arrival of associational governance would lead to a cull of inspectorates, audit commissions and the rest. The point of empowering the members of associations with strong voice and exit rights is precisely to make them self-regulating; government does not set minimum standards for the services that unions provide to their members – and nor would we want it to. The regulatory apparatus of the state has extended precisely because existing users of welfare services have little or no power over producers.

Finally, if social inequality were addressed primarily through a universal guaranteed minimum income, supplemented by positive-action associational vouchers for those Hirst defines as having 'specific welfare needs' (Hirst 1994: 179–84), then such a strategy – if properly implemented – could overcome the need for a redistributive grant system. The remaining forms of direct government funding could then be performance-related, thus leaving government with some limited but important power to steer behaviour through the use of incentives.

Political methods of state intervention

There are two forms of particularism which threaten to undermine more universalistic notions of the common good. The first kind – the one which appears to preoccupy Hirst, Cohen and Rogers – might be called the particularism of minorities. However the second kind, of which Nimbyism is a local example, refers to the particularism of majorities. 'The majority' is a fluid and contingent phenomenon which 'transcends particular kinds of difference only to the extent that it can constitute and recoil from a greater difference' (Burns *et al.* 1994: 281). The majorities which oppose a site for local travellers or a residence for adults with learning difficulties will always be different amalgams of diverse interests.

In Britain it has been the particularism of majorities which has provided the primary basis for the objections of many socialists and social democrats to any democratic devolution of a localist or associational form. Essentially, and without too much simplification, from this perspective it is believed that communities of any form are simply not to be trusted to act in ways which do not have regressive distributive effects, as their members are either too selfish or lack the expertise to make informed decisions. In contrast we want to argue that, if the rights of minorities are to be preserved, government must become much more proactive in representing the public interest through engagement and dialogue, instead of hiding behind technocratic intervention and regulation. In this way, we believe, it could adjudicate between the competing claims of different minority interests, protect minority communities from majoritarian aggression, and represent the claims of a common good, which is necessarily abstract and may include the needs of future generations against the concrete demands of citizens demanding solutions to problems in the here and now. In other words, a dialogical state could embody a spirit of universalism without disempowering its own citizens, who necessarily mobilise around their own particular needs and perspectives.

There is currently a widespread debate within political science, involving feminists and critical theorists among others, which asks whether it is possible to generate practices through which differences and conflicts between citizens in highly pluralistic societies can be negotiated and, in some respects, overcome. Originating with the work of Jürgen Habermas, the concept of 'communicative action' has been developed by writers influenced by feminism, such as Benhabib (1992), to describe modes of human interaction which facilitate understanding between separate and different subjects. Benhabib suggests that communicative action is 'a moral conversation in which the capacity to reverse perspectives, i.e., the willingness to reason from another's point of view, and the sensitivity to hear their voice is paramount' (Benhabib 1992: 8).

Clearly, if places existed within the public sphere which were designed to promote the possibility of communicative action, then actors speaking for the various goods (general, majority and minority) could be capable of a dialogue from which reasonable agreements and mutual learning could emerge. Benhabib is careful to speak in terms of 'open-ended processes of moral argumentation' (Benhabib 1992: 169) rather than 'consensus', for the former includes 'agreement to differ' and thereby a commitment to continue interaction in spite of conflicts which are, for the time being, irresolvable. As Schlosberg (1995) points out, it is possible to disagree and yet enjoy an experience of solidarity if one's standpoint has been recognised by the other.

How then could government use its power to facilitate communicative action? Let us just mention three possibilities here: the diffusion of a communicative ethos, the construction of spaces for dialogue, and the development of dialogic techniques. Such possibilities are not simply abstract ideas: they have already found forms of realisation in the practices of some of the more innovative local and regional governments in Britain, the USA and Western Europe – particularly those that have been open to ideas emerging from the new social movements.

The development of an ethos of communicative action would require a citizenry which was genuinely committed to a spirit of enquiry. Local and regional governments could contribute to the diffusion of such an ethos by modelling active forms of listening in their own practices. The best public authorities in Britain and elsewhere already do this by practising open government and effective forms of citizen consultation around planning, health, environmental and other issues. Unfortunately most public authorities still lack any awareness of how their interventions may promote either co-operation or competition between different communities. The new ethos would require government to be much more reflexive than in the past. It would also need to be proactive in identifying win-win solutions and in gaining the commitment of different communities to them (Harrison *et al.* 1995).

The design of spaces for dialogue is also something which has been subject to much recent experimentation. We are speaking here of the role of public authorities in contributing to the development of local forums, in which political representatives and citizens can debate issues of concern regarding the relationship between government and communities and/or relationships between communities – neighbourhood or estate-based forums, youth forums, forums for people with disabilities, facility management committees, citizens' juries, etc. (Beresford and Croft 1993; Burns *et al.* 1994). The design of dialogic spaces which are able to contain powerful feelings without being exploded apart is a key challenge in the coming years (Jeffers *et al.* 1996).

Finally, we are seeing the emergence of new techniques for facilitating dialogue – ones which can often be traced back to the environmental and peace movements. Conflict-resolution strategies have been applied to intercommunal conflict within inner-city areas (Norman 1995) and to neighbour and other kinds of interpersonal dispute (Schlosberg 1995). In Britain the development of networks such as Mediation UK has also been instrumental in creating forms of structured dialogue between disputants.

CONCLUSION

In this chapter, we have tried to apply the 'thought experiments' of Hirst, Cohen and Rogers to the practicalities of creating a society in which responsibility for our common welfare would fall neither primarily upon the state nor upon individuals and their families. We believe such a model does enable us to transcend the false polarities of exit and voice and could provide for an immensely rich and diverse range of approaches for meeting human needs without undue fragmentation. Between those who only see 'a dead hand' in the state and those who only see parochialism and factionalism within civil society, we believe there is a third way, one in which the relationship between the local state and civil society could be symbiotic rather than destructive. The task of generating such a symbiosis is one germane both to practice in the here-and-now and to the challenge of building a distinctively new welfare society.

NOTES

1 Note that, depending on how control is defined, it may imply a stronger voice right than those proposed in either of the two main schemes under consideration here.
2 For more on this dilemma, seen in terms of a choice between the liberal values of toleration and autonomy, see Kymlicka (1995: 15).
3 Could there be an exclusively white housing association? Here, we would argue, it is necessary to invoke a theory of structural disadvantage in order to argue that only social groups who have suffered or are suffering such disadvantages can be allowed to form associations along particularist lines as part of a way of overcoming such disadvantage.

BIBLIOGRAPHY

Anthias, F. and Yuval-Davis, N. (1992) *Racialized Boundaries: Race, Nation, Gender, Colour and Class and the Anti-racist Struggle*, London: Routledge.
Banks, M. (1996) *Ethnicity: Anthropological Constructions*, London: Routledge.
Benhabib, S. (1992) *Situating the Self: Gender, Community and Postmodernism in Contemporary Ethics*, Cambridge: Polity Press.
Beresford, P. and Croft, S. (1993) *Citizen Involvement: A Practical Guide for Change*, Basingstoke: Macmillan.
Burns, D., Hambleton, R. and Hoggett, P. (1994) *The Politics of Decentralization: Revitalizing Local Democracy*, Basingstoke: Macmillan.
Clarke, J. and Stewart, J. (1994) 'The local authority and the new community governance', *Regional Studies* 28, 2: 201–7.
Cohen, J. and Rogers, J. (eds) (1995) *Associations and Democracy: The Real Utopias Project. Vol. 1*, London: Verso.
Committee on Standards in Public Life (1995). *Standards in Public Life: First Report of the Committee on Standards in Public Life*, Chairman Lord Nolan, London: HMSO.
Di Maggio, P. and Powell, W.W. (1983) 'The iron cage revisited: institutional isomorphism and collective rationality in organisational fields', *American Sociological Review* 48, 2: 147–60.
Dryzek, J. (1996) 'Political inclusion and the dynamics of democratization', *American Political Science Review* 90, 1: 475–87.
Habermas, J. (1994) 'Struggles for recognition in the democratic constitutional state', in A. Gutmann (ed.) *Multiculturalism: Examining The Politics of Recognition*, Princeton NJ: Princeton University Press.
Harrison, L., Hoggett, P. and Jeffers, S. (1995) 'Race, ethnicity and community development', *Community Development Journal* 30, 2: 144–57.
Hirschman, A. (1970) *Exit, Voice and Loyalty*, Cambridge MA: Harvard University Press.

Hirst, P. (1994) *Associative Democracy: New Forms of Economic and Social Governance*, Cambridge: Polity Press.

Hoggett, P. (1994) *The Future of Civic Forms of Organisation: The Future of Charities and the Voluntary Sector*, Working Paper 4, London: Demos.

Hoggett, P. (1996) 'New modes of control in the public service', *Public Administration* 74, 1: 9–32.

Hood, C. (1991) 'A public management for all seasons?', *Public Administration* 69, 1: 3–19.

Jeffers, S., Hoggett, P. and Harrison, L. (1996) 'Race, ethnicity and community in three localities', *New Community* 22, 1: 111–26.

Kikert, W. (1993) 'Autopoiesis and the science of (public) administration: essence, sense and nonsense', *Organisational Studies* 14, 2: 261–78.

Kikert, W. (1995) 'Steering at a distance: a new paradigm of public governance in Dutch higher education', *Governance* 8, 1: 135–57.

Kymlicka, W. (1995) *Contemporary Political Philosophy: An Introduction*, Oxford: Oxford University Press.

Le Grand, J. (1989) 'Markets, welfare and equality', in J. Le Grand and S. Estrin (eds) *Market Socialism*, Oxford: Oxford University Press.

Lewis, J. (1993) 'Developing the mixed economy of care: emerging issues for voluntary organisations', *Journal of Social Policy* 22, 2: 173–92.

Moyser, G., Day, N. and Parry, G. (1992) *Political Participation and Democracy in Britain*, Cambridge: Cambridge University Press.

Norman, A. (1995), 'Building multiethnic coalitions within public sector organisations: an expanded dialogue model', in E.-Y. Yu and E. Chang (eds) *Multiethnic Coalition Building in Los Angeles*, Claremont, CA: Regina Books.

Perri, 6 and Vidal, I. (eds) (1994) *Delivering Welfare: Repositioning Non-profit and Co-operative Action in Western European Welfare States*, Barcelona: CIES.

Pestoff, V. (1994) 'Beyond exit and voice in social services: citizen as co-producers', in 6 Perri and I. Vidal (eds) *Delivering Welfare: Repositioning Non-profit and Co-operative Action in Western European Welfare States*, Barcelona: CIES.

Pratchett, L. and Wingfield, M. (1996) 'The demise of the public service ethos', in L. Pratchett and D. Wilson (eds) *Local Democracy and Local Government*, Basingstoke: Macmillan.

Rhodes, R. (1996) 'The new governance: governing without government', *Political Studies* 44, 4: 652–77.

Rosenblum, N.L. (1994) 'Democratic character and community: the logic of congruence', *Journal of Political Philosophy* 2, 1: 67–97.

Schlosberg, D. (1995) 'Communicative action in practice: intersubjectivity and new social movements', *Political Studies* 42, 2: 291–311.

Schmitter, P.C. (1995) 'The irony of modern democracy and the viability of efforts to reform its practice', in J. Cohen and J. Rogers (eds) *Associations and Democracy*, London: Verso.

Taylor, M. and Hoggett, P. (1994) 'Trusting in networks? The third sector and welfare change', in 6 Perri and I. Vidal (eds) *Delivering Welfare: Repositioning Non-profit and Co-operative Action in Western European Welfare States*, Barcelona: CIES.

Thompson, S. and Hoggett, P. (1996) 'Universalism, selectivism and particularism: towards a postmodern social policy', *Critical Social Policy* 16, 1: 21–43.

Unger, R.M. (1987) *False Necessity: Anti-necessitarian Social Theory in the Service of Radical Democracy*, Cambridge: Cambridge University Press.

Williams, F. (1989) *Social Policy: A Critical Introduction*, Cambridge: Polity Press.

Young, I.M. (1990) *Justice and the Politics of Difference*, Princeton NJ: Princeton University Press.

Chapter 16

Globalisation, fragmentation and local welfare citizenship

Allan Cochrane

INTRODUCTION: WELFARE CITIZENSHIP

Debates about welfare citizenship have generally been dominated by the ghost of T.H. Marshall, whose approach defined the terrain (in Britain at least) for much of the period after 1945. Rarely can a single academic have summarised so effectively the dominant understandings of a particular age as Marshall did in his discussions of citizenship. At the risk of oversimplification, Marshall's position can be summarised relatively briefly.

Marshall saw capitalism as an inherently unequal system characterised by fundamental social tensions. But he also believed that inequality was a necessary price to pay for the operation of a successful market economy. For Marshall, citizenship was both a challenge to and a necessary aspect of capitalist development. 'It is clear,' he wrote, 'that in the twentieth century, citizenship and the capitalist class system have been at war' (Marshall 1950: 29). But it was a war whose outcome was generally positive. Marshall stressed the gradual extension of basic rights (civil, political and social) which were won within states for citizens. He identified a progressive growth of citizenship which paralleled the development of capitalism and the increased social divisions (class inequality) which accompanied it. Citizenship, he argued, offered the possibility of 'class abatement'. It promised the means of managing capitalism's inherent social tensions. His model of 'welfare capitalism' was one which 'functioned through markets subject to adjustment by a government which at the same time made full scale provision for (minimum) social security and (optimum) health and welfare, with the co-operation of industry and commerce' (Marshall 1975: 105).

Marshall's notion of citizenship is a powerful one which links civil, political and social rights. The first of these 'rights' relates to individual freedom (and includes such aspects as freedom of speech), the second embodies the right to participation in public power, as politician, or, more frequently as elector, while the third relates to economic and social welfare. Each is associated with specific state institutions: civil rights with the courts and judiciary; political rights with government (local and parliamentary); social rights with the health service, education departments and social services.

The interrelationship between these different rights and their emergence at different historical moments (civil rights first, then political rights and finally social rights) define twentieth-century welfare citizenship.

This conception of citizenship implies the existence of obligations as well as rights. Citizens have the responsibility to obey the law, participate in democracy and contribute financially through taxation. So, for example, the provision of elementary education by the state was accompanied by the duty of children to attend, as education became compulsory. In contrast to neo-liberal thinkers and theorists of the 'new right', who tend to concentrate on the first two of the 'rights' identified by him (and particularly the first, which may be understood as 'negative' freedom – that is, freedom from interference by others and the state in particular), Marshall explicitly incorporated social rights into his conception of citizenship.

It was on this basis, Marshall argued, that modern societies were able to sustain the allegiance of their citizens, despite the inequality inherent within market capitalism. For him, citizenship was a crucial element in helping to legitimate the existence of social inequality, since full membership of the community might be achieved through shared citizenship, rather than eco-nomic equalisation. In this context, Marshall maintained, equalisation of status was more important than equalisation of income. He stressed the importance of equal rights and duties for full members of the community (citizens) existing alongside forms of economic and social inequality. However poor an individual citizen might be, s/he would have the same civil, political and social rights as those who were more wealthy – including access to a 'universal' system of welfare services and benefits.

In recent years Marshall's approach has faced increasing criticism (see e.g. Hay 1996: 66–81; Lister 1995; Pascall 1993; Roche 1991: particularly Pt I) after a long period in which its conclusions were rather too easily taken for granted as part of the dominant academic common sense. The conception of history which underpinned Marshall's arguments seems to have been predicated on the assumption of some sort of inevitable (albeit contested) progress of human society towards 'welfare capitalism' and social citizenship. The emergence in the 1980s and 1990s of approaches to welfare which sought to reverse the commitment to a comprehensive system, and encouraged the growth of a wel-fare 'underclass' (that is, one effectively excluded from the forms of citizenship Marshall identified), must call key aspects of his analysis into question. More important, despite its breadth and clarity, Marshall's analysis is based on a homogeneous model of citizenship, which fails to acknowledge some impor-tant tensions and differences between those labelled as citizens.

'Citizenship' itself becomes a universal category within which many groups fail to recognise their experience. So, for example, the role played by many 'black' and 'Asian' people within the British welfare state is difficult to locate within Marshall's broad notion of citizenship, since many of them have effec-tively been excluded from most of the 'rights' identified by Marshall, even while some of them have been employed within the welfare institutions which underpin the social rights of others. Similarly, although Marshall did identify the significance of women's suffrage, he failed to recognise that while women had political rights as individuals, their social rights depended on access through their husbands, male partners or children. His belief that equality of 'status' somehow compensated for fundamental (structural) inequalities in access to resources also looks increasingly difficult to sustain. The universalism of his approach fits uneasily with the recognition that the universal categories he identifies effectively exclude large parts of the population (see e.g. Williams 1993). Lister (1995) directly poses the question whether a universal notion such as citizenship can ever adequately incorporate women, when its initial definition was largely based on their exclusion from it.

Marshall has moved from icon to villain in a relatively short space of time, and some of the criticisms made of him are less convincing than others. So, for example, Hay suggests that Marshall was wrong to identify a conflict between citizenship and the inequalities of capitalism. On the contrary, Hay (1996) argues, Marshallian citizenship can be seen as a necessary element in the political legitimation of an inherently unequal (and unstable) capitalist regime. In some ways, however, this criticism is misplaced since Marshall, too, saw the rise of citizenship as a necessarily stabilising feature of capitalism. More important, perhaps, Marshall's approach implies (at least) an active process of challenge and contestation as part of the process of the construction of welfare citizenship, which is a valuable corrective to views which simply see it as something which can be taken for granted. Similarly, because it draws so heavily on the uniqueness of the British experience, paradoxically perhaps, Marshall's approach also makes it easier to identify the differences between various national welfare systems.

CHALLENGES AND CHANGES: THE NEW CONTEXT

This, however, is not the place to engage in a (even a critical) defence of some aspects of Marshall's work, however (see Bulmer and Rees 1996 for one attempt to do so). The purpose of this chapter is rather a different one. Despite its fundamental flaws, Marshall's analysis summarised the dominant understandings of welfare citizenship in the period after 1945. The coming together of these sets of rights seemed to define important aspects of the welfare regimes which emerged in most 'western' countries in the first half of the twentieth century, and were consolidated in the twenty-five years after 1945. Above all, they appeared to underpin politically the way in which the national welfare regimes of the various Keynesian welfare states operated. The undermining of these national systems has been accompanied by an increased questioning of Marshall's approach to citizenship, but as it disappears into the sunset, it is important to ask what is replacing it, both in practice and in terms of dominant understandings.

One crucial aspect of the changes which have been taking place is the more (explicitly) globalised context which is emerging. It is increasingly difficult to believe in a world of highly autonomous states within whose boundaries political decisions can be made about welfare, without any wider repercussions being apparent. It is no longer possible to pretend that states can have domestic policies which are hermetically sealed from their foreign policies. There is broad agreement about this across the political (and academic) spectrum, although there is some disagreement about the room for manoeuvre which remains for states within the broader context (see e.g. Anderson 1995), and the notion of 'globalisation' (in which we might be moving towards a 'borderless' world: Ohmae 1990) is increasingly being questioned (Hirst and Thompson 1996). More important, perhaps, it is apparent (as David Held's work in particular has stressed) that we are seeing the emergence of multiple and overlapping networks of power operating through a series of global and regional connections.

In this context, Held sets out to explore the possibilities of what he calls 'cosmopolitan governance' through a range of self-regulating associations within civil society (Held 1996). Drawing on Marshall, Held identifies the principle of 'autonomy' as a key normative aspect of citizenship, by which he means 'an equal capacity to act across key political institutions and sites of power' (Held 1996: 71), and sets out to identify ways in which it might be achieved within the new global order. He identifies institutional spaces appropriate to particular activities, at a range of different scales, to take account of the most appropriate level of intervention, spelling out the need for 'cosmopolitan democracy' relating to 'the different power systems which constitute the interconnections of different peoples and nations' (Held 1996: 271). What Held offers is a powerful attempt to reconstruct citizenship (and democracy) in global terms. It is, however, less clear that moves in that direction are actually taking place. Held's arguments are as much a normative claim about what ought to happen if democracy is to survive in a more globalised world as an attempt to identify arrangements which might be emerging in practice.

If one aspect of the new world points to the need for a 'globalisation' of democracy and citizenship, another seems to highlight the need to respond to processes of 'localisation', in the context of a break-up of universalism. The local welfare state was always an important aspect of the construction of welfare citizenship more broadly, as it was located at the core of the national system, particularly in the UK. Local citizenship was particularly important because of the role of local states in shaping rights and entitlements to key aspects of welfare and social services, which themselves helped to define social rights in Marshall's sense. It was also always (in principle at least) a key arena in which the exercise of political rights was undertaken. The taken-for-granted and day-to-day aspects of citizenship are those which find their expression through locally based institutions and activities. Cooke (1990:

135–6) has argued that localities act as important laboratories for social and political innovation, and in the 1970s and 1980s in the UK local government was certainly one of the key sites on which the contests over the nature of political and social life took place (see e.g. Cochrane 1993b). Cooke suggests that precisely because of the processes associated with globalisation the scope (and need) for localised initiative has also increased. This is, perhaps, clearest in the competition for economic welfare expressed through place marketing and related activities, but similar pressures also exist in more traditional areas of welfare. The fragmentation of the supposedly monolithic welfare states has been associated with a move towards the redefinition of welfare in terms which stress the importance of enterprise and economic competitiveness (see e.g. Jessop 1994).

The reshaping of local politics in the UK since the late 1970s may also be interpreted as an attempt to define or redefine the nature of welfare citizenship. However inadequate the traditional Marshallian model, even in its heyday, its significance as a symbolic representation should not be discounted. The different aspects appeared to come together in a reasonably straightforward manner around the structures of the local welfare state. In principle, civil rights were guaranteed since councils were subject to the rule of law. Political rights were clear cut and expressed through regular elections. In some of the more effusive statements of local democracy, it was suggested that local government was inherently more open than other levels of government (councillors were closer to electors, and even officials were necessarily much closer to those they served than civil servants ever could be: see e.g. SAUS 1983). Social rights apparently found their expression through access to a whole range of locally delivered services (from housing to education, social services and local infrastructure). Of course, this did not mean that all was perfect. On the contrary, as Gyford neatly points out in his – not unsympathetic – summary of municipal labourism, 'Usually it did the right things for people; but sometimes it could do the wrong things to people; and only rarely had it previously discussed either of those things with people' (Gyford 1985: 10).

LOCAL CITIZENSHIP AND LOCAL ACCOUNTABILITY

The model of citizenship associated with the high period of the local welfare state came under severe challenge in the 1980s and 1990s. Some of the challenges and questioning came from those who might have been expected to benefit from their social inclusion as citizens. This was a time in which claims to individual rights encouraged direct legal challenges to the decisions taken by councils and their officers: in social work, for example, it was a time of regular judicial reviews of one sort or another, particularly in the field of child protection (see e.g. DoH 1991). The courts were used to challenge decisions on housing allocations, on the provision of support to disabled people and on the admission of children to particular schools (see e.g. Loughlin 1996 for a discussion of the changing legal and constitutional position of local government at this time). Law centres (often funded by councils) became a focus for cases which highlighted the responsibility of councils to supply particular services to individuals and groups (see e.g. Taylor 1993 for a review of challenges to dominant practice in social services departments).

As far as political rights are concerned, the practice has rarely been quite as impressive as the more exaggerated claims might suggest. Only relatively small numbers of those eligible (around 30–40 per cent) take their responsibilities seriously enough to vote, many citizens remain unclear precisely what service is the responsibility of which authority (Young 1986), and the satisfaction ratings for the services which receive the highest budgetary allocations remain relatively low (at 42 per cent for schools, 30 per cent for housing and 30 per cent for social services: Rallings et al. 1996: Tables 4.3 and 4.4). The social rights associated with the local welfare state were too often seen as exclusionary rather than inclusionary (for example, in the allocation of council housing) and associated with social control rather than opportunity.

It is important not to exaggerate the extent of popular disenchantment with local government, even in the early 1980s, since surveys continued to show more favourable attitudes to local than to central government and levels of satisfaction with some services (such as education) remained high. Nevertheless, there can be no doubt that the political atmosphere was changing. Despite the often dramatic ideological differences between them, the critics all focused on the problems associated with a local government system dominated by bureaucracy and professionalism, which excluded and patronised those reliant on the services provided through it (see e.g. Blunkett and Green 1983). They questioned the old assumptions about what local welfare citizenship had to offer; they questioned the existing rules of the game.

But the most immediately apparent outcome of all the challenges and questioning was not a revaluation of citizenship in inclusive and participative terms. On the contrary, under the influence of successive Conservative governments (but with the implicit support of many Labour councils) there was a move towards the notion of citizen–consumer, linking citizenship to market-based approaches to local service delivery and the allocation of resources at local level. The approach redefines electors as citizen–consumers able to influence resource allocation through their choices (for example, of the schools to which to send their children) and their preparedness to pay for services (whether individually or through tax-benefit packages: see e.g. Le Grand 1990). Increasingly emphasis has been placed on 'accounting', rather than 'accountability', with passive consumers receiving what is best for them. Accounting offers the possibility of summarising complex organisational relationships in a single figure (Humphrey et al. 1993: 17), while at the same time, 'By offering to bring intangible, intractable matters under managerial control and giving contentious issues a technical appearance, any opposition seemed illogical and irrational' (Humphrey and Scapens 1992: 142–3). As Miller notes, 'a distrust of experts is to be countered by a trust in numbers, particularly financial numbers. One particular body of expertise – accountancy – is to be made the expertise of expertise' (Miller 1996: 60).[1]

The principles underlying this shift reflect a particularly narrow notion of citizenship. The implicit assumption is that there is a general – and unproblematic – agreement on what services are needed, so that the only issue is how to deliver them most economically and efficiently. This is usually simply translated into an emphasis on cheapness, although effectiveness is the third in the trinity (of economy, efficiency and effectiveness) of management accounting as expressed in the gospel according to the Audit Commission. The universalism of Marshall is translated into a new universalism which even more effectively questions the notion that there might be differences of priority, as well as access to power and resources, between different groups. The role of local citizens in this model is principally to limit the profligacy of local politicians and officials (either through their voting behaviour or by moving to areas with low levels of local taxation: see e.g. Foster *et al.* 1980). The government's introduction of the 'poll tax' or community charge as the main form of local taxation at the end of the 1980s was largely intended to reinforce the relationship between local spending and local taxes, so that voters would be more aware of these issues. But even after the failure of that initiative, this remains the dominant official view. In a speech made while he was Chancellor of the Duchy of Lancaster (and responsible for overseeing the government's Citizen's Charter initiative), William Waldegrave argued that the search for democratic accountability was irrelevant to the operation of the local welfare state: what mattered to people was the quality of the services they received (Waldegrave 1993).

Once accountability is redefined in these terms, the notion of citizenship loses any potentially transformative power it might have had. A technical process apparently replaces a political one, and once the aim has been identified it is possible to judge how well it has been achieved according to some universal template applied by external experts, such as the Audit Commission with its continuing series of authority profiles. Spatial differentiation seems irrational in the context of the universal language of accounting. In the end, therefore, the notion of the 'citizen–consumer' makes it difficult to envisage the possibility of active citizenship.

DEMOCRACY AND PARTICIPATION

Another way of capturing (or renewing) the notion of local citizenship might be to build on the idea of active citizenship, particularly by picking up on ideas such as participation or 'empowerment'. In principle one might expect such ideas to make it easier to acknowledge the importance of difference, rather than imposing a universal template into which 'citizens' are then expected to fit. In principle, participation itself can be seen to be a good thing, which encourages the 'empowerment' of those who were previously merely defined as passive recipients of initiatives developed by experts of one sort or another. But precisely what this might mean in practice is perhaps rather more elusive.

In the past, citizen participation has not always been viewed very positively by those who have been involved. It has too often been seen as little more than a process of 'consultation' over issues whose outcomes have already been determined. So, for example, participation on planning matters often amounts to little more than the possibility of responding to planning applications on 'planning' grounds (rarely the grounds which interest those apparently being consulted). Participation might also be a euphemism for incorporating some local residents into the political process, while excluding others. Instead of empowering people, it might rather be a means of delegating responsibility to them (for example, through a contract for housing management, or membership of a school governing body) without also providing the necessary financial base.

A more radical approach to the problem, however, might be to start from somewhere else completely. Most of the discussion of local welfare states and citizenship has tended to start from the existing local government system as a base. Theoretically, at least, however, other starting points are possible, and may highlight alternative possibilities, some of which may even already be developing. It may be that the appropriate arena for political action by citizens is not electoral politics, but the wide range of formal and informal 'voluntary' organisations, to which most people already belong in some capacity or another. Some of these will be based on local communities, while others may be based on the shared interests of service users. Hirst's discussion of associative democracy is one of the most developed versions of this approach, redefining politics in terms which question the centrality of 'governments' and 'states' (Hirst 1994; see also Cohen and Rogers *et al.* 1995). Hirst builds on the notion that society is made up of a plurality of associations, through which individuals come together in a complex variety of ways reflecting their multiple identities (at work, in leisure, at home, as consumers and so on). In other words, these associations start from assumptions about difference, rather than homogeneity. Although the associations are not necessarily local, many of them will be locally based and come together in ways which help to define places in terms which recognise the significance of local diversity – differences between places as well as between groups and individuals. It is important to recognise the overlapping nature of these associations, since many people are likely to belong to more than one, confirming that they define themselves in multiple ways, but also allowing for more differentiated forms of politics and, by implication, more differentiated notions of citizenship.

This offers the prospect of developing 'intermediate forms of governance', beyond the local welfare state (as well as beyond the individual and beyond simple models of the market). Building on the traditions of guild socialism, for example, Hirst is particularly interested in the ways in which the associations might operate to provide a significant alternative to the centralising and bureaucratic forms taken by the welfare state. In a rather different context, Amin and Thrift stress the importance of 'networks of intermediate institutions in between market and state' (Amin and Thrift 1995: 50) as a basis on which it should be possible to generate 'a process of collective governance of the socioeconomy', which should also make it possible to broaden 'the arena of institutions involved in guiding economic outcomes at diverse spatial scales' (Amin and Thrift 1995: 55). In other words, they offer the prospect of a widespread social involvement in influencing the direction of the regional and local economy, through involvement in a diffuse and dispersed set of associations (or institutions).

The arguments of the associationalists make it possible to imagine a society with widespread participation in decision making over a wide range of issues. They make it possible to move towards radical notions of pluralist democracy like those espoused by Mouffe (1992). She questions notions of citizenship (like Marshall's) which are universalist and undifferentiated. Like Hirst she stresses the importance of differences between individuals and groups, and highlights the extent to which individual citizens themselves have multifaceted political and social identities, which rarely find expression in the formal world of electoral politics. Approaches like these allow theorists to recognise and celebrate the political importance of a range of agencies which are frequently overlooked in more orthodox approaches.

This way into the problem is potentially exciting because it opens up alternative agendas for citizenship, as well as suggesting ways of developing wider welfare agendas at local level. But it raises problems of its own, too. One, which is recognised by Hirst (1995) (and is familiar from more orthodox pluralist writing), is that all associations do not start out equal. Power is distributed differentially and this is bound to be reflected in the way in which associations operate. It is not always clear how differences in power between associations can be dealt with, or indeed quite what will happen to those whose involvement is likely to be severely limited, whether through choice or through necessity. Research on urban regimes and growth coalitions makes it clear that some agendas are likely to dominate at the expense of others (indeed the importance of non-decision making in simply excluding some issues from business-led agendas is hard to ignore: see e.g. Harding 1995).

There is a related concern about the way in which groups are formed: that of who is able to join which. Hirst sets out some 'ground rules' on group formation but it is still all too easy to see how the balance is likely to operate in favour of some at the expense of others. Despite the optimism of the associationalists, it is just as likely that the process of forming associations and of coalition building will be used to exclude some groups and some people from influence, instead of opening up the process. One way of dealing with this might be to allow some scope for the state to intervene with a claim to have some overarching responsibility for managing relations between associations (possibly relying on a legitimacy drawn from electoral representation). Hirst (1994) sets out a fairly complex structure of regional assemblies with different forms of representation (mixing functional and electoral principles), and allocates them significant roles in terms of managing inequalities of power. Amin and Thrift (1995) follow a different line. They set out a programme for democratising existing (state) networks and building alternative networks in civil society. In this way they hope to overcome what they see as a democratic deficit both in the operation of representative government and in the potential power dynamics of associationalism.

A further problem with much of the debate about associationalism from whatever perspective is that (however attractive the prospect may be) the mechanism of transition is difficult to identify: in other words it is difficult to see quite how to get from here to there. Leaving it to organic change seems likely to take too long – by the time it happens a neo-liberal agenda may already have been implemented. It is unclear who the agents of change will be. The outcome may be desirable, but the transition is less clear. In his discussion of the arguments developed by Cohen and Rogers (1995), Offe notes that they fail to identify the 'reformist agents and political promoters' who can catalyse the necessary change. He asks if it is legitimate to conclude that associationalism is 'an arrangement of the greatest functional, but at the same time very limited normative appeal, which for this very reason is quite unlikely to be adopted in contexts in which it does not already find favourable conditions due to historical antecedents' (Offe 1995: 126). Although these comments apply particularly strongly to the formulation developed by Cohen and Rogers, they also highlight broader difficulties with the approach. It is possible to present the blueprint of a complex institutional model of cross-cutting representation, as Hirst (1994) does, without it ever being quite clear how one might get from here to there.

Paradoxically, despite the non-statist starting point of the theory, it looks as if only state action can generate moves towards an associationalist future. Hirst acknowledges that the state needs to be involved in the 'orchestration of social consensus' (Hirst 1994: 118). Unfortunately, however, once that is recognised, it becomes difficult to see quite why the state should be expected to involve itself in moves which were likely to undermine its position in the longer term. However, the continued survival of the local state may offer genuine opportunities, since local government is already under severe pressure and is being forced to look for ways out of the dead end of existing institutional arrangements.

In this context the notion of 'community government' may offer a way out because it promises the possibility of managing and influencing the wider networks of which local councils are only a part. A radical version of this approach is adopted by Burns *et al.* (1994: 279), who suggest that new approaches to democracy and the public sphere are needed, based on 'a much greater plurality of democratic provider organisations' which are 'collectively accountable or controlled'. But they also stress that strong local representative institutions are required alongside these agencies, because there are likely to be substantial inequalities of power and influence between them. In this model, although elected local governments would not any longer be able to act as monopoly providers of welfare services, they would retain a key role in helping to overcome the fragmentation of civil society.

This also implies a commitment to supporting and underpinning the development of active associations which involve citizens across a range of issues and interests, even when their activities may be embarrassing to the councils which support them. It represents a substantial move beyond the complex set of 'contractual and quasi-commercial relationships between the council, acting on behalf of the community, and other agencies whose links to the community are limited to the point at which they deliver services to it' (Alexander 1991: 73). Within such relationships, Alexander notes that 'There is a danger that the argument in favour of democracy and accountability will be lost by default as the energy of managers is directed exclusively to the technical issues raised by fragmentation and politicians continue to behave as if nothing, or nothing much, has changed' (Alexander 1991: 76). The 'community government' model has the potential to turn this on its head because it emphasises the importance of associations as political agencies rather than agencies for the delivery of services under contract.

From the perspective of community and voluntary organisations (which are so far about the closest to the forms of association which Hirst and others discuss), of course, the new world of local politics offers the prospect of careful negotiation, a tight-rope walk between satisfying the demands of those who issue the contracts and the demands of their members or those whom they seek to represent. There is a tension between accepting the rules of the powerful, to ensure that resources are made available for activities which fit with the aims of community and voluntary organisations, and losing touch with the members or supporters of those organisations. This is particularly the case when levels of activism begin to fade as the work of organisations becomes routinised and professionalised (see e.g. Cochrane 1986; Gutch and Young 1988). Any expanded notion of welfare citizenship (which continues to incorporate social rights) depends on the possibility of a continuing process of renewal, in which there is always access to the emerging institutions or new ones can be created and recognised relatively easily. In this context it may be possible to move beyond 'citizenship', recognising that groups and individuals, their demands and needs cannot be reduced to a simple formula, while making it possible for them to influence welfare outcomes.

CONCLUSION

The role of elected local government in Britain has certainly changed dramatically since the early 1970s. It would be easy to conclude that local politics have declined in importance and that the locally based institutions of the welfare state have lost their significance. However, drawing such a conclusion would be premature. Increasingly tight, centrally imposed controls over council spending and pressures to move away from direct service provision by local authorities have been accompanied by a proliferation of other locally based institutions outside electoral control. There has been an apparently inexorable rise in the number and range of institutions of non-elected local government (see e.g. Greer and Hoggett 1996). Attempts to capture the new world have used notions such as networks, partnerships, mixed economies and governance rather than government.

Some of the main features of change have had fundamental implications for understandings of local citizenship. Local welfare states in the UK have been transformed as new agencies (such as Training and Enterprise Councils) have been created, older agencies (such as health authorities) have taken on new responsibilities, the voluntary sector has expanded to take a leading role in some policy areas (such as in the shape of housing associations), the private sector has been given new responsibilities and interagency working has become the norm across the board. John Stewart (1996), in particular, has noted the rise of what he calls the 'new magistracy' running many of these organisations, and facing little or no electoral accountability. The relationship between citizen and government has become increasingly opaque in a world of multiple stakeholders, including businesses, hybrid public–private organisations and public sector agencies as well as individuals. It is not clear who is accountable to whom for what, and it is still less clear what the relationship is between citizen and agency on many issues (not least because it is not always clear which agency is responsible for what, since there are frequently cross-cutting lines of subsidy, financial support and membership).

The old models of political accountability – however inadequate and misleading – have gone, without any clear alternatives yet having emerged, or been created. The old promises of citizenship have never been met: the new possibilities remain highly contested and uncertain. The danger is that as the old models collapse, the new ones will be defined by the powerful, rather than those seeking change and substantive forms of social justice. Associationalism offers one alternative model, but is unlikely to emerge organically from the existing relations around welfare. It looks as if the state will have to be actively involved in achieving its own redefinition. There may be scope for moves in this direction because of the way in which local politics has been reshaped since the early 1980s. If elected local government is able to take up the opportunities which present themselves, then change is possible, but it will require a fundamental rethinking of their role by local politicians and officials.

NOTE

1   Similar claims are, of course, also being made for the equally arcane mysteries of managerialism, with their visions, mission statements and purchaser/provider splits (see e.g. Cochrane 1993a, 1994).

BIBLIOGRAPHY

Alexander, A. (1991) 'Managing fragmentation: democracy, accountability and the future of local government', *Local Government Studies* 17, 6: 63–76.

Amin, A. and Thrift, N. (1995) 'Institutional issues for the European regions: from markets and plans to socioeconomics and powers of association', *Economy and Society* 24: 41–66.

Anderson, J. (1995) 'Beyond the nation state', in J. Anderson, C. Brook and A. Cochrane (eds) *A Global World? Re-ordering Political Space*, Oxford: Oxford University Press.

Blunkett, D. and Green, G. (1983) *Building from the Bottom: The Sheffield Experience*, Fabian Tract 491, London: Fabian Society.

Bulmer, M. and Rees, A. (1996) *Citizenship Today: The Contemporary Relevance of T.H. Marshall*, London: UCL Press.

Burns, D., Hambleton, R. and Hoggett, P. (1994) *The Politics of Decentralization: Revitalizing Local Democracy*, Basingstoke: Macmillan.

Cochrane, A. (1986) 'Community politics and democracy', in D. Held and C. Pollitt (eds) *New Forms of Democracy*, London: Sage.

Cochrane, A. (1993a) 'From financial control to strategic management: the changing faces of accountability in British local government', *Accounting, Auditing and Accountability Journal* 6, 3: 31–52.

Cochrane, A. (1993b) *Whatever Happened to Local Government?*, Buckingham: Open University Press.

Cochrane, A. (1994) 'Managing change in local government', in J. Clarke, A. Cochrane and E. McLaughlin (eds) *Managing Social Policy*, London: Sage.

Cohen, J. and Rogers, J. (eds) (1995) *Associations and Democracy: The Real Utopias Project. Vol. 1*, London: Verso.

Cooke, P. (1990) *Back to the Future?*, London: Unwin Hyman.

DoH (Department of Health) (1991) *Child Abuse: A Study of Inquiry Reports 1980–1989*, London: HMSO.

Foster, C.D., Jackman, R. and Perlman, M. (1980) *Local Government Finance in a Unitary State*, London: Allen & Unwin.

Greer, A. and Hoggett, P. (1996) 'Quangos and local governance', in L. Pratchett and D. Wilson (eds) *Local Democracy and Local Government*, Basingstoke: Macmillan.

Gutch, R. and Young, K. (1988) *Partners or Rivals? A Discussion Paper on the Relationship between Local Government and the Voluntary Sector*, Luton: Local Government Training Board.

Gyford, J. (1985) *The Politics of Local Socialism*, London: Allen & Unwin.

Harding, A. (1995) 'Elite theory and growth machines', in D. Judge, G. Stoker and H. Wolman (eds) *Theories of Urban Politics*, London: Sage.

Hay, A.C. (1996) *Re-stating Social and Political Change*, Buckingham: Open University Press.

Held, D. (1996) *Democracy and the Global Order: From the Modern State to Cosmopolitan Governance*, Cambridge: Polity Press.

Hirst, P. (1994) *Associative Democracy: New Forms of Economic and Social Governance*, Cambridge: Polity Press.

Hirst, P. (1995) 'Can secondary associations enhance democratic governance?', in J. Cohen and J. Rogers (eds) *Associations and Democracy: The Real Utopias Project. Vol. 1*, London: Verso.

Hirst, P. and Thompson, G. (1996) *Globalisation in Question*, Cambridge: Polity Press.

Humphrey, C. and Pease, K. (1991) 'After the rainbow', *Local Government Studies* 17, 4: 1–5

Humphrey, C. and Scapens, R. (1992) 'Whatever happened to the liontamers? An examination of accounting change in the public sector', *Local Government Studies* 18, 3: 141–7.

Humphrey, C., Miller, P. and Scapens, R. (1993) 'Accountability and accountable management in the UK public sector', *Accounting, Auditing and Accountability Journal* 6, 3: 7–29.

Jessop, B. (1994) 'The transition to post-Fordism and the Schumpeterian workfare state', in R. Burrows and B. Loader (eds) *Towards a Post-Fordist Welfare State?*, London: Routledge.

Le Grand, J. (1990) *Quasi-Markets and Social Policy*, Studies in Decentralisation and Quasi-Markets 1, Bristol: SAUS.

Lister, R. (1995) 'Dilemmas in engendering citizenship', *Economy and Society* 24, 1: 1–40.

Loughlin, M. (1996) *Legality and Locality: The Role of the Law in Central–Local Government Relations*, Oxford: Oxford University Press.

Marshall, T.H. (1950) *Citizenship and Social Class and Other Essays,* Cambridge: Cambridge University Press.

Marshall, T.H. (1975) *Social Policy in the Twentieth Century*, 4th edn, London: Hutchinson.

Miller, P. (1996) 'Dilemmas of accountability', in P. Hirst and S. Khilnani (eds) *Reinventing Democracy*, Oxford: Political Quarterly/Blackwell.

Mouffe, C. (1992) *Dimensions of Radical Democracy: Pluralism and Citizenship*, London: Verso.

Offe, C. (1995) 'Some skeptical considerations on the malleability of representative institutions', in J. Cohen and J. Rogers (eds) *Associations and Democracy: The Real Utopias Project. Vol. 1*, London: Verso.

Ohmae, K. (1990) *The Borderless World: Power and Strategy in the Interlinked Economy*, London: Collins.

Pascall, G. (1993) 'Citizenship – a feminist analysis', in G. Drover and P. Kerans (eds) *New Approaches to Welfare Theory*, London: Edward Elgar.

Phillips, A. (1996) 'Feminism and the attractions of the local', in D. King and G. Stoker (eds) *Rethinking Local Democracy*, London: Macmillan.

Pratchett, L. and Wilson, D. (eds) (1996) *Local Democracy and Local Government*, Basingstoke: Macmillan.

Rallings, C., Temple, M. and Thrasher, M. (1996) 'Participation in local democracy', in L. Pratchett and D. Wilson (eds) *Local Democracy and Local Government*, Basingstoke: Macmillan.

Roche, M. (1991) *Rethinking Citizenship. Welfare, Ideology and Change in Modern Society*, Cambridge: Polity Press.

SAUS (School for Advanced Urban Studies) (1983) *The Future of Local Democracy*, Bristol: SAUS.

Stewart, J. (1996) 'Reforming the new magistracy', in L. Pratchett and D. Wilson (eds) *Local Democracy and Local Government*, Basingstoke: Macmillan.

Taylor, G. (1993) 'Challenges from the margins', in J. Clarke (ed.) *A Crisis in Care? Challenges to Social Work*, London: Sage.

Waldegrave, W. (1993) *The Reality of Reform and Accountability in Today's Public Service*, London: Public Finance Foundation.

Williams, F. (1993) 'Gender, "race" and class in British welfare policy', in A. Cochrane and J. Clarke (eds) *Comparing Welfare States: Britain in International Context*, London: Sage.

Young, K. (1986) 'Attitudes to local government', in *The Conduct of Local Authority Business: Committee of Inquiry into the Conduct of Local Authority Business. Research Vol. III: The Local Government Elector* 'Widdicombe Report', Cmnd 9797–9801, London: HMSO.

Chapter 17

Postmodernity and Social Europe

Norman Ginsburg

INTRODUCTION

This chapter opens with a discussion of modern social policy and its post-modernisation and then attempts to apply these ideas to analysing the development of the notion of Social Europe, focusing in particular on the Green and White Papers on social policy published by the European Commission in 1993 and 1994 respectively.

SOCIAL POLICY, MODERNITY AND POSTMODERNITY

Williams (1992: 204–5) makes a useful distinction between postmodernity 'as a condition' and 'as a particular shift in theory and analysis'. In order to get to grips with Social Europe the focus will be on postmodernity as a condition; that is, a collection of economic, political and social shifts and transformations. These may be linked in such a way that we can talk about a transition taking place from the modern era to a postmodern one, or perhaps a more modest shift to late modernity. In terms of social policy it is reasonably clear that modernity, in Northwestern Europe at least, is represented by the Keynesian welfare state as developed since Bismarck under a diversity of national regimes. Modern social policy is driven by the mission of combining capitalist economic efficiency with social and national cohesion. It recognises the primacy of social class divisions within the social structure and its corporatist political basis is the solidarity between the social partners, the representative organisations of capital and labour. It began as a conservative response to socialist agitation in Germany and it arguably reached its peak during the Cold War as a counter to the apparently socialist regimes in Eastern Europe. In Sweden modern social policy was seen by many as the centrepiece of its transition to socialism.

Modern social policy was originally founded on the rock of the stable, patriarchal nuclear family in which a male breadwinner brought home a family wage to meet many of the basic needs of his dependents. This has of course been supplanted by the dual-earner family, but by no means entirely. The basic needs from which modern social policy provides protection are universal and reasonably predictable. Social insurance is the central element of social security and health-care funding. The system is predicated on the continuous and full-time paid employment of the breadwinner(s). The core welfare collectivity is the nation state, which underwrites social citizenship juridically and financially. Delivery of benefits and services is frequently devolved to local or regional government and non-governmental organisations.

It may be a contradiction in terms to refer to postmodernist social policy since the idea of 'social policy' may be intrinsically modernist, focusing on universal, basic needs and collective means of meeting them (Williams 1992: 208). At the very least, however, postmodern ideas offer insight into the limitations of modernity and suggest visions of the future. In trying to summarise the essential elements of a postmodernist perspective on social policy, a diversity of sources has been drawn upon here, fusing perhaps uncomfortably elements from theories of post-Fordism, postindustrialism and late modernity.

Postmodernism calls into question every element of modern social policy as summarised above. For postmodernists, socialism, like other universalising, Enlightenment ideologies, is dead; if socialism is dead, collectivising social policy is no longer appropriate or needed as a response. Class divisions and the corporatist structures of capital and labour are also no longer central to the socio-political landscape. Diversity and fragmentation of identities, communities and associations in contemporary society is a central feature of postmodernity. The postmodern politics of social policy is radically pluralist, with pressures coming from the new social movements upholding the diversity of needs and associations. Giddens (1994: 6) talks of the 'expansion of social reflexivity' brought about by the wider availability of information which empowers individuals, enabling them to be far more critical of received wisdoms. Theorists of postindustrialism and post-Fordism note that the standard employment contract is disappearing and that paid employment in the future will be casualised and intermittent, with short-term, temporary contracts and flexitime contracts the norm. Family structures also appear to be diversifying quite rapidly with the growth of serial monogamy, absent fatherhood, single motherhood and childlessness. Caring responsibilities and obligations are negotiated individually within these structures, often without much support from the state. Fundamental risks such as the loss of a home, permanent unemployment, environmental hazards, marriage break-up or care in old age may be uninsurable, privately or socially for the great majority. Giddens (1994) has argued that in the late modern era the fundamental issue for social policy is no longer insurance against predictable risks but the 'management of risk'; that is, the task of prevention of risk occurrence. Of course there is nothing necessarily new in this: public health measures, social housing and active labour-market policies are all 'positive welfare' programmes in Giddens's sense of the term. None the less the postmodern perspective highlights the inappropriateness of modern social policy in managing the 'new' risks. The idea of a citizens' income, a guaranteed minimum income for individuals underwritten by the state, addresses this issue directly and gathers considerable support from analysts embracing elements of a postmodern perspective. In the era of postmodernity, the nation state, however, is no longer at the centre of social policy making and delivery. These processes may be devolved both upwards and downwards, upwards to supra-national organisations and downwards to associations, employers and individual consumers. Social Europe is clearly one such supra-national organisation, but one of its core principles, particularly in the social policy field, is that of subsidiarity, the devolution of responsibility to the most local level feasible. Hence the issue of Social Europe is highly relevant to the discussion of postmodern social policy.

THE NEO-LIBERAL MOMENTUM

Before moving on to that issue, however, some reflection on the relationship between postmodernisation and neo-liberalism is appropriate. Taylor-Gooby (1994: 388) has argued that 'postmodern approaches' are directly opposed to 'economic liberalism'. He suggests that economic liberalism 'is the nearest approximation to a universal theme in world affairs'. Hence postmodernism's rejection of universal ideology puts it in fundamental opposition to neo-liberalism. This is a problematic argument for at least two reasons. First, it is probably going too far to suggest that neo-liberal macroeconomic thought has achieved universal, hegemonic status in the west, particularly if one considers regimes like Sweden and Germany. Nevertheless it may be approaching the status of a universal ideology, viz. Chancellor of the Exchequer Gordon Brown's approach to fiscal and monetary policy. Secondly, versions of the postmodernisation thesis seem to have much in common with neo-liberalism. Hence Crook *et al.* (1992: 38) describe some of the effects of post-modernisation on the state as involving 'a horizontal redistribution of power and responsibility to autonomous bodies' and 'the marketisation and privatisation of previously state-run enterprises'. They also envisage 'the generation of inequality [being] progressively displaced into the arenas of consumption' (p. 39). There are, however, very significant contrasts between the nationalism, commercialism, individualism and patriarchal familism associated with the neo-liberal view and the associationism, multi- and inter-culturalism, familial pluralism, environmentalism and empowerment ideas associated with postmodern views. The latter hold out some hope for challenging the neo-liberal consensus, which seems to have prevailing influence in EU policy making at the moment.

SOCIAL EUROPE

Recent comparative studies of European welfare states barely mention the European Union or the Commission (George and Taylor-Gooby 1996; Esping-Andersen 1996). Instead, in harmony with a postmodern view, they reinforce an impression of the enormous diversity of social policies in terms of legislation, welfare rights, sources of finance, forms of administration and delivery, status of professionals, industrial relations, and relationships with the private sectors including the family. There is a structured diversity (Ginsburg 1992: 23–4) amongst the European welfare states, in which the elements of diversity do not appear to be diminishing despite the common structural pressures. So how should we assess the meaning and relevance of Social Europe in the context of postmodernisation and the structured diversity of welfare in the late 1990s?

On the face of it, the idea of Social Europe seems intrinsically modernist. It suggests the development of a uniform social policy for Europe, responding to the common incidence of welfare risks and needs across the Union developed by the internal market. Indeed it has been and still is seen by the Commission as an engine of social cohesion, much as the Bismarckian and Keynesian welfare states were once seen by governments as engines of national cohesion. The social divisions which Social Europe principally addresses are class divisions, particularly the increased insecurity and unemployment of workers since the late 1970s. Much of the policy making has dealt with industrial relations issues – health and safety at work, industrial democracy, equal opportunities in the workplace, etc.

The 1980s saw the full emergence of the idea of Social Europe. Newman (1996) traces its origins to the incoming French socialist government in 1981 which promoted the idea at the Fontainebleau summit in 1984. The rationale was that 'the Community would not be able to compete internationally unless it also strengthened its social cohesion' (Newman 1996: 83). This was reinforced with the appointment in that year of Jacques Delors as Commission president. He immediately declared that his goal was not only economic and monetary union (EMU) but the creation of a 'Social Europe'. The notion of social cohesion and its contribution to economic competitiveness and growth are a matter that needs careful consideration. If the principal global competitors of the EU are Japan and the United States, they offer contradictory indications on this issue. While Japan certainly stands out as socially cohesive, the United States is surely at the other end of the spectrum on many parameters of cohesion. Yet according to most commentators the US has improved its global economic competitiveness over the past decade, especially compared to the EU. Nevertheless recent North American analyses have put new life into the argument that social inequality and declining social protection undermine economic flexibility and growth (Blank 1994; McFate *et al.* 1995).

For the European Commission social cohesion is achieved by 'full employ-ment'; social inclusion or integration is equated with paid employment. As Levitas (1996: 8) has pointed out, quoting from the EU White Paper on European social policy, 'the cause of exclusion is not the fundamental nature of capitalism (which never gets discussed) but "contemporary economic and social conditions" which "tend to exclude some groups from the cycle of opportunities"'. The principal means of developing social cohesion is there-fore through supply-side employment policies. By the early 1990s policy analysts broadly sympathetic to the Social Europe project, such as Leibfried and Pierson (1992) and Kleinman and Piachaud (1993), were extremely scep-tical about the feasibility of the modernist, Delors vision of Social Europe. Hantrais (1995: 19–37) has charted in detail the Commission's retreat from the original, active harmonisation of social policy towards the more passive one of convergence.

THE NEW SOCIAL EUROPE

Newman (1996) suggests that the high point in the development of Social Europe occurred in 1989 with the adoption of the Social Charter, since when the general hiatus over further European integration has left Social Europe in 'an acutely difficult position'. However, the Green Paper and the White Paper (EC 1993, 1994) on social policy '*may* represent a significant new stage in EU social policy making' (Newman 1996: 85). These documents certainly mark a shift from the modernism of the 1980s model of Social Europe discussed above. 'Social Europe' has now become a looser 'European social model' merely founded on shared liberal democratic values. The White Paper intro-duces an element of postmodernity in asserting policy 'convergence which respects diversity' (EC 1994: 12) as a new norm. Although the Green Paper in fact hardly mentions policy convergence, the responses to it clearly generated controversy on the issue, not just from neo-liberals. Hence in the White Paper it is noted that 'all the comments on the Green Paper stress the need to respect the diversity of European societies', though 'convergence of goals and policies over a period of time by fixing common objectives is vital' (EC 1994: 12). It is therefore conceded that common policy objectives can be reached by different routes. Given the diversity of economic development and resources of the member states, it is also recognised that policy should focus on 'the establishment of a framework of basic minimum standards' (p. 12). This is quite some way from the high-quality welfare system implied in the Delors vision of Social Europe, reflecting an almost Beveridgean emphasis on the social minimum.

The tone of the White Paper in particular is almost a plea for recognition of the role of social policy in economic integration. This reflects an anxiety that social policy is in fact playing 'second string' to the development of the internal market and EMU. An underlying debate with neo-liberalism which would accord social policy a marginal role is near the surface, particularly in the White Paper. Vobruba (1995: 304) has pointed out that 'the differences between the Green Paper and the White Paper ... reveal how social policy projects are pared away to almost nothing in the complex negotiation process'. In the Commission's view, the role of social policy has to shift further from income and status maintenance towards investment in human capital through education and training, particularly preparing and encouraging unemployed people to contribute to economic activity. This is very much in tune with recent New Labour thinking with its echoes of 'workfare'. Equally, though, it has to be said that 'active labour-market policy' in Sweden, for example, has always intervened in a fairly authoritarian manner in the lives of unemployed people.

Hence the principal emphases in both documents are first the role of social policy in the drive for economic competitiveness – that is, productivity gains – and secondly the need to reduce unemployment through active labour-market or supply-side policies. Obviously these two policy aims may be incompatible because productivity gains frequently imply the shedding of labour, but this is not recognised anywhere in the documents, as Vobruba (1995: 308) notes. In terms of the legitimation and delivery of policy the overwhelming emphasis in the papers is corporatist. The principal actors are the 'social partners', trade unions and employers in 'social dialogue' – somewhat exclusionary structures. This sits rather uncomfortably alongside the other emphasis on social cohesion and inclusion. Despite these emphases, the papers show the Commission beginning to come to terms with aspects of postmodernisation on a number of issues, if only to a very limited extent. These issues include the following.

Paid employment

The White Paper (EC 1994: 30) recognises the rapid development of 'more flexible forms of work contract (fixed-term, temporary and part-time)'. Perhaps betraying some hostility to such developments, it merely comments that 'if these flexible forms of work are to be generally accepted, it is important to ensure that such workers are given broadly-equivalent working conditions to standard workers'. The Green Paper confines itself to some important reflections on the possibilities of work sharing, which 'can make considerable sense when linked to new patterns of working time, more flexible working hours, more alternation between work and training and more flexible retirement' (EC 1993: 37). The only concrete policy proposal, mooted in both documents, is a possible directive to facilitate the spread of part-time work. The Green Paper is also deeply concerned about the intensification and decentralisation of the labour process and the use of a 'contingent' or casualised labour force to complement and/or replace the 'core'. It identifies the central problem as being 'how to adapt labour law and practices in such a way as to constitute a positive incentive towards the adoption of new techniques and processes while seeking to preserve ... workers' rights and social progress' (EC 1993: 41). In the submissions to the Commission on these issues of 'labour standards' subsequent to the Green Paper, 'there is no clear consensus', with member states 'divided in their opinions about the need for further legislative action on labour standards at European level' (EC 1994: 31).

Family and gender issues

The White Paper dedicates a whole chapter to 'equality of opportunity for women and men', and as one would expect from the Commission there is a strong emphasis on making gender equality in the workplace a reality. The Green Paper acknowledges that 'social and labour market structures' continue to uphold traditional patriarchal values, which 'conflicts with the new reality [in which] dual income and lone parent families are increasingly common' (EC 1993: 25). In this context the Green Paper suggests 'encouraging more flexibility in careers and working hours' and 'promoting innovative ways to combine household and working responsibilities' (EC 1993: 57). This is taken up in the White Paper, which trails the possibility of a directive 'covering the issues of reconciling professional and family life, including career breaks such as parental leave ... It would set minimum standards within a framework designed to encourage competitive solutions in a changing world' (EC 1994: 31). The document also recognises the need for 'positive policy action ... to promote a more nearly-equal sharing of parental responsibilities' (p. 43). Although it is not clear what all this might mean in policy terms beyond improved child care and parental leave, it is a clear recognition of the postmodernisation of the family and of parenting.

Social divisions

Both documents give some specific attention to the 'social integration' of elderly people, disabled people and people of minority ethnic origin. The Green Paper also discusses briefly the integration of young people through job guarantees, apprenticeships and 'lower entry wages', but this is not carried forward into the White Paper. The discussion of elderly people in both documents is both brief and vague, with no comment on flexible pensions and retirement ages, or care and support of infirm elderly people. The White Paper recognises the 'need to build the fundamental right to equal opportunities [for disabled people] into Union policies' (EC 1994: 51) but does not propose fundamental reform such as directives or treaty amendments. On third-country nationals, most of whom are of minority ethnic origin, the White Paper recognises that the internal market must permit their free movement, which is far from being the case at the moment. As a very modest first step the Commission proposes that 'Member States give priority to third-country nationals permanently and legally resident in another Member State, when job vacancies cannot be filled by EU nationals or nationals of third countries legally resident in the Member State' (EC 1994: 39). What does this mean? It seems to imply a European network between job centres or at least an active labour-market policy unheard of in the UK. The White Paper envisages the 'realisation of full free movement rights' as a very long-term prospect which 'will depend on the labour market situation' (EC 1994: 39). On combating racism and xenophobia, the White Paper notes that the Commission is pressing for 'powers to combat racial discrimination to be included in the Treaty' (p. 39). The documents have nothing to say about equal opportunities and anti-discrimination policies for gays and lesbians. In contrast with the discussion of gender divisions, these documents are hesitant and uninformed in response to the pressures coming from 'new' social movements and identities.

Participation and democratising processes

Both documents express serious concern about the relative exclusion of women both from the collective bargaining and negotiation processes of the social partners and from the wider arenas of public and political bodies. In the White Paper, the Commission says it will seek 'proposals for action' on this front. At a broader level, the Green Paper acknowledges the postmodernisation of political processes. Hence 'within the Member States there has been over the past decade a strong movement towards local and regional initiatives, in which diverse groups have taken part', but 'the relationship between this micro-level action and government policy has not yet been clearly worked out' (EC 1993: 71). In a break with the corporatist tradition, the White Paper says that 'voluntary and other representative organisations have a right to be consulted by the Union and to play their role in the process of change ... the Union needs to develop partnerships with a wider range of institutions' (EC 1994: 57). As Conroy (1996: 16) puts it, 'if the employers and unions have a social dialogue, then non-governmental organisations (NGOs) seek a civil dialogue on the future of social policy'. The Commission has now established a forum for non-governmental organisations to present their views on social policy. In late 1995 the European Platform of NGOs was established, embracing a huge network of social and welfare organisations, and the first forum was held in March 1996.

This analysis of the texts of the Green Paper and the White Paper on social policy hopefully demonstrates that postmodernisation processes are seeping through into the thinking of the Commission and that the idea of Social Europe is moving in more realistic directions. However, these modest shifts cannot disguise the reality that European social policy is currently being driven by economic considerations, principally the drive for monetary union. The arguments in favour of EMU are, firstly, that it will create a more stable macroeconomic environment (an anti-inflationary discipline) and, secondly, that eliminating unnecessary transaction costs will add up to 0.4 per cent to GDP. As the Green Paper puts it, EMU implies that 'all social groups and in particular the social partners are aware of what is feasible in terms of wage rises and other social improvements and act accordingly' (EC 1993: 58). Thus it is hoped in effect that the funding of the welfare state can be depoliticised and reified across the Union. While the Green Paper acknowledges that EMU will require 'social policy adjustments', the White Paper, amazingly, makes no reference to EMU at all.

In order to achieve EMU, the convergence criteria for economic policy established by the Maastricht Treaty have to be achieved by each qualifying member state. The key criteria for social policy are that states must have a maximum budget deficit of 3 per cent of GDP per annum and a maximum total public sector debt of 60 per cent of GDP. Forecasts suggest that a clear majority of member states will fulfil the criteria by 1999, when the single currency is due to be launched. One estimate suggests that meeting the criteria by 1999 could 'temporarily reduce employment in the EU by 0.5 million' and 'would reduce growth in Italy, Sweden and Greece by 0.5, 0.7 and 2.5 per cent respectively' (Begg and Nectoux 1995: 292). This would increase demand for social benefits while their funding is being diminished, possibly creating significant political opposition. Nevertheless, in the run-up to 1999 the French and German governments have been using the Maastricht criteria as a convenient external pressure with which to legitimate programmes of public expenditure cuts, particularly in social protection and health care. These measures have provoked strong public opposition led by the trade union movements in both countries. Although the Juppé reforms of social security initiated in November 1995 have largely been implemented, the resistance they met with may have provoked some second thoughts on further retrenchment.

POSTMODERN VIEWS OF THE EU STATE

With the realisation that a supra-national, federal EU welfare state will never happen, attempts have been made by political scientists to theorise the nature of EU social policy now and in the future. As Streek (1996: 65) puts it, 'the political and economic regime that is developing in Western Europe, whatever it may be, is a new kind of animal that is altogether different from the national state'. This new animal is characterised by 'neo-voluntarism', in which member states are enjoined to participate in policies but cannot be compelled to do so. Streek (1996: 77) argues that the European social policy regime will be differentiated from traditional, national welfare states 'by its low capacity to impose binding obligations and the high degree to which it depends on various kinds of voluntarism'. This view implicitly shares much with elements of a postmodernist perspective, but it also has something in common with that of Majone (1993: 156), who sees the EU functioning simply as a regulatory state, reflecting the neo-liberal economics which he sees as pervasive in the three treaties (Rome, the Single European Act and Maastricht). Hence the role of the EU for Majone (and for neo-liberals) is confined to the regulation of markets to ensure fair competition, environmental and consumer protection, equal treatment for men and women and so on. For Majone, this regulatory role does not appear to extend to the enforcement of either minimal or adequate standards of human welfare, but, of course, it could do. Finally, Caporaso (1996: 45–7) identifies 'three aspects of the postmodern polity' in the EU: its weak core institutions, especially in social policy; its numerous spatial locations (the Parliament, Council, Commission and Court); and its 'multilevel polity'. This last is characterised by 'networks of interaction' between different layers of government (national, supra-national, regional, local) rather than just formal structures of accountability and responsibility. What that means in practice is obviously problematic, but it is certainly plausible to see the EU developing into a postmodern form of the state, quite different from the conventional, national forms of the recent past.

CONCLUSION

This chapter has argued that the notion of a modernist, supra-national European welfare state, which was on the Commission's agenda until quite recently, has been abandoned. Aspects of postmodernisation are having an impact on the Commission's thinking and on political scientists analysing the future of European social policy. Social policy in Europe is, however, being driven hard by economic policy, notably the Maastricht convergence criteria, which arguably reflect more of a neo-liberal agenda and the narrow economic interests of capital. Great concern is expressed about social cohesion, but it is not sufficient to be translated into effective policies. EMU is quite likely to step up the processes of social exclusion and increasing inequality if, as promised, it contributes to increased economic efficiency. Increased economic efficiency in Britain since the late 1970s has produced the reverse of the trickle-down effect. Yet the Commission continues in effect to cling to trickle-down in arguing that EMU can contribute to social progress. Whether this is possible without a commitment to a Social Europe in which effective measures are adopted to reverse increasing social inequalities is highly questionable.

BIBLIOGRAPHY

Begg, I. and Nectoux, F. (1995) 'Social protection and economic union', *Journal of European Social Policy* 5, 4: 285-302.
Blank, R. (ed.) (1994) *Social Protection versus Economic Flexibility: Is there a Trade-off?*, Chicago: University of Chicago Press.
Caporaso, J. (1996) 'The European Union and forms of the state', *Journal of Common Market Studies* 34, 1: 29–52.
Conroy, P. (1996) 'Europe – desperately seeking citizens', plenary address to the Social

Policy Association Conference, Sheffield, 17 July.

Crook, S., Pakulski, J. and Waters, M. (1992) *Postmodernization: Change in Advanced Society*, London: Sage.

Esping-Andersen, G. (ed.) (1996) *Welfare States in Transition*, London: Sage.

EC (European Commission) (1993) *European Social Policy: Options for the Future*, Green Paper, Luxembourg: European Commission.

EC (European Commission) (1994) *European Social Policy: A Way Forward for the Union*, White Paper, Luxembourg: European Commission.

George, V. and Taylor-Gooby, P. (eds) (1996) *European Welfare Policy*, Basingstoke: Macmillan.

Giddens, A. (1994) *Beyond Left and Right: The Future of Radical Politics*, Cambridge: Polity Press.

Ginsburg, N. (1992) *Divisions of Welfare*, London: Sage.

Hantrais, L. (1995) *Social Policy in the European Union*, Basingstoke: Macmillan.

Kleinman, M. and Piachaud, D. (1993) 'European social policy: conceptions and choices', *Journal of European Social Policy* 3, 1: 1–19.

Leibfried, S. and Pierson, P. (1992) 'Prospects for Social Europe', *Politics and Society* 20, 3: 333–66.

Levitas, R. (1996) 'The concept of social exclusion and the new Durkheimian hegemony', *Critical Social Policy* 16, 1: 5–20.

McFate, K., Lawson, R. and Wilson, W.J. (eds) (1995) *Poverty, Inequality and the Future of Social Policy*, New York: Russell Sage Foundation.

Majone, G. (1993) 'The EC between social policy and social regulation', *Journal of Common Market Studies* 31, 2: 153–70.

Newman, M. (1996) *Democracy, Sovereignty and the European Union*, London: Hurst.

Streeck, W. (1996) 'Neo-voluntarism: a new European social policy regime?', in G. Marks, F. Scharpf, P. Schmitter and W. Streeck (eds) *Governance in the European Union*, London: Sage.

Taylor-Gooby, P. (1994) 'Postmodernism and social policy: a great leap backwards?', *Journal of Social Policy* 23, 3: 385–404.

Vobruba, G. (1995) 'Social policy on tomorrow's euro-corporatist stage', *Journal of European Social Policy* 5, 4: 303–15.

Williams, F. (1992) 'Somewhere over the rainbow: universality and diversity in social policy', in N. Manning and R. Page (eds) *Social Policy Review 4*, Nottingham: Social Policy Association.

Index

abandonment 43, 172, 205, 206–8, 214
accountability 195, 196, 240, 242;
  'accounting' rather than 257; collective 262;
  electoral 263; local 256–8; political 263
addiction 204, 206–8, 209, 210, 213, 214, 215
aesthetics 39, 197, 201
affinities 50, 51, 190
affluent people 93, 94, 95, 128
age 52, 58, 61, 160; individual's 'being' in
  relation to 148; populations managed on the
  basis of 208; relationships between 'race',
  gender, class, region and 63–4; retirement
  273; sexuality and 122, 123, 124, 130;
  struggles around 60
ageism 62
Ahmad, B. 59–60
AIDS (acquired immune deficiency
  syndrome) 103, 105, 122; public health
  concerns surrounding 213
alcohol(ism) 204, 209, 229; policy initiatives
  214
Alexander, A. 262
alienation 141, 142
ambivalence 33, 34, 110
anomie 98
anthropology 28, 139, 145
anti-discrimination 58, 128, 133, 274
anti-foundationalism 35, 38, 75
anti-oppression 3, 50, 57, 58–64, 74
anti-racism 55, 58, 59, 61; campaigns 97;
  competencies 63; debates within 148; self-
  proclaimed 96; sustained critique of
  welfare state 110
architecture 20, 39, 49, 50, 164; postmodern
  146
argument(s) 33, 34, 143, 181, 240, 261; moral
  and political 87; needs-based 113
art(s) 19, 36, 49, 50, 104, 164; purity and
  autonomy of 20
Asian people 132, 242, 253
associationist vision 5, 237–51, 269
assumptions 59, 61, 105, 115, 253, 257;

actuarial 92; of difference 259; difficult to
  sustain 108; family and motherhood 127;
  foundational 172, 181; of heterosexuality
  129–30; humanist 205; normative 57;
  rationalist 103, 110; social, conservative 21;
  statist 246; taken-for-granted 130
Australia 128, 209, 210
authority 210, 211; discretionary 176;
  occupational 172; professional 172, 207,
  212, 227; sharing 77; traditional 172, 173
autonomy 62, 105, 188, 190; art 20;
  associational 244; budgetary 198; clinical
  211, 224; connecting with personal
  responsibilities 91; group, local and
  institutional 44; individual 44, 54, 61, 230,
  239, 242, 243; local communal 145;
  professional 74; state 255; sufficient
  condition for 246; voice 144

Baker, John 15, 27–8
Ball, Stephen J. 5, 12
Barthes, Roland 9, 11
Baudrillard, J. 7, 8, 29, 40, 50, 86, 87, 138;
  critique of Marxism 140; ludic or 'spectral'
  postmodernism 52; symbolism of
  consumer culture 53
Bauman, Z. 1, 3, 32, 35, 43, 86, 87, 89–90, 97,
  99
Beck, Ulrich 1, 4, 19, 32, 153–4, 158–9, 208
Beck-Gernsheim, E. 158–9
beliefs: cornerstone 112; foundational 34;
  spiritual 107
Bell, Bernard Iddings 39
Bell, Daniel 10, 39
benefits 94, 122, 127, 238; assuming
  heterosexuality in order to obtain 132;
  delivery of 268; demand for 275; eligibility
  and entitlement 160; getting pregnant in
  order to obtain 131; personal information
  for 227; tax 257
Benetton 223, 224
Benhabib, S. 248